FLUID AND ELECTROLYTE METABOLISM IN INFANTS AND CHILDREN

FLUID AND ELECTROLYTE METABOLISM IN INFANTS AND CHILDREN: A UNIFIED APPROACH

WILLIAM B. WEIL, JR., M.D.
Professor and Chairman
Department of Human Development
Michigan State University
East Lansing, Michigan

with

MICHAEL D. BAILIE, M.D., PH.D.
Associate Professor
Departments of Human Development
and Physiology
Michigan State University
East Lansing, Michigan

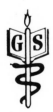

GRUNE & STRATTON

A Subsidiary of Harcourt Brace Jovanovich, Publishers
New York □ San Francisco □ London

Library of Congress Cataloging in Publication Data

Weil, William B
  Fluid and electrolyte metabolism in infants and
children.

  Bibliography: p.
  Includes index.
  1. Water-electrolyte imbalances in children.
  2. Water-electrolyte balance (Physiology)
  I. Bailie, Michael D., joint author. II. Title.
  [DNLM: 1. Water-electrolyte balance—In infancy and
childhood. 2. Water-electrolyte imbalance—In infancy
and childhood. WD220 W422f]
  RJ399.W35W44   612'.01522   77-21064
  ISBN 0-8089-1028-0

Grune & Stratton, Inc.
111 Fifth Avenue
New York, New York   10003

Distributed in the United Kingdom by
Academic Press, Inc. (London) Ltd.
24/28 Oval Road, London NW 1

Library of Congress Catalog Number 77-21064
International Standard Book Number 0-8089-1048-5

Printed in the United States of America

This book is dedicated first to William McLean Wallace, M.D., who guided, nurtured, and refined my interest and knowledge in the field of fluid and electrolyte metabolism; and second to my wife and daughters who with their encouragement, forbearance, and patience created the environment in which this work could be done.

PREFACE

One might well ask why another book on fluid and electrolyte metabolism is needed. Beginning with James L. Gamble's paperbound syllabus, there have been numerous books, monographs, and brochures produced in this field. Generally these works have been directed toward either students or physicians. This book has been designed with students, residents, and physicians in mind. It is hoped that the beginning medical student, the resident in pediatrics or in family practice, and the physician in clinical practice will all find this discussion of benefit.

For a book to be useful on a broad scale, it should contain some of the underlying physiology of fluid and electrolyte metabolism, a reasonable description of the more common clinical disorders, and a variety of practical examples of how this information can be used in treating patients. The format of this book is designed with these goals in mind. The basic physiology is in Part I, the clinical disorders are described in Part II, and cases illustrating specific problems are in Part III. In addition, there are numerous illustrative case examples throughout Parts I and II so that the reader can use this material for self-assessment, as is appropriate for any self-instructional medium, and certainly the book is still the most common self-instructional form available to us.

There are two approaches employed in this volume that separate it from many others. The first of these is an attempt to present the material from a unitary viewpoint. General principles that apply to most types of fluid and electrolyte problems are stressed throughout. The concept is that if one comprehends these basic facts, one can then analyze the majority of cases with the same fundamental approach: the body's homeostatic processes are concerned primarily with maintaining the *volume* of body fluids, secondarily with preserving the *composition* of these fluids, and lastly with regulating *acid–base balance*. In the management of patients, the same priorities apply: one's first concern should be volume preservation, then composition correction, and finally improvement in acid–base status.

The second approach involves presentation of the material on acid–base balance from the position that one is working with hydrogen ion concentrations, not pH. For most of us, pH is an abstraction with which it has been difficult to work; hydrogen ions are cations, and these are substances with which we have learned to be somewhat more comfortable.

Thus this book will attempt to present the problems created by water, electrolyte, and acid–base disorders as physiologic problems rather than as separate, specific disturbances associated with specific disease states. The advantage of this approach is that the majority of problems found in patients can be considered from a unitary point of view, not as a series of unrelated clinical entities. Thus, if one sees an infant with diarrhea, an adolescent with diabetes mellitus, an 8-year-old child with bowel obstruction, or a 3-year-old child with a burn, the same approach to management of their deranged body fluids can be utilized; one will not have to remember specific formulae or fluid calculations for each situation. Instead, one can consider the various physiologic problems involved and apply the same principles in determining the necessary therapeutic intervention.

Much of the confusion prevalent today in the literature and in the minds of many physicians is a result of our rapidly increasing understanding of renal physiology, cardiovascular dynamics, and endocrine interactions in disturbed body fluid equilibrium. One result of this proliferation of information is more and more detailed description of the mechanisms involved in individual diseases. With this propensity for scientific exactness, we have been better able to evaluate and manage such complex cases as the child who has had open-heart surgery followed by postoperative renal shutdown. However, in the process we have tended to forget that the problems of the great majority of children requiring fluid therapy are not so complex and must be cared for with more limited laboratory resources and less time. Thus we are creating a small cadre of highly skilled investigators and therapeuticians and leaving a vast number of physicians with little to assist them in the day-to-day difficulties that constitute the majority of fluid problems seen in practice. It is partially to redress this situation that this book has been undertaken.

Some ideas for this approach to the subject were first considered when the senior author was working with William M. Wallace, then chairman of the Department of Pediatrics at Case–Western Reserve University. Many years passed before there was an opportunity to develop those ideas into a manuscript. Although many new concepts and hypotheses were developed between the initial period of planning and the final writing, the basic plan for presentation did not change.

For whatever success this book may have, much of the credit should go to William M. Wallace, who had one of the finest minds among the workers in this field. Any failure can be attributed to the fact that he was no longer alive to provide counsel, criticism, and correction when the writing took place.

Appreciation must also be expressed to many others, including Andrew D. Hunt, dean of the College of Human Medicine, Michigan State University; Arthur F. Kohrman, associate chairman of the Department of Human Development; Pamela Watkins, secretary; Peter Barre, graduate assistant; and the staff of the Biomedical Communications Center in the College of Human Medicine. Thanks are also due to Waldo E. Nelson,

M.D., and Robert W. Winters, M.D., for help and constructive criticism in the development of two papers that formed the basis for parts of this book, and to the C.V. Mosby Co., publishers of the *Journal of Pediatrics*, for permission to use material that previously appeared in that journal.

William B. Weil, Jr., M.D.

CONTENTS

LIST OF TABLES

LIST OF FIGURES

PART I

Physiologic Considerations

1
Body Fluids

Successful application of a unitary approach to body fluid problems requires some basic understanding of the underlying physiology of body fluids, and therefore this physiology will be our first consideration.

The body fluids are a heterogeneous mixture of fluids; they differ in quantity, in quality, in their rapidity of change, and in their responses to adverse situations. To facilitate communication, several conventions and definitions have come into general use. Total body water (TBW) is a term used to indicate all the fluids of the body, with the exception of those that exist within the gastrointestinal and genitourinary tracts. TBW may be subdivided into the fluid within cells, intracellular fluid (ICF), and that

external to cells, extracellular fluid (ECF). The ECF can be further par-
titioned into that fluid within the vascular system, the blood volume, and
that outside the blood vessels, the interstitial fluid. The volumes of these
so-called body fluid compartments are difficult to measure with precision,
and to some extent they depend on the method used to measure them.

TOTAL BODY WATER

Lean Body Mass and Body Fat

Man's body has a remarkably constant composition, with the exception of the proportion of body fat. This constancy of all but fat has led to
the concept of lean body mass (LBM), or the fat-free body, as a useful
reference point. The composition of the LBM has been a subject of investigation for many years, and much has been learned about the changes
that occur with age and the stability that is maintained at particular
periods of life. Unfortunately, it is not yet practical to measure either
LBM or body fat content in every patient; so our clinical evaluations of
body composition must include body fat, and therefore they are approximations. When discussing body composition, the water, the dry solids
(soft tissue and bone solids together), and the fat are considered as distinct
quantities, even though they are mixed in various ways in individual
tissues and organs. Furthermore, the fat is considered separate from the
water and the cell proteins that encompass the lipid deposits. The LBM of
a typical adult male is composed of about 75% water and 25% solids.
Added to the LBM is the fat, which is equal to about 15% of total weight.
Since the amount of fat in the body is variable and the fat is assumed to
contain no water itself, the percentage of water in the whole body (including the fat, in contrast to LBM) will vary inversely with the fat content.
The absolute amount of water in the body does not vary with the amount
of fat; however, the proportion of the body that is water will decrease as
"dry" fat is increased in the body.

Using a child as an example, if the LBM is 20 kg and the body water
is 75%, or 15 liters, the percentage of water in the total body will vary
from 68% to 60% for body fat content of 10% and 20% of whole body
weight, respectively.

Whole body weight = LBM + body fat*
For 10% fat, in this example:
  whole body weight = LBM + 10% of whole body weight

---

* Body fat contains small amounts of lean tissue (protein, ash, and water) in the fat
cell protoplasm. For clinical purposes, this can be ignored.

whole body weight $-$ 0.10 whole body weight = LBM
0.90 whole body weight = 20 kg
whole body weight = 22.2 kg
and since TBW = 75% LBM = 15 liters,

$$\text{percentage water in whole body weight} = \frac{15}{22.2} \times 100$$

$$= 67.6\%$$

For 20% fat, in this example:
whole body weight = LBM + 20% whole body weight
whole body weight $-$ 0.20 whole body weight = 20 kg
0.80 whole body weight = 25.0 kg

$$\text{therefore, percentage water} = \frac{15}{25} \times 100$$

$$= 60\%$$

In an adolescent female, body fat can vary from 15% to 30%, and using similar calculations for a girl with LBM of 42.5 kg, body fat would vary from 7.5 kg to 18 kg. The percentage water in the total body would vary from 64% to 53%.

Changes in Total Body Weight with Age

The percentage of water in the lean body decreases slightly with age, but the percentage of water in the whole body decreases still more because of the increasing proportion of fat in the body as the child matures. For clinical purposes one can reasonably assume that the infant's body is about two-thirds water (67%) and that the older child and adult have TBWs of 60%. In emaciated or obese individuals these values will vary more widely; they can range from 70% to 75% of the body as water in the emaciated and from 40% to 50% of the body as water in the obese.

Body Water Compartments

As was previously noted, it has been convenient to divide TBW into several categories, based on its location in the tissues. There have been extensive investigations of this compartmentalization of TBW, as well as characterization of the transfers between these compartments and determinations of their sizes under varying conditions. The basic problem with each of these studies is inherent in the compartment concept itself. In this concept, there is tacit assumption that all the fluid in any one compartment has the same composition and that all the fluid follows the same physicochemical reactions.

The two major divisions of body water are the intracellular fluid (ICF) and the extracellular fluid (ECF). The ICF, as its name implies, refers to

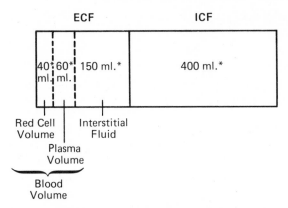

*Values are approximate volumes/kg. of body weight in an adult male.

Fig. 1-1.   Body water compartments. Diagrammatic representation of the body water compartments in 1 kg of body weight for a typical adult male. In the adult female each of the values is slightly lower because of the greater amount of body fat in the average female: the fat is essentially a water-free solid. In children, the volume of the ICF is somewhat smaller, and the volume of the ECF is somewhat larger: the largest differences are in the premature infant. The values gradually approach those of the adult during childhood.

the water inside cells. The more we learn about subcellular particles in the cytoplasm and the constituents of the nucleus, the more apparent it becomes that the ICF cannot be considered as a homogeneous "bag" of chemicals in solution.

The ECF is also heterogeneous, even when the intravascular fluid is considered separately. Attempts to measure the ECF with a variety of chemical agents have given quite different values in the same individual. This has led to the golf-score notion, i.e., the lowest volume measured is the correct one. It is based on the assumption that all larger volumes represent varying degrees of penetration of the measuring substance into the ICF. Even this idea becomes untenable when it is seen that studies with inulin, which gives one of the smaller volume measurements, have demonstrated varying penetrations into the water of noncellular connective tissue depending on time, density of the tissue, and the animal species being studied.

Similar problems can be cited for each compartment or "space" that has been proposed. In spite of this, there is still some utility in dividing body water into several categories for the purpose of discussing fluid physiology. In doing this, it must be kept in mind that these categories cannot be rigidly defined or precisely measured, nor can they be expected to behave as discrete physicochemical entities, even though they are assigned numerical values. Chemical compositions and transfers of various substances between compartments are described in the remainder of this work. Such descriptions should always be considered approximations that indicate qualitative phenomena, not exact quantitative changes.

With this caveat, plasma volume, blood volume,* ECF, interstitial fluid (the difference between ECF and blood volume), and ICF will be described and used to discuss general responses of body fluids to a variety of disturbances (Fig. 1-1). The ECF and the ICF are the two major divisions of body water to be considered. The plasma volume is included in the ECF because the ionic composition of plasma is similar to that of the interstitial fluid (the part of the ECF that is outside the vascular system). Because the plasma proteins are confined primarily to the vascular space, there are certain characteristics of this space that will be considered separately.

EXTRACELLULAR FLUID

Volume

The volume of the ECF has been measured using inulin, sulfate ions, chloride ions, and related substances that appear to be excluded from cells. Each substance tends to yield a different value for the ECF volume. Whether the inulin space,† the sulfate space, or the chloride space is used to represent the ECF, there is good agreement that this volume decreases with age. For clinical use, 25% of body weight is a good approximation for the volume of ECF in infancy, and 20% is appropriate for older children and adults. As an example, a 7-kg infant has an ECF of 1750 ml $(0.25 \times 7 = 1.75 = 1750$ ml). A 70-kg adult has an ECF of 14,000 ml $(0.20 \times 70 = 14 = 14,000$ ml). The very small premature infant has an ECF equal to 30% of its body weight.

---

* The water of the blood cells is intracellular in the strictest sense, but by convention this fluid is usually considered part of the ECF. The red blood cells are not characteristic of the other cells in the body, and this fact supports the use of the ECF convention for blood cells.

† In the sense used here, the term *space* indicates the volume of distribution within the body of the particular chemical substance used as a modifier of the term *space;* i.e., the inulin space is the volume of distribution of inulin in the body after equilibrium has been reached.

Composition

DEFINITION OF TERMS

Before describing the composition of the ECF, several terms need to be defined and understood:

milligram (mg)
milligrams/deciliter (mg/dl)
milliequivalent (mEq)
milliequivalents/liter (mEq/liter)
millimole (mM)
millimoles/liter (mM/liter)
milliosmole (mOsm)
milliosmoles/liter (mOsm/liter)
solute

When a substance is measured in terms of its weight, this is traditionally expressed in a weight/volume relationship. If the amount is small, the milligram (mg) is used as the unit of weight; for larger amounts, the unit is the gram (g). The volume used for the weight/volume relationship is 0.1 liter. In the past, the weight/volume terms have been expressed in two ways: either milligrams/100 ml (mg/100 ml) or milligrams percent (mg%). Recently, the more appropriate term for 0.1 liter, the deciliter (dl), has come into wider use, and the weight/volume relationship is given in milligrams/deciliter (mg/dl). As an example, normal plasma calcium concentration is given as $Ca^{++} = 10$ mg/100 ml $= 10$ mg% $= 10$ mg/dl.

When using terminology reflecting molarity or equivalency, decimal figures have essentially been eliminated by using millimolar and milliequivalent values: 1 mole = 1000 millimoles (mM); 1 equivalent = 1000 milliequivalents (mEq). The volume is then expressed in terms of 1 liter as milliequivalents/liter (mEq/liter) or millimoles/liter (mM/liter).

The term milliequivalent is used to represent the amount of any positively or negatively charged substance (e.g., Na^+, K^+, Cl^-, HCO_3^-, NH_4^+, Ca^{++}, Mg^{++}, HPO_4^{--}) when the electrical property of that substance is the important consideration. Since this is the property of greatest concern in body fluid physiology, milliequivalent is now the term in general use for such ions.

$$mEq = \frac{mg \times net\ charge}{atomic\ or\ molecular\ weight}$$

In terms of concentration, milliequivalents are expressed per liter of fluid:

$$mEq/liter = \frac{mg/liter \times net\ charge}{atomic\ or\ molecular\ weight}$$

Nonionized substances are frequently important because they can become ionized or because the number of molecules present (rather than the weight) is the property of physiologic importance. The osmotic pressure of body fluids is one such property, because it determines the transfer of water from one fluid space to another; and the osmotic pressure depends on the number of molecules present in a solution, not their weight. Thus the terms millimole (mM) and milliosmole (mOsm) are frequently used interchangeably for substances such as H_2CO_3, glucose, and urea; again, concentrations are expressed per liter. As an example, for a blood glucose of 90 mg% = 90 mg/dl = 900 mg/liter and molecular weight = 180,

$$\text{glucose mM/liter} = \frac{\text{mg/liter}}{\text{molecular weight}} = \frac{900}{180} = 5 \text{ mM/liter}$$

For conversion of a concentration that is expressed on a weight/volume basis to a concentration expressed as milliequivalents/liter (mEq/liter) or millimoles/liter (mM/liter), the concentration in milligrams/deciliter (mg/dl) is multiplied by 10 to yield milligrams/liter (mg/liter); that value is then divided by the atomic or molecular weight to obtain millimoles/liter (mM/liter). If the substance is an ion, the millimoles/liter are multiplied by the number of charges on the ion to determine the milliequivalents/liter. As an example, calcium has an atomic weight of 40, and since an ion has two positive charges (Ca^{++}), Ca^{++} = 10 mg/dl (an average value for serum Ca^{++}).

10 mg/dl × 10 = 100 mg/liter

$\dfrac{100 \text{ mg/liter}}{40}$ = 2.5 mM/liter (40 is the atomic weight of Ca^{++})

2.5 × 2 = 5.0 mEq/liter (2 is the number of charges on Ca^{++})

All particles in a solution, ions and uncharged molecules, contribute to the chemical properties or colligative properties of the solution. The ions and the other molecules are collectively termed the solute. One important effect of solute in body fluids is that it creates the osmotic pressure of a solution. The solute, for these considerations, is the sum of all osmotically active substances, and the value of this sum is expressed as the solute concentration in milliosmoles/kilogram (mOsm/kg).

Technically, the solute concentration responsible for the osmotic pressure, or any other colligative property (such as the freezing point depression), is correctly expressed as osmolality, which is the solute con-

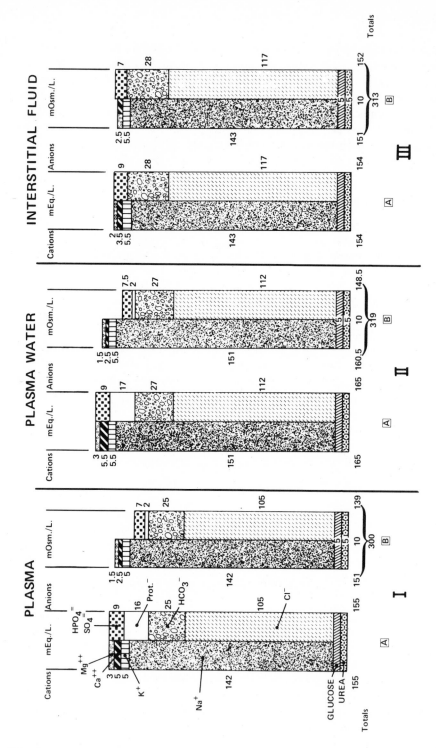

centration per kilogram of solvent. Physiologic processes are concerned with osmolality. However, because of ease in measurement, the term osmolarity is often used; osmolarity is solute concentration per liter of solution. In body fluids the two values are so close that there is little clinical significance to the difference. The two terms can usually be interchanged if the units are given correctly. This book will generally use osmolarity: milliosmoles/liter (mOsm/liter).

Plasma, Plasma Water, and Interstitial Fluid

The compositions of plasma and of interstitial fluid, which contains very little protein, can be examined in terms of ionic composition as well as osmolar content (Fig. 1-2). The following items are most pertinent to an interpretation of the representations in Figure 1-2:

1. The numerical values given in Figure 1-2 are average values for the older child and adult. They are not absolute, as the normal value will have a definable range, and the mean, as well as the range, will depend on the analytic method used. These values are for illustrative purposes, and although they approximate the normal mean values, they should not be used in that sense.

2. In each of the three fluids (I, II, III), A represents the composition in terms of ionic equivalence, and B represents the composition in terms of solute concentration or osmolarity.

3. Section I represents the plasma, and column IA represents the

---

Fig. 1-2. Composition of ECF. The figure is divided into three parts representing the composition of plasma, plasma water, and the interstitial fluid; in each part there are two pairs of columns. The pair on the left shows the composition of the fluid in milliequivalents/liter, and the cation column on the left is equivalent to the anion column on the right. The right-hand pairs of columns in each part show the same ions and substances expressed as milliosmoles/liter. The major difference is that protein, which has a value of 16 mEq/liter, has a concentration of only 2 mOsm/liter because of the large size of these molecules and the multiple charges on each molecule. The concentrations in plasma water have been increased roughly 5%–6% to account for the presence of the solids in plasma. The concentrations in interstitial fluid have been corrected by the Gibbs-Donnan factor for anions and cations, which results in approximately a 5% decrease in the concentration of the cations and a 5% increase in the concentration of the anions over those in plasma water. This is the result of the interstitial fluid being essentially protein-free.

ionic values (in mEq/liter) as they come from laboratory determinations.* Column IB diagrams the same constituents in terms of their solute concentrations in plasma.

4. In all sections, the ionic values, as shown in the A columns, are equal for total cations and anions, as there can be no net charge in the fluids. Although there are situations in which isolated shifts of cations or anions occur in the body and produce a net electric charge, these changes are transitory and of small magnitude. One reason that these shifts are minimal is that the electromotive force (voltage potential) generated by unequal charges leads either to transmission of a neuronal or muscular impulse (with subsequent return of the ions to their original state) or to a compensatory shift of ions to return the potential difference to baseline.

5. In the B columns, only the number of "particles" present is important; the charge is not important. Therefore the anions and cations need not be equal. The totals in these columns are given for cations, anions, and uncharged substances together, as osmolarity does not involve charges.

The plasma proteins themselves, because of their high molecular weights, represent relatively few molecules in the solution. Thus 6.5 g of protein per 100 ml (dl) of plasma will have 16 mEq/liter of negative charge but will equal only 2 mOsm/liter of solute.

6. Although theoretically the solute concentration or osmolarity of plasma is 300 mOsm/liter, the normal mean value, as determined in the laboratory, is about 280 mOsm/liter. This results from the fact that proteins bind a major portion of the divalent ions but also bind a fraction of the monovalent cations and anions. Although plasma proteins have net negative charges, they are amphoteric (having both positive and negative charges) and thus can bind both cations and anions. Ions bound to protein have no effective osmolar activity, and thus they are not measured using general laboratory procedures for determining osmolarity.

7. The second part (II) of Figure 1-2 represents the values in plasma water. Plasma may be considered a solution composed of a solvent (water) and solute (protein, electrolytes, urea, glucose, etc.). Most of the lipids in plasma are dispersed rather than dissolved. Therefore they do not affect the osmolarity or ionic equilibria in the body fluids. However, since a sample of plasma for laboratory analysis includes the lipids, the presence of large amounts of lipids in the plasma can give a distorted reading of the actual concentration of solutes present in the solvent of plasma (the plasma water). Thus a correction for any large amounts of fat present in the serum can be used to modify the reported laboratory values to provide

---

* Glucose and urea, which are not ionized, are included for comparative purposes, but they do not contribute numerically to the ionic composition, and no numeric values are given for them in the A columns. However, since they are solutes, numeric values are given in the B columns.

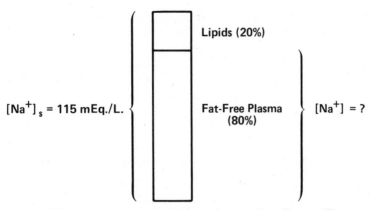

$[Na^+]_s$ = 115 mEq./L. $\big\{$ **Lipids (20%)** / **Fat-Free Plasma (80%)** $\big\}$ $[Na^+]$ = ?

Fig. 1-3. Sodium concentration in fat-free plasma. The diagram illustrates the concept of hyponatremia secondary to hyperlipidemia. The apparent concentration of sodium in the serum is actually found to be within the normal range when the concentration is calculated on the basis of fat-free plasma. Just as in the body as a whole, the lipids are essentially water-free and thus contain few electrolytes. However, when plasma is sampled for chemical analysis, an aliquot of the plasma will contain whatever fat is present. In nonhyperlipidemic states the small amount of fat in the plasma has little effect on the concentration of sodium. However, when the lipids in plasma are markedly elevated, the sodium value may appear to be pathologically decreased.

a value that would be representative of fat-free plasma. As an example, a plasma with 20% lipids, as might occur in diabetic ketoacidosis, has a reported serum Na^+ concentration of 115 mEq/liter. If the lipids were not present, what would the $[Na^+]_s$ be?* See Figure 1-3. In actuality, the Na^+ that was analyzed exists in only 80% of a liter, or 800 ml, even though a liter of fluid is used to report the value. To obtain a corrected, or fat-free, value, the 115 mEq of Na^+ in 800 ml of fat-free plasma is multiplied by a factor (in this case 1000/800) to give a "true" value of $(1000/800) \times 115 = 144$ mEq/liter.

The correction used for a high lipid content in plasma is of value in assessing clinical situations. If one wishes to examine the equilibrium between the plasma and the interstitial fluid (the extravascular portion of the ECF), the electrolyte concentrations must be calculated in terms of concentrations in the solvent of the plasma (the plasma water). The serum proteins are present in much higher concentrations in plasma than in interstitial fluid. Since the capillary walls are essentially impermeable to

* Brackets around a symbol are used to indicate "the concentration of." $[Na^+]$ should be read as "the concentration of sodium." Subscripts are used to indicate the fluids for which the concentrations are given: s is for serum, p is for plasma, e is for ECF, and i is for ICF. When no subscript is used, it may be assumed that the concentration is for serum. $[Na^+]_s$ is read "the concentration of sodium in the serum."

the proteins, and since the proteins have net negative charges, the equilibria across the capillary wall must be corrected for the semipermeable characteristics of the vascular membrane. These corrections are made on the basis of the concentrations in the plasma water. Serum proteins occupy about 6% of plasma, and thus electrolyte concentrations in plasma water will be about 6% higher than in plasma.

8. The interstitial fluid (part III) differs from plasma (and plasma water) in that it has negligible protein content. As a result, the protein anions are not represented. To compensate for this and to preserve electroneutrality, the concentrations of the other anions increase and the concentrations of the cations decrease, in comparison to their concentrations in plasma water. The alterations in concentrations of anions and cations follow the Gibbs-Donnan rule.* In the case of the plasma interstitial fluid, the absence of protein in the interstitial fluid also reduces the amount of divalent ion present in the interstitial fluid, since some of the divalent ions are quite strongly bound to protein.

9. The theoretical osmolarity of the interstitial fluid is lower than the theoretical osmolarity of plasma water. Therefore water ought to move into the plasma from the interstitium, but this is prevented by the greater hydrostatic pressure in the vascular system, which in health balances the difference in osmotic pressure and results in no net transfer of water.†

Implications

There are several clinically useful ways in which the foregoing information may be used:

1. Since $[Na^+]$ represents almost all of the cation in the ECF, doubling $[Na^+]$ gives a value approximating the solute concentration: If $[Na^+] = 140$ mEq/liter, $140 \times 2 = 280$; thus the osmolarity can be estimated as 280 mOsm/liter.

If urea or glucose concentrations are increased, then the osmolarity cannot be estimated on the basis of $[Na^+]$ alone. In such situations, the

---

* If two solutions of ions are separated by a membrane that is permeable to all but one of the ions, e.g., protein^{n-}, the concentration of the other ions, e.g., Na^+ and Cl^- will be related as: $\dfrac{Na^+_A}{Na^+_B} = \dfrac{Cl^-_B}{Cl^-_A}$ or $Na^+_A Cl^-_A = Na^+_B Cl^-_B$

† The effective osmotic pressure of plasma water can be assumed to be 6% higher than the effective osmotic pressure of plasma, or about 298 mOsm/liter. The effective osmotic pressure of interstitial fluid is unknown. Although there is a very low protein concentration in interstitial fluid, the fixed connective-tissue proteins do bind anions and cations; thus the effective osmotic pressure will be somewhat less than the theoretical osmotic pressure.

osmolarity for glucose (molecular weight 180) is

$$
\begin{aligned}
\text{glucose} = &\quad 90 \text{ mg/dl} = \;\; 5 \text{ mOsm/liter} \quad (90 \times 10)/180 \\
= &\quad 180 \text{ mg/dl} = 10 \text{ mOsm/liter} \\
= &\quad 500 \text{ mg/dl} = 28 \text{ mOsm/liter} \\
= &\quad 750 \text{ mg/dl} = 42 \text{ mOsm/liter} \\
= &\; 1000 \text{ mg/dl} = 56 \text{ mOsm/liter} \\
= &\; 1500 \text{ mg/dl} = 83 \text{ mOsm/liter}
\end{aligned}
$$

and for urea (molecular weight 60)

$$
\begin{aligned}
\text{BUN*} = &\;\; 10 \text{ mg/dl}; \quad \text{urea} = \;\;\; 21 \text{ mg/dl} = \;\; 3.5 \text{ mOsm/liter} \\
= &\;\; 15 \text{ mg/dl}; \qquad\qquad\; = \;\;\; 32 \text{ mg/dl} = \;\; 5 \text{ mOsm/liter} \\
= &\;\; 20 \text{ mg/dl}; \qquad\qquad\; = \;\;\; 43 \text{ mg/dl} = \;\; 7 \text{ mOsm/liter} \\
= &\;\; 50 \text{ mg/dl}; \qquad\qquad\; = \; 107 \text{ mg/dl} = 18 \text{ mOsm/liter} \\
= &\; 100 \text{ mg/dl}; \qquad\qquad\; = \; 214 \text{ mg/dl} = 36 \text{ mOsm/liter} \\
= &\; 150 \text{ mgPdl}; \qquad\qquad = \; 321 \text{ mg/dl} = 53 \text{ mOsm/liter}
\end{aligned}
$$

Serum osmolarity can then be estimated by converting the glucose or urea concentration to mOsm/liter and then adding that figure to twice the $[Na^+]$.

2. In plasma or serum, since the variations in $[Mg^{++}]$, $[Ca^{++}]$, $[K^+]$, $[Prot.^-]$, and $[HPO_4^{--}, SO_4^{--}, Org. Ac.^-]$ are usually relatively small in comparison to the variations in $[Na^+]$, $[Cl^-]$, and $[HCO_3^-]$, a simple relationship normally exists among the last three ions:

$$[Na^+] = [Cl^-] + [HCO_3^-] + (12 \pm 3)$$

Thus, if the laboratory provides the information

$$
\begin{aligned}
[Na^+] &= 135 \text{ mEq/liter} \\
[Cl^-] &= 101 \text{ mEq/liter} \\
[HCO_3^-] &= \;\; 21 \text{ mEq/liter}
\end{aligned}
$$

then

$$[Na^+] = [Cl^-] + [HCO_3^-] + (12 \pm 3)$$

becomes

$$135 = 101 + 21 + 13$$

which meets the equality, since the last term is between 9 and 15.

* Since blood urea nitrogen (BUN) measures only the nitrogen content of urea, the osmolarity can be calculated by dividing the BUN (in mg/liter) by 28 (two nitrogen atoms of atomic weight 14 in each molecule of urea) or by converting [BUN] to [urea] by multiplying BUN by 60/23 (the molecular weight of urea divided by twice the atomic weight of nitrogen) and dividing the [urea] (in mg/liter) by 60.

If the laboratory returns

$$[Na^+] = 143 \text{ mEq/liter}$$
$$[Cl^-] = 100 \text{ mEq/liter}$$
$$[HCO_3^-] = 18 \text{ mEq/liter}$$

then

$$143 = 100 + 18 + 25$$

The last term is too large, and therefore either there is a laboratory error or there is an increase in [Prot.$^-$] or in the [HPO$_4^{--}$, SO$_4^{--}$, Org. Ac.$^-$] fraction. In cases of multiple myeloma, for example, the proteins could be increased; in cases of diabetic acidosis, renal failure, etc., the HPO$_4^{--}$, SO$_4^{--}$, Org. Ac.$^-$ fraction could be increased. Further evaluation of the patient would be necessary to distinguish between laboratory error and unexpected problems in the patient.

The contribution of protein to the anionic column can be estimated by multiplying the concentration in grams/deciliter by the factor 2.43. This factor has been determined experimentally and is the net charge per gram of serum protein. Serum proteins have both positive and negative charges, but the negative charges exceed the positive in the amount of 0.243 mEq/liter for each gram of protein. Thus, with a normal serum protein concentration of 6.5 g/dl, the net anionic equivalence = $0.243 \times 6.5 = 1.6$ mEq/dl. Since equivalent values are given per liter, the 1.6 mEq/dl = 16 mEq/liter. For simplicity, the values of protein per deciliter are multiplied by 2.43 to give the equivalent in milliequivalents/liter. For example, in the nephrotic syndrome the [Prot.$^-$] may be 2.0 g/dl; then the anionic value would be $2.0 \times 2.43 = 5$ mEq/liter instead of the normal 16 mEq/liter. As a result, the difference between [Na$^+$] and [HCO$_3^-$] + [Cl$^-$] would decrease by about 10 mEq/liter, since either the concentration of one or more of the anions would have had to increase or the [Na$^+$] would have had to decrease or both of these changes would have had to occur so that the total concentration of anions and the total concentration of cations would remain equal. Thus knowledge of the relationships among the ionic constituents of the plasma can be useful in evaluation of the patient and evaluation of the laboratory results.

Example

A 10-year-old boy with severe dehydration, oliguria, hyperpnea, and a fruity odor to his breath had the following values reported by the laboratory:

$$[Na^+] = 115 \text{ mEq/liter}$$
$$[Cl^-] = 87 \text{ mEq/liter}$$
$$[HCO_3^-] = 6 \text{ mEq/liter}$$

$$[K^+] = \quad 7 \text{ mEq/liter}$$
$$BUN = \quad 40 \text{ mg/dl}$$
$$\text{plasma protein} = \quad 6.5 \text{ g/dl}$$
$$\text{blood sugar} = 900 \text{ mg/dl}$$
$$\text{total lipid} = \quad 10 \text{ g/dl}$$

How should these values be interpreted?

$[Na^+] = 115$ mEq/liter (a low value; normal $= 135–145$ mEq/liter).

$[Cl^-] = 87$ mEq/liter (a low value; normal $= 95–105$ mEq/liter).

$[HCO_3^-] = 6$ mEq/liter (a low value, compatible with the metabolic acidosis of diabetic ketoacidosis).

$[K^+] = 7$ mEq/liter (a high value, seen at times initially in diabetic ketoacidosis, especially in dehydration with diminished renal function).

$BUN = 40$ mg/dl (a high value, compatible with diminished renal function as seen in serious dehydration).

Total plasma Protein $= 6.5$ g/dl (a normal value).

Blood sugar $= 900$ mg/dl (a high value, expected in diabetic ketoacidosis).

Total lipid $= 10$ g/dl (a very high value, but seen occasionally in severe diabetic ketoacidosis; this would produce a very turbid plasma).

The low values for $[Na^+]$ and $[Cl^-]$ remain unexplained. How does one proceed to appreciate the total plasma pattern?

In a complex situation such as this, where some abnormal values are not easily explained, it is frequently helpful to diagram the findings as in Figure 1-4 and estimate or calculate the unknown values.

1. To calculate the anion equivalence of protein, the concentration (in g/dl) is multiplied by 2.43: $6.5 \times 2.43 = 16$ mEq/liter.

2. With no reason to assume any marked change in calcium or magnesium, normal values can be used: $[Ca^{++}] = 5$ mEq/liter; $[Mg^{++}] = 3$ mEq/liter.

3. The sum of cations (in mEq/liter) $= [Na^+] + [K^+] + [Ca^{++}] + [Mg^{++}] = 115 + 7 + 5 + 3 = 130$ mEq/liter.

Since the sum of anions must equal the sum of cations, $[Cl^-] + [HCO_3^-] + [Prot.^-] + [HPO_4^{--}, SO_4^{--}, Org. Ac.^-] = 130$ mEq/liter. Values can be substituted for the first three terms and the fourth calculated: $87 + 6 + 16 + [HPO_4^{--}, SO_4^{--}, Org. Ac.^-] = 130$; then $[HPO_4^{--}, SO_4^{--}, Org. Ac.^-] = 21$ mEq/liter. Although this value is higher than normal, it is not surprising for ketosis and/or mild azotemia.

4. Since the low Na^+ and Cl^- values may be related to the total osmolarity of the serum, the osmolar values for urea and glucose are determined, and then the total osmolarity can be estimated. The osmolar value for urea is calculated either by converting BUN to urea and then dividing by the molecular weight of urea:

$$BUN = 40; \text{urea} = BUN \times \frac{60}{28} = 86 \text{ mg/dl}$$

$$86 \text{ mg/dl} = 860 \text{ mg/L}$$

$$\frac{860}{60} = 14 \text{ mOsm/L}$$

or, more simply, by multiplying BUN by 10 to obtain milligrams/liter and then dividing by 28 (the atomic weight for the two nitrogens that are measured as BUN): (40 × 10)/28 = 14 mOsm/liter.

5. The osmolar value for glucose is obtained by multiplying the value in milligrams/deciliter by 10 to obtain milligrams/liter and then dividing by the molecular weight (180): (900 × 10)/180 = 50 mOsm/liter. The total osmolarity for the plasma is as follows:

Cations:	Na^+	115.0	
	K^+	7.0	
	Ca^{++}	2.5	(half as many milliequivalents as there are two charges per ion)
	Mg^{++}	1.5	
Anions:	Cl^-	87	
	HCO_3^-	6	
	Prot.$^-$	2	(because of the high molecular weight, the serum proteins exert an osmolarity of about 2 mOsm/liter for a serum protein level of 6 g/dl)
	Org. Ac.$^-$	21	(assuming a net charge of one per anion.)
Non-ions:	glucose	50	
	urea	14	
Total osmolarity =		306	mOsm/liter

Since this is a value that is within the normal range for serum osmolarity, it can be assumed that the low $[Na^+]$ and $[Cl^-]$ are the result of total osmolar regulation. After control of body fluid volume has been attempted, the regulating mechanisms act to maintain normal total solute concentration. In this case the glucose level cannot be lowered immediately; thus sodium and chloride reabsorption is reduced until the concentrations of these ions are such that total osmolarity (solute concentration) is within a nearly normal range.

6. Finally, correction should be made for the high fat content of the plasma. Fat is like protein in that it occupies space; plasma with 10% fat and 6.5% protein is only 83.5% water. In order to compare these values with later ones in the same patient or in other patients without hyper-

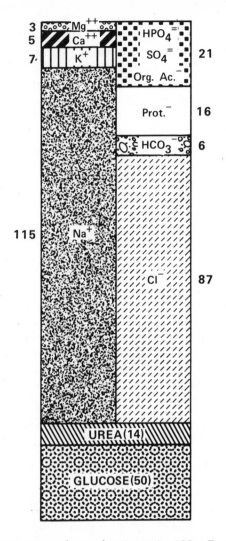

Total cations (anions) estimated = 130 mEq./L.

Fig. 1-4. Serum values in diabetic ketoacidosis. These values illustrate what may occur to the measured electrolyte concentrations in the presence of hyperglycemia. Since regulation of total osmolarity of the plasma is the dominant regulating system for solute concentrations, the presence of 50 mOsm/liter of glucose in the plasma (as in this example) will often result in a concomitant decrease in the concentrations of the ionic substances also present is plasma.

19

lipidemia, the values should be corrected to the normal water content of plasma, which is 94%. Thus all the values obtained in this patient would be greater in plasma that has a normal lipid content by a factor of 94/83.5, which equals 1.12, or a 12% increase over the reported laboratory results.

Figure 1-5 is a representation of values corrected for lipid content. These are what would be found if the plasma had a normal lipid concentration. The urea will be 15.7 mOsm/liter and the glucose 56 mOsm/liter (1008 mg/dl). The total solute concentration will be the sum of the cations, anions, and nonionized compounds (all in mOsm/liter): $306 \times 1.12 = 343$ mOsm/liter, which is somewhat increased but is commensurate with the clinical picture of dehydration described for this child. Therefore the laboratory values are entirely consistent with the clinical findings.

INTRACELLULAR FLUID

The fluid that is within the cells of the body is even more heterogeneous than the ECF. Much less is known about the physiology of the ICF than about the physiology of the ECF because access to the ICF is technically limited. Nevertheless, since some characteristics of the ICF are known, and since most of the critical chemical reactions of the body take place in this environment, there are valid reasons, at times, to consider this volume as if it were homogeneous and were divided into millions of little bags of water, all doing the same thing at the same moment.

Volume Change with Age

The volume of the ICF varies less as the body develops than does the volume of the ECF. The ICF increases slightly as a percentage of the LBM with increasing age. Although the change in ICF as a percentage of LBM is relatively constant and stable, the change in ICF as a percentage of *total* body weight is unpredictable because of the variability introduced by body fat.* If body fat increases markedly with age, the ICF as a percentage of total body weight will fall (Fig. 1-6). Thus the ICF, as a portion of the total body, may decrease, may not change, or may increase over a period of time, depending on the rate and extent of accumulation of body fat. For purposes of calculation in the clinical setting, the ICF can be considered to represent 40% of body weight throughout the human life span. This may overestimate the volume in the infant and underestimate it in the elderly, but the error is small and not of practical importance.

---

* Adipose tissue consists of cells with a small amount of cytoplasm and thus small amounts of intracellular water. However, the accepted approach for examining most body water problems is to assume that body fat is protein-free and water-free, i.e., pure fat.

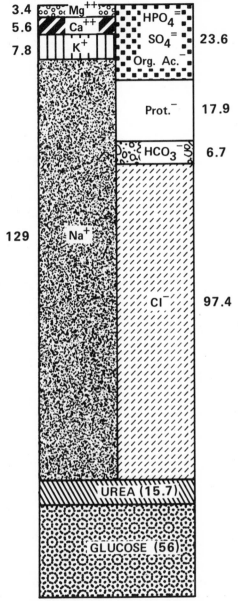

Fig. 1-5 Serum values corrected for 10% plasma lipids. As in Figure 1-3, the presence of excessive lipids in the plasma may result in an apparent reduction in the concentration of all other substances. To obtain a true measure of the concentrations of the ionic solutes and of glucose, it is necessary to correct the values for the amount of lipid present whenever the lipid concentration is abnormally elevated. These values represent correction for a lipid concentration of 10% in the plasma that is illustrated in Figure 1-4.

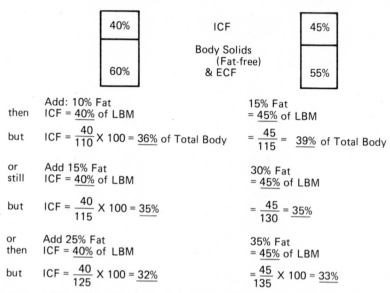

Fig. 1-6.   ICF and total body fat. The calculations shown in this figure illustrate the effect of varying amounts of total body fat on the concentration of intracellular fluid in the total body for young adults and for elderly individuals, who generally have somewhat larger percentages of intracellular fluid. As the percentage of fat in the young adult varies from 10% up to 25%, the apparent volume of ICF decreases from 36% of total body mass to 32% of total body mass. In the elderly adult, where the ICF is 45% of the LBM, the percentage of ICF in the total body (including fat) decreases from 39% to 33% as total body fat increases from 15% to 35%.

Ionic Composition

The cell wall is a membrane that is relatively impermeable to cations and almost impermeable to anions, and it contains a variety of active transport systems. In addition to these different membrane transport characteristics encountered, the composition of the ICF is markedly different from that of the ECF. The primary univalent cation is K^+; the primary divalent cation is Mg^{++}. The anion pattern is less clear; phosphate in organic form represents the major anion, and proteinates furnish the next highest amount of anion. Sulfates are present to some extent; HCO_3^- concentration is about one-half its concentration in plasma, and there is negligible Cl^- in most body cells. Since cells of different organs and different tissues and in different locations in the body appear to have differing compositions, and since direct analyses of cell fluid are not available, any diagrammatic representation of ICF is speculative and an approximation at best; however, it can be used to indicate the relative contents of the ions as well as to indicate that the total cation concentration (and therefore the anion concentration as well) is greater than that of the ECF. This does not indicate any difference in the osmolarity of the two fluids, since large proportions of the ions are divalent, some ions are bound, and many ions represent multiple charges on single large molecules. Osmotic equality is assumed to exist across the cell membrane in stable physiologic states (Fig. 1-7).

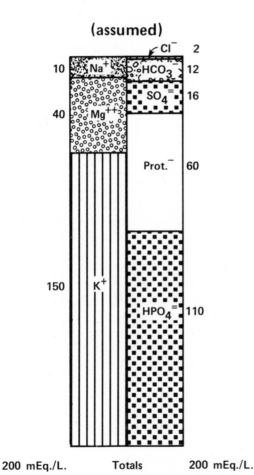

200 mEq./L.   Totals   200 mEq./L.

Fig. 1-7.   Composition of intracellular water. Since the fluid within cells is compartmentalized into many subdivisions (such as nuclear water, mitochondrial water, etc.), one can only make assumptions about an overall composition of intracellular water. These assumed, or average, composite values are given as milliequivalents/liter.

Implications

The almost exclusively extracellular positioning of the Cl^- provides a reasonably accurate method of estimating the volume of the ECF.* If the ECF can be estimated, and if there is a measurement of the TBW, then the ICF can be obtained by subtraction:

$$TBW = ECF + ICF$$
$$TBW - ECF = ICF$$

Generally, the absolute volume is not known, and the change in volume from an estimated normal state is what is sought.

Once the volumes of the ECF and ICF have been calculated on the basis of the extracellular positioning of Cl^-, changes and transfers of other ions into and out of the ECF can be estimated.

Example

A 10-year-old boy who was previously healthy and well nourished developed carditis with cardiac failure and edema. He was admitted to the hospital weighing 45 kg. Analysis of his serum provided the following information: $[Na^+] = 130$ mEq/liter; $[Cl^-] = 95$ mEq/liter. Over the next 72 hours he was given diuretics and non-salt-containing fluids. During that period he excreted a total of 7500 ml of urine with a $[Cl^-]$ of 56.8 mEq/liter, and his weight stabilized at 40 kg. At the end of 72 hours his serum values were $[Na^+] = 140$ mEq/liter and $[Cl^-] = 100$ mEq/liter.

What were the changes in volume of the TBW, ICF, and ECF? Assuming his body composition was average after his diuresis was complete,

$$TBW = 60\% \text{ of body weight} = 24 \text{ liters}$$
$$ICF = 40\% \text{ of body weight} = 16 \text{ liters}$$
$$ECF = 20\% \text{ of body weight} = 8 \text{ liters}$$

The total Cl^- in the ECF equals the volume of the ECF multiplied by the $[Cl^-]$ in the ECF. The serum $[Cl^-]$ must be corrected for the water content of plasma, as well as corrected by the Gibbs-Donnan factor, to obtain the ECF $[Cl^-]$:

$[Cl^-]_s = 100$ mEq/liter
$[Cl^-]$ plasma water $= [Cl^-]_s \times (100/\%\ H_2O \text{ in plasma})$
$\phantom{[Cl^-] \text{ plasma water}} = 100 \times (100/94) = 106$ mEq/liter of plasma H_2O

---

* The errors in such a calculation include the fact that Cl^- is present in higher concentration in the gastric parietal cells (and in connective tissue) and in lower concentration in some other cells than is predicted by the Gibbs-Donnan equilibrium.

$$[Cl^-]_{ECF} = [Cl^-] \text{ plasma } H_2O \times \text{Gibbs-Donnan factor}$$
$$= 106 \times 1.05 = 111 \text{ mEq/liter of interstitial fluid}$$

For practical purposes these corrections can be combined and calculated by increasing the serum $[Cl^-]$ by 10%. Since 10% of serum $[Cl^-]$ in this patient $= 0.10 \times 100 = 10$, the ECF $[Cl^-] = 100 + 10 = 110$ mEq/liter. Then the ECF Cl^- content $=$ ECF volume $\times$ ECF $[Cl^-] = 8$ liters $\times 110$ mEq/liter $= 880$ mEq of Cl^-. The loss of Cl^- from the body in the previous 72 hours $=$ urine volume $\times$ urine $[Cl^-] = 7.5$ liters $\times 56.8$ mEq/liter $= 426$ mEq of Cl^-.

Thus the amount of Cl^- present in the body at the time of admission equals the amount present after 72 hours plus the amount lost;* 880 mEq + 426 mEq = 1306 mEq of Cl^- present in the body on admission.

The volume of distribution of the Cl^- on admission is obtained by dividing the total amount of Cl^- by its concentration in the ECF. The $[Cl^-]$ in the ECF equals the serum $[Cl^-] + 10\% [Cl^-] = 95 + 9.5 = 104.5$ mEq/ liter. Thus the initial ECF volume $= 1306/104.5 = 12.5$ liters.

The weight gain of 5 kg can therefore be divided into a 4.5-liter $(12.5 - 8)$ expansion of the ECF, and the remaining 0.5 liter may be considered as a gain in the ICF.

Once the volume of the ECF has been estimated in this manner, changes in the distributions of other ions can be evaluated, and any shift of the body water between compartments can be calculated. If the intake of Na^+ in the example were 0, and if the urinary output had a $[Na^+] = 60$ mEq/liter, the changes in Na^+ would be derived as follows: final Na^+ in the ECF $=$ ECF volume $\times$ ECF $[Na^+]$. The ECF $[Na^+]$ can be considered equal to the serum $[Na^+]$, since the correction for water and the Gibbs-Donnan factor for cations tend to cancel each other out.†

Therefore, final ECF $Na^+ = 8.0$ liters $\times 140$ mEq/liter $= 1120$ mEq. Initial ECF Na^+ content $=$ initial ECF volume $\times$ initial ECF $[Na^+]$. Initial ECF $= 12.5 \times 130$ mEq/liter $= 1625$ mEq.

$$\text{loss of } Na^+ = \text{urine volume} \times \text{urine } [Na^+]$$
$$= 7.5 \text{ liters} \times 80 \text{ mEq/liter}$$
$$= 600 \text{ mEq}$$

The difference in ECF Na^+ between the initial situation and the final situation $=$ initial ECF $Na^+ -$ final ECF $Na^+ = 1625 - 1120 = 505$ mEq.

* If there had been any Cl^- intake in this period, the amount of the intake would have to be subtracted from the output to obtain the net amount lost (or gained, if the patient were in "positive balance").

† The plasma water correction $= [NA^+]_{serum} \times (100/94)$, and the Gibbs-Donnan factor cations $= [Na^+]_{plasma\ water} \times (95/100)$. Combining the two factors, $[Na^+]_{serum} \times (100/94) \times (95/100) = [Na^+]_{ECF}$. Thus, $[Na^+]_{serum}$ is essentially equal to $[Na^+]_{ECF}$.

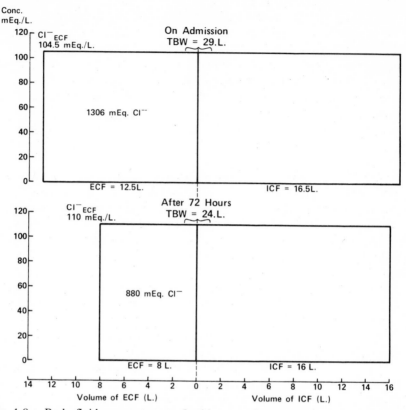

Fig. 1-8. Body fluid compartments. In this type of representation the volume of each fluid compartment (the extracellular and the intracellular) is given along the abscissa, and the concentration of solute is given on the ordinate, either in milliequivalents/liter or in milliosmoles/liter. The area defined by the volume and the concentration is equivalent to the quantity of the solute being represented. The volume of the TBW is equivalent to the sum of the ECF and the ICF. The quantity of solute is the sum of the area under the ECF curve and the area under the ICF curve. The concentration of solute in the TBW is assumed to be equal to the concentration of solute in each body water compartment. The concentrations of any individual solute would rarely be identical in the two compartments, whether the concentration were reported in milliequivalents/liter or in milliosmoles/liter. However, when one is considering an ion that is present in only one compartment (in this example, the chloride ion) the concentration may be shown as equivalent in the ICF for simplicity of representation. This does not imply the presence of chloride at any particular level in the ICF.

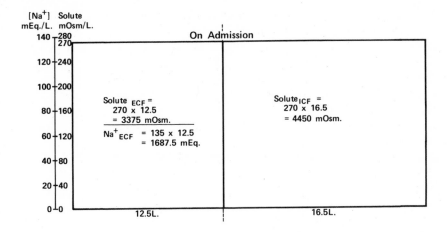

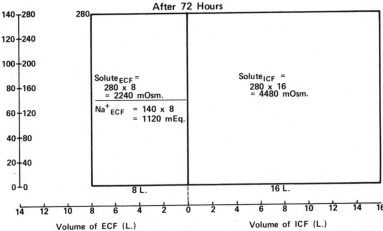

Fig. 1-9. Body fluid solute. The method of representation of volume and concentration is similar to that shown in Figure 1-8. In this example, it is assumed that the total solute concentration is equivalent to twice the sodium concentration in the ECF. It is also accepted that the solute concentration in the ICF will be the same as that in the ECF. In this example, after 72 hours the patient has lost water in excess of solute, so that the volume of the TBW is reduced but the concentration is increased. In the ICF there has been little change in total solute content, but the loss of water (by shifting it to the ECF) has increased the solute concentration.

27

Since the loss of Na^+ in the urine (600 mEq) exceeded the change in ECF Na^+ from the initial situation to the final situation (decrease of 505 mEq) by 95 mEq (600 − 505), these 95 mEq of Na^+ can be assumed to have come from the ICF.* However, if there were a loss of Na^+ from the ICF to the ECF there would have to be some corresponding change in the anions or a change in another cation in the opposite direction (ECF → ICF) or a combined anion–cation change in order to preserve electroneutrality in both ECF and ICF. However, the information presented in the example is insufficient to determine what changes might have occurred in other ions.

The changes in volume and changes in ionic concentration can be shown diagrammatically as a graph in which the horizontal axis represents volume of fluid, the vertical axis represents concentration of an ion, and the area under the curve is equivalent to the total amount of the ion present (Fig. 1-8). Once the volumes for TBW, ECF, and ICF have been calculated using Cl^-, the same kind of diagram can be used to show changes in other ions or in total solute. In Figure 1-9 the total solute is calculated as $2 \times [Na^+]$. From the calculations shown in Figure 1-9 it is apparent that loss of body water was primarily from the ECF and loss of solute was almost exclusively from the ECF. (It has been assumed, as mentioned earlier, that the osmolar concentration of the ICF equals the osmolar concentration of the ECF.)

---

* If there had been any Na^+ intake in this period, it would have to be subtracted from the total output to obtain the net output. If Na^+ intake had exceeded output, then there would have been a net intake or a positive balance of Na^+. In this example, which had a decrease in ECF Na^+, there would have had to have been a large shift of Na^+ into the ICF to account for a decrease in ECF Na^+ in the presence of a positive Na^+ balance for the whole body.

2

Fluid Balance

The turnover of fluids by the body can be separated into those processes that deliver fluid to the body (intake) and those that release fluid from the body (output). Intake and output processes, whose physiologic roles are to maintain the constancy of the body fluids, greatly influence each other, and each can, to some extent, correct for deficiencies in others.

Fluids entering and leaving the body do so by entering or leaving the plasma volume. Although the fluid in the vascular system is brought into equilibrium with the total ECF relatively quickly, a finite period of time is required for the exchange. It is quite possible for the intake or output to be large enough and to occur quickly enough to produce cardiac failure (volume overload) or peripheral vascular collapse and shock (volume depletion). Overloading the vascular system with an excessive rate of intake or total quantity of intake is a much greater danger when output mechanisms are disturbed, and an excessive rate of output or total quantity of output is much more likely to produce shock when a disorder of intake is also present. Thus there is an extensive interrelationship between intake and output, but to simplify discussion they will first be considered separately.

INTAKE

Characteristics

Traditionally, an ingested substance has been classified as solid or liquid, but this is based on its physical state rather than on its composition. For purposes of evaluating fluid and electrolyte problems, other properties are more important: (1) the total amount of the substance, (2) water content (as percentage water or water measured in grams), (3) ionic composition, and (4) "solute load." The first two properties are straightforward, although it is often surprising to learn how much water is present in most "solid" foods. The water content of an average diet provides about 40–50 ml of water per 100 kcal.* In addition, metabolism of foodstuffs generates water as one of the end products. On the average, there is about 0.1 ml of water generated for each kilocalorie metabolized, or 10 ml/100 kcal. The fluids in solid food represent about half of the total fluid intake of an individual who is on a normal diet.

The ionic composition is also relatively simple, until the problem of acid–base balance arises. Although acid–base phenomena will be described later, it is important to remember that the majority of ingested foods (especially proteins) release relatively large quantities of H^+ during their metabolism. It is also important to keep in mind that fresh fruits, when metabolized, produce H^+ acceptors and are therefore alkalinizing—contrary to common belief.

The solute load of an ingested or administered substance refers to the amount of solute that will result from metabolism of the substance and will require removal by renal excretion. In this context, the usual amounts

---

* The kilocalorie will be abbreviated 1 kcal herein; 1 kcal is equivalent to 1000 calories. (Another system of notation uses the term 1 Cal; thus 1 Cal = 1000 cal = 1 kcal.)

of carbohydrate and fat are metabolized to CO_2 and H_2O and thus do not require renal excretion for their removal. Therefore carbohydrates (except for their ionic content) and fat are not generally considered contributors to the solute load. In contrast, protein foods, which are cellular in nature, contain the ions of the tissue fluids and tissue protein that will be metabolized to urea or related nitrogenous compounds that will then require renal excretion for their removal from the body.

EXAMPLE.   One kilogram of meat (75% water, 25% protein) yields about 1653 mOsm of solute. This figure is derived by assuming that the solute concentration in tissue fluid is 300 mOsm/liter; 0.75 liter × 300 mOsm = 225 mOsm. The protein (25% or 250 g) is 16% nitrogen (N), or 40 g (40,000 mg). If all the nitrogen is converted to urea (with 2 N/molecule), 40,000 mg N_2 will yield 1428 mOsm of urea (40,000/28 = 1428); 1428 + 225 = 1653 mOsm/kg of meat.

Control

Control of intake of food and fluids depends primarily on two subjective drives: hunger and thirst. The stimuli and the receptor sites for these reactions are numerous and not well defined. Dryness of the oral mucous membranes appears to be a major stimulus for thirst. In turn, the regulatory system for mucous membrane dryness is complex. It is known that these regulatory systems appear to involve both hypothalamic and cortical centers. When functioning well, they are superb regulators, maintaining weight, body water volume, and osmolarity with remarkable constancy. The control systems can be overridden by conscious input and by emotional input. The thirst mechanism appears to be responsive to both volume and concentration variables. In many animal species the control of intake is more closely attuned to meet physiologic needs than it is in man. With the extensive development of man's higher central nervous system (CNS) centers, he has more extraneous inputs into his regulatory systems, and therefore his fluid intake is less immediately related to fluid needs than is the case in other animals.

Quantity as a Function of Size

In spite of the variability in intake of fluid and calories, average values can be assigned to intake as a function of body size or age. It is obvious that intake does vary with size, but the exact relationship is not immediately apparent. That the relationship is not a direct function of weight becomes obvious by comparison of a 3-year-old child weighing 15 kg and an adult weighing 75 kg. The adult does not consume five times what the 3-year-old child does.

RELATION TO METABOLIC RATE

The fluid intake of an individual must be adequate to replace fluid losses. The losses, in turn, are functions of metabolic rate. Therefore it is necessary to consider the factors that affect metabolic rate in order to understand fluid requirements. A certain intake of calories is necessary to support the metabolic processes that produce tissue for growth and replacement and to provide energy for work and regulatory processes.

METHODS OF CALCULATION

The metabolic rate* (measured as calories per unit of time), as an indicator of the total metabolism of the individual, can be measured directly and is mathematically related to size. When the relationship of metabolic rate to size is examined, the metabolic rate is found to be a function of weight: $\sqrt[3]{weight^2}$ or $weight^{2/3}$. Height may also be used to express this relationship, but it correlates less well than weight. $Weight^{2/3}$ is not a convenient term to use in medical practice; thus other relationships have been sought. The surface area of the body is also a function of $weight^{2/3}$, and thus metabolic rate can be rather directly related to surface area.

The most commonly used values for metabolic rate in terms of calories per surface area (square meter) are 1800–2000 $kcal/m^2$. The use of 1800 $kcal/m^2$ yields somewhat low values in infancy, and 2000 $kcal/m^2$ yields high values in adolescence. Many other empirical formulas have been derived to predict kilocalories from body size in a linear relationship. One such formula relates kilocalories directly to $weight^{2/3}$ ($kg^{2/3}$). Over the range of weights seen in children, a good fit is obtained by using the formula 200 kcal $\times$ $weight^{2/3}$ = total kilocalories required; 200 kcal $\times$ $weight^{2/3}$ yields values that are slightly high in adolescence, but otherwise it provides reasonable figures. Table 2-1 provide values for kilocalories at various ages for boys. The values for girls are similar until adolescence, when the size differences become larger. The values in this table were calculated by several methods. The values in columns 5 and 7 were derived using arbitrary figures of 2000 $kcal/m^2$ and 200 kcal $\times$ $weight^{2/3}$. These represent reasonable values up to 14–15 years of age for healthy children eating an average diet. The values are almost double the basal metabolic rate. Although the values in the table are somewhat high for a child who is inactive, the unpredictable effects of illness on metabolic rate make these figures reasonable for clinical use.

---

* The term *metabolic rate* refers to total caloric expenditure. Basal metabolic rate is the rate at rest; it represents the minimal rate for maintenance of body function. The rate at which energy is required for growth and for activity must be added to the basal rate to give the total metabolic rate.

The effects of illness on metabolic rate are unpredictable in general, be-cause fever will increase metabolic rate, but inactivity will reduce it. In any particular illness the amount of fever and amount of inactivity cannot be foreseen, and the effects of one may be greater than, equal to, or less than the effects of the other in an individual ill child.

Unfortunately, weight$^{2/3}$ is not easily calculated, and surface area cannot be measured routinely. Although the use of surface area to esti-mate metabolic processes in individuals of different size is common and is occasionally used in this text, a table or graph must be used to estimate metabolic rate from weight or height (see Appendix). The simplest refer-ence base for metabolic processes would be some expression using only weight or age as the variable, and several formulas have been proposed. Four such formulas are shown in Table 2-1 and Figure 2-1 and are com-pared with calculations based on surface area and on weight$^{2/3}$. One of the formulas that is easy to use is that first suggested by Priscilla White: total kilocalories/day = 1000 + (100 × age in years). This simple formulation provides values that are somewhat high in infancy and a bit low in the early teens, especially for boys. There is modification of this formula that gives somewhat closer approximation to other estimations [total kilocalories = 800 + (125 × age in years)], but this lacks some of the simplicity of the original. Calculations of total kilocalories for boys 0–18 years of age and calculations of kilocalories/kilogram using each of these formulas are given in Table 2-1 (columns 9–12) and in Figure 2-1. One of the characteristics of formulations based solely on age is that all persons (light or heavy) at any age have the same caloric requirement, and there-fore the heavier person is provided fewer kilocalories/kilogram than the lighter person of the same age. The reverse situation obtains with formula-tions based on weight, such as that suggested by William Wallace. These are shown in columns 13–16 of Table 2-1. In the Wallace-type calculation the heavier person, at any age, gets a higher total of kilocalories than the lighter person, but they get the same kilocalories/kilogram at any particu-lar age.

If the variations in weight at any age were all due to differences in LBM or, alternatively, to differences in total body fat, there would be a rational basis for choosing one type of formulation over the other. How-ever, the differences may be of either type at any age, so that either type of formulation can result in inappropriate values for specific children.

There is a simple formulation that lies between the White type and the Wallace type: kilocalories/kilogram = 100 − weight (kg). In such a calcu-lation the heavier child receives fewer kilocalories/kilogram than the thin one, but the heavier child receives somewhat more in total calories. The main disadvantage with this last equation is that it does not hold true for weights in excess of 40 kg or ages greater than 13 years. The relationship

Table 2-1

Caloric Requirements for Boys Determined by Several Methods*

Age (years) (1)	Average Weight (kg) (2)	Average Height (cm) (3)	Average Skin Area (m^2) (4)	Total Kilocalories = 2000/m^2 Total kcal (5)	kcal/kg (6)	Total Kilocalories = 200 × Weight$^{2/3}$ Total kcal (7)	kcal/kg (8)
0	3.4	50.6	0.21	420	124	432	127
0.5	7.6	66.4	0.36	720	95	774	102
1.0	10.1	75.2	0.44	880	87	932	92
1.5	11.4	81.8	0.49	980	86	1016	89
2	12.6	87.5	0.54	1080	86	1080	86
3	14.6	96.2	0.61	1220	84	1196	82
4	16.5	103.4	0.68	1360	82	1296	79
5	18.8	110.0	0.75	1500	80	1424	76
6	21.9	117.5	0.84	1680	77	1566	72
7	24.5	124.1	0.92	1840	75	1688	69
8	27.3	130.0	0.99	1980	73	1812	66
9	29.9	135.5	1.06	2120	71	1930	65
10	32.6	140.3	1.13	2260	69	2040	63
11	35.2	144.2	1.20	2400	68	2144	61
12	38.3	149.6	1.27	2540	66	2270	59
13	42.2	155.0	1.35	2700	64	2426	57
14	48.8	162.7	1.50	3000	62	2670	55
15	54.5	167.8	1.60	3200	59	2880	53
16	58.5	171.6	1.68	3360	57	3020	51
17	61.8	173.7	1.73	3460	56	3120	50
18	63.1	174.5	1.74	3480	55	3172	50

* Average weights, heights, and surface areas for boys 0–18 years of age and total kilocalories and kilocalories/kilogram on the basis of six methods of calculation. If only weight and height are known, and they differ from the values given in the table, as estimate of surface area may be obtained by interpolation. Thus a boy who is 4 years old, who weighs 17 kg, and who is 110 cm tall could by interpolation be estimated to have a surface

Total Kilocalories = 1000 + (100 × Age)		Total Kilocalories = 800 + (125 × age)		Kilocalories/ Kilogram = 95 − (3 × age)		Kilocalories/ Kilogram = 100 − Weight (kg)	
Total kcal (9)	*kcal/kg (10)*	*Total kcal (11)*	*kcal/kg (12)*	*Total kcal (13)*	*kcal/kg (14)*	*Total kcal (15)*	*kcal/kg (16)*
1000	294	800	235	323	95	330	97
1050	138	862	114	710	93.5	698	92
1100	109	925	92	930	92	909	90
1150	101	987	86	1030	90.5	1025	89
1200	95	1050	83	1120	89	1095	87
1300	89	1175	80	1250	86	1240	85
1400	85	1300	79	1370	83	1370	83
1500	80	1425	76	1500	80	1520	81
1600	73	1550	71	1690	77	1710	78
1700	69	1675	68	1810	74	1840	75
1800	66	1800	66	1940	71	1990	73
1900	63	1925	64	2030	68	2100	70
2000	61	2050	63	2120	65	2190	67
2100	60	2175	62	2180	62	2290	65
2200	57	2300	60	2260	59	2380	62
2300	54	2425	57	2370	56	2450	58
2400	49	2550	52	2590	53	2490	51
2500	46	2675	49	2730	50	2450	45
2600	44	2800	48	2770	47	2410	41
2700	44	2925	47	2720	44	2350	38
2800	44	3050	48	2590	41	2330	37

area of approximately 0.72 m². For the formula listed above columns 5 and 6, his total kilocalories would be expected to be approximately 1400 and his kilocalories/kilogram would be 81. For the formula listed above columns 9 and 10, his total kilocalories would be expected to be 1450 and his kilocalories/kilogram would be 82.

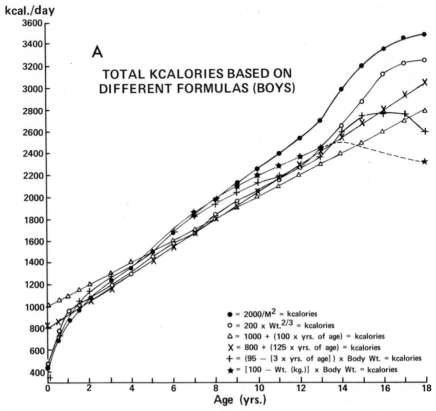

Fig. 2-1A.   Total kilocalories using a variety of formulas to calculate the caloric requirement of boys ages 0–18 years. It is apparent that between the ages of 2 and 13 years there are minimal differences, depending on which formula is used. Below 2 years and above 13 years of age these different formulas yield considerable differences.

between   kilocalories/kilogram = 95 − (3 × age)   and   kilocalories/kilogram = 100 − weight (kg) is shown in Figure 2-2.

A summary of the problems encountered with each of the suggested formulations for determining metabolic needs is given in Table 2-2. From such a tabulation it can be seen that there is no one formulation that is appropriate under all circumstances. Because of the author's familiarity with the Wallace-type formulation, it will be used for most purposes in this text. In so doing, it is recognized that the values for infants under 6 months of age are somewhat low, and the values of 110 kcal/kg for newborns and 100 kcal/kg at 3 months of age will be substituted. In addition, the formula will not be used past 16 years of age. With the same qualifications for the infant and an arbitrary cutoff at 40 kg, the formula

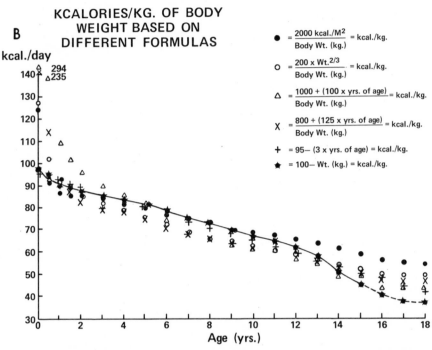

KCALORIES/KG. OF BODY WEIGHT BASED ON DIFFERENT FORMULAS

$\bullet = \dfrac{2000 \text{ kcal.}/M^2}{\text{Body Wt. (kg.)}} = \text{kcal./kg.}$

$\circ = \dfrac{200 \times Wt.^{2/3}}{\text{Body Wt. (kg.)}} = \text{kcal./kg.}$

$\triangle = \dfrac{1000 + (100 \times \text{yrs. of age})}{\text{Body Wt. (kg.)}} = \text{kcal./kg.}$

$\times = \dfrac{800 + (125 \times \text{yrs. of age})}{\text{Body Wt. (kg.)}} = \text{kcal./kg.}$

$+ = 95 - (3 \times \text{yrs. of age}) = \text{kcal./kg.}$

$\star = 100 - \text{Wt. (kg.)} = \text{kcal./kg.}$

Fig. 2-1B.   Kilocalories/kilogram body weight based on different formulas. The values shown in Figure 2-1A are divided by the median weight for boys at each age to obtain the values shown in this figure. Again, it is apparent that between the ages of 2 and 13 years the various formulas give comparable values. However, below 2 years and above 13 years of age there is considerable disparity. The values shown by the single line drawn through the figure are those generally accepted on the basis of other studies.

kilocalories/kilogram = 100 − weight (kg) could also be used, and it would be somewhat better for thin or obese children.

Returning to the general question of intake, in the healthy state the caloric intake will slightly exceed the metabolic requirements for growth and energy, as there are small losses of calories in urine and stool. Fluid intake is proportional to metabolism, for reasons that will be discussed later in the section Output, but it is equivalent to 1–1.5 ml per kilocalorie metabolized. For an infant on a milk diet, the value will be 1.5 ml/kcal, as milk contains 20 kcal per ounce, or approximately 30 ml/20 kcal = 1.5 ml/kcal. The older child receiving most of his calories from solid food will have a fluid intake closer to 1.0 ml/kcal. Infants receiving parenteral fluids, as will be discussed later, will also have intakes of about 1 ml per kilocalorie metabolized. The number of kilocalories *metabolized* is used here because the infant on parenteral fluids rarely receives enough

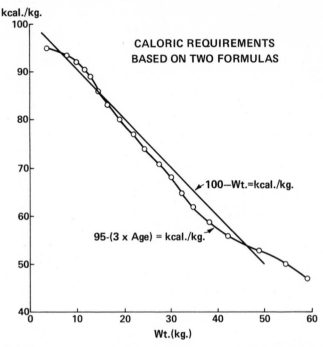

Fig. 2-2. Caloric requirements based on two formulas. These formulas appear to be the most useful of those shown in the previous figures over the weight range shown on the abscissa. The formula 95 − (3 × age) is used throughout this book.

calories to meet his total metabolic requirement; thus he uses his own body fat and other tissues to meet his caloric requirements, and fluid must be provided on the basis of his total energy expenditure, not on the basis of what is provided from external sources.

OUTPUT

Since the input side of man's fluid balance varies over relatively wide ranges, for both intentional and unintentional reasons, and since man's internal environment remains relatively constant, the output side must be relatively precise and well controlled. Fluid output from the body occurs through three mechanisms: evaporative losses from the skin and lungs, urinary excretion, and loss from the gastrointestinal tract, primarily as stool water. To some extent, all of these losses are related to metabolic rate.

Table 2-2

Comparison of Formulations for Caloric Requirements*

Age Period (years)	Kilocalories = 2000/m²	Kilocalories = $200 \times \text{Weight}^{2/3}$	Kilocalories = 1000 + (100 × Age)	Kilocalories/kilogram = 800 + (125 × Age)	Kilocalories/kilogram = 95 − (3 × Age)	Kilocalories/Kilogram = 100 − Weight
0–2			Very high	High-6 months / Slightly low	Low–NB	Slightly low–NB
2–5						Slightly high
5–10	Slightly high					
10–13	High		Slightly low			Low
13–15	High	Slightly low	Low		Low	Very low
15–18	Very high	High	Low			
Variations for individuals of different weights at same age:						
in total kilocalories	Yes	Yes	No	No	Yes	Yes
in kilocalories/kilogram	Yes	Yes	Excessive	Excessive	No	Yes

* There are some difficulties encountered in the use of each of the formulas listed in Table 2-1. For example, the formula kilocalories = 2000/m² provides increasingly high values from the age of 10 years onward, but it does allow for variation on the basis of weight at the same age in both total kilocalories and kilocalories/kilogram. The formula in the third column, kilocalories = 1000 + (100 × age in years), gives values that are very high in the first 2 years of life and low in late adolescence. This formula does not allow for variation between individuals with different weights at the same age, and it yields excessive variation on the basis of kilocalories/kilogram for individuals of different weights at the same age.

Insensible Water Loss

Evaporative loss from the skin and lungs is termed insensible water loss (IWL) and is distinguished from sweat loss, which is termed sensible water loss. The IWL occurs because the vapor pressures of the skin, pulmonary mucous membranes, and alveoli differ from the vapor pressure of the environment. The vapor pressures of the respiratory mucous membranes and alveoli are relatively constant, but that of the skin varies with skin temperature. Environmental vapor pressure variation is not great unless it is altered by artificial means.

HEAT DISSIPATION

On the average, about 25% of the heat generated by the body is dissipated by evaporation as IWL. Conversion of 1 ml of water to vapor requires 0.58 kcal. Thus, for every metabolic increment of 100 kcal, 25 kcal are dissipated by IWL, and this requires evaporation of $25/0.58 = 43$ ml of water. About one-third of these kilocalories (or water) are lost from the lungs and about two-thirds from the skin. The pulmonary losses will increase markedly with hyperventilation, but skin losses will decrease to some extent under these circumstances and will partially offset the increased respiratory loss. It should also be noted that if the environmental vapor pressure is raised to that of the body,* essentially preventing IWL, body temperature will rise as a result of the blocking of this important source of heat dissipation.

VARIATION WITH METABOLIC RATE

The rate of IWL varies as the metabolic rate. Thus, whatever alters the metabolic rate will also proportionately change the amount of water lost through the skin and lungs.

Most illnesses, especially when associated with fever, increase the metabolic rate. A 1°C rise in body temperature increases the metabolic rate and the IWL by 10%. Hyperthyroidism, salicylism, hyperactivity, the spasms in tetanus, and shivering are among a variety of conditions that increase caloric expenditure and thereby increase heat production and IWL.

Hypothyroidism, prolonged sedation, hypothermia, and coma are among the factors that will lower heat production and lower IWL. In the basal metabolic state the caloric requirements are about half of those shown in Table 2-1 and Figure 2-1.

EXAMPLE. What is the IWL for a 2-year-old child? From the formula for caloric expenditure [95 − (3 × age)], the kilocalories/kilogram

---

* This could occur if the environment contained air at 37°C and 100% humidity.

are found to equal $95 - (3 \times 2) = 89$ kcal/kg. Since IWL $= 43$ ml/100 kcal, the IWL per kilogram for this child $= 43 \times (89/100) = 38$ ml/kg. If the 2-year-old child is of average weight (12.6 kg), the total IWL $= 38 \times 12.6 = 478.8$, or 480 ml/day.

   EXAMPLE.   What is the IWL for a 10-year-old child weighing 30 kg? Kilocalories/kilogram $= 95 - (3 \times \text{age}) = 95 - (3 \times 10) = 65$ kcal/kg. IWL $= 43$ ml/100 kcal. For 65 kcal, $43 \times (65/100) = 28$ ml. IWL $= 28$ ml/kg. For 30 kg, IWL $= 30 \times 28 = 840$ ml of water per day.

   Using an alternative formula for metabolic rate/kilogram, $100 - \text{weight} = 100 - 30 = 70$ kcal/kg, and IWL $= 43 \times (70/100) = 30.1$ ml/kg; IWL $= 30.1 \times 30$ kg $= 900$ ml/day.

   The difference between the two methods of calculation is of no clinical significance, since both figures represent clinical approximations.

SWEATING

   When environmental temperature exceeds 80°F–95°F (27°C–35°C) sweating usually occurs. Sweat losses are very difficult to estimate, but a rough approximation may be made:

   Mild sweating: 5–10 ml/100 kcal metabolized.
   Moderate sweating: 20–30 ml/100 kcal metabolized.
   Severe sweating: 75–100 ml/100 kcal metabolized.

   In the examples given previously, it was necessary to convert the water losses per 100 kcal to losses per kilogram in each case. However, since the formula that has been chosen to represent kilocalories/kilogram is a straight-line function, it is possible to develop a straight-line relationship for any water loss that is proportional to metabolic rate. For this purpose, two representative ages, one at each end of the linear function, will provide the information necessary for interpolation of the value for any intermediate age. A 7-kg infant 5–6 months of age and a 60-kg child of 16 years will be used (Table 2-3). One of the obvious advantages of selecting these two ages and weights is that the values per kilogram for the 16-year-old child will be exactly half the values per kilogram for the 5–6-month-old infant. This will be true for all the fluid losses that are related to metabolic rate, and therefore it will be true for all the fluid required as input to replace output losses.

Renal Water Loss

   The amount of water lost from the body as urine varies, principally because of two factors: the solute content and the solute concentration in the urine.

Table 2-3

Maintenance Fluid Requirements: IWL*

	7 kg (5 months)	60 kg (16 years)
Kilocalories/kilogram	95 kcal	47 kcal
IWL/kg†	40 ml	20 ml
Moderate sweating/kg‡	20 ml	10 ml

* Water losses from skin and lungs, with values for IWL per kilogram of body weight and sweat losses under conditions in which moderate sweating occurs. The losses per kilogram for a 7-kg infant are double those for a 60-kg child of approximately 16 years. Values for weights or ages intermediate between these two points can be determined approximately by interpolation.

† IWL = 43 ml/100 kcal = 43 × (95/100) = 40 ml/kg at 0.5 years; IWL = 43 × (47/100) = 20 ml/kg at 16 years.

‡ Assume moderate sweating = 21 ml/100 kcal = 21 × (95/100) = 20 ml/kg at 0.5 years; moderate sweating = 21 × (47/100) = 10 ml/kg at 16 years.

SOLUTE CONTENT

The solute content is a function of the metabolic rate, since the solute to be excreted is the solute that results from the production of calories. As mentioned earlier, carbohydrate metabolism and fat metabolism generally do not result in solute that must be excreted. Protein catabolism and ingested ionic substances are the primary sources of the constituents of the urinary solute. As mentioned previously, there are about 1650 mOsm of solute per kilogram of meat, or 660 mOsm/100 g protein (as part of a diet).* Carbohydrate by itself ordinarily produces no solute for excretion; but dietary carbohydrate is derived principally from fruits and vegetables, which are cellular substances, and their plant tissues contain ionic constituents similar to those of animal tissue. About 15% of dietary solute comes from such sources. The total solute load of an ordinary 3000-kcal diet is about 1200 mOsm, or 40 mOsm/100 kcal metabolized.

In the fasting state, body protein and fat are catabolized for calories, since the small amount of stored carbohydrate is rapidly depleted. In this situation the rate of fat metabolism exceeds the body's ability to complete the oxidation of the keto acids, and these accumulate in body fluids and are excreted as solute in the urine. Nevertheless, the total solute load produced during fasting is lower than that produced on a regular diet, primarily because there are fewer calories metabolized and the solute load

* This assumes that the dry protein content of meat is 25% of the fresh weight. Thus, if 250 g of protein contains all the solute of meat, 100 g of protein would contain (100/250) × 1650 = 660 mOsm.

per 100 kcal metabolized is essentially unchanged. For an adult the solute load during fasting is about 800 mOsm/day. In work published in the 1940s by Gamble and his associates it was shown that administration of 100 g of carbohydrate to an adult who was otherwise fasting would reduce the urinary solute load 50% (400 mOsm/day). This occurs for two reasons: first, the amount of body protein catabolized is almost halved; second, the addition of this amount of carbohydrate essentially eliminates excessive production of keto acids; thus there is no urinary solute load resulting from fat catabolism. These studies have never been duplicated exactly in infants, but what information is available suggests that the infant and child respond comparably to the adult. The amount of glucose required by an infant to prevent ketosis is approximately 3 g/kg/day. In the adult, the value is 1.5 g/kg/day, or about 100 g for most adults.

Using this information and making several assumptions, it is possible to predict the solute load in several clinical situations and for any age from birth to 16 years. The assumptions are the following:

1. The caloric requirement for each age can be calculated as $95 - (3 \times age) = $ kilocalories/kilogram.

2. A normal diet produces 40 mOsm of solute per 100 kcal.

3. In the fasting state, for the factors mentioned previously, caloric expenditure is about two-thirds of "normal," but the solute load remains at 40 mOsm of solute per 100 kcal.

4. For the usual child receiving parenteral fluids, caloric expenditure is the same as during fasting (two-thirds of "normal"), but adequate glucose (2–3 g/kg) prevents production of excess keto acids.

5. The basal metabolic state is at half the "normal" caloric level, and the solute load is 25 mOsm/100 kcal.

The solute loads per kilogram of body weight per day that are produced by regular diet, by fasting, and by parenteral fluids with adequate glucose, as well those produced in the basal metabolic state, are shown in Figure 2-3 for ages 0–16 years.

EXAMPLE. A 5-year-old child on a full diet weighs 18 kg. To calculate his solute output, one can proceed in two ways:

1. His caloric requirement = $95 - (3 \times 5) = 80$ kcal/kg. The solute load of a full diet = 40 mOsm/100 kcal. His solute load per kilogram = $40 \times (80/100) = 32$ mOsm/kg. His total solute load = 32×18 kg = 576 mOsm.

2. From Figure 2-3, using the full-diet line, his solute load reads 32 mOsm/kg at 5 years of age; and $32 \times 18 = 576$ mOsm.

If the same child had been admitted to the hospital with gastroenteritis and was receiving parenteral fluids containing at least 3 g of glucose per kilogram (or $3 \times 18 = 54$ g; this amount of glucose is present in approximately 1 liter of 5% glucose or in approximately 2 liters of 2.5% glucose):

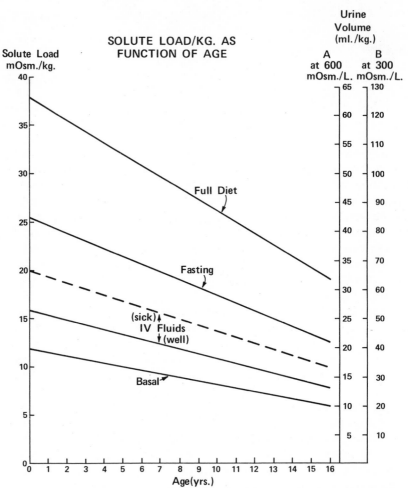

Fig. 2-3.   Solute load per kilogram as a function of age. The solute loads created under five sets of conditions are illustrated for individuals 0–16 years of age. The solute load for a well child on a full diet is approximately three times that under basal conditions. The solute load produced during prolonged fasting, because of the increased protein catabolism, is approximately twice the basal value. For children receiving intravenous fluids containing at least 3 g of carbohydrate per kilogram of body weight per day, the solute loads are intermediate between those of the basal state and those in prolonged fasting. Because of the catabolism associated with illness, the solute loads for sick children on intravenous fluid are slightly greater than the solute loads for otherwise well children receiving intravenous fluids. The ordinate scales on the right illustrate the volume of urine required to excrete the solute load produced by the body at two different urine concentrations. Column A represents the volume of fluid required when the urine concentration is 600 mOsm/liter, and column B shows the urine volume required when the concentration of urine is 300 mOsm/liter, or essentially an isotonic urine.

1. His caloric utilization would be about half that required when well; one-half of 80 = 40 kcal/kg. The solute generated remains the same, at about 40 mOsm/100 kcal; 40 × (40/100) = 16.0 mOsm/kg. His total solute load = 18 × 16.0 = 288 mOsm.

2. From Figure 2-3, the intravenous fluids (sick) line reads 16.0 mOsm/kg at 5 years of age. Total solute load = 18 × 16.0 = 288 mOsm.

SOLUTE CONCENTRATION

The second factor involved in urine volume is urinary solute concentration. Solute concentration (mOsm/liter) is dependent on the renal concentrating mechanism, which in turn is controlled by several factors that will be discussed later. If the glomerular filtrate, which is essentially a plasma ultrafiltrate, is neither concentrated nor diluted when it reaches its final form as urine, the osmolarity will be about 300 mOsm/liter. This corresponds to a specific gravity of 1.008–1.012.* The extent to which the human kidney can dilute urine is 50–60 mOsm/liter (specific gravity 1.001), and maximum concentration is about 1400 mOsm/liter (specific gravity 1.035–1.040). At maximum dilution, the urine is one-fifth as concentrated as a plasma ultrafiltrate; at maximum concentration, the urine is almost five times as concentrated as plasma ultrafiltrate.

In persons with normal kidney function, the concentration of the urine will depend on the state of hydration of the body fluids. A person who has consumed a large volume of fluid and is overhydrated will produce a urine of low osmolarity (300 mOsm/liter, specific gravity 1.010). A person who is dehydrated will produce a urine low in volume and high in concentration. For people who are neither overhydrated nor underhydrated, the urine concentration will usually fall between 300 and 1000 mOsm/liter (specific gravity 1.010–1.030). In other words, in the presence of healthy kidneys, urine volume tends to be a function of the intake of fluids. In the presence of diseased or pathologic states, when the concentrating power and/or diluting power of the kidney are limited, the volume of the urine becomes more dependent on the concentrating (or diluting) ability of the kidney for any specific solute load. Under these circum-

* Specific gravity has no physiologic basis, but it is used as an approximation of urine concentration because it is relatively easy to measure. Specific gravity reflects the weight of dissolved substances relative to the weight of an equal volume of water. Osmolarity reflects the number of particles in solution. If the composition of the particles is more or less the same from one time to the next, specific gravity will be proportional to the osmolarity. When a heavy compund such as an iodinated hippuric acid derivative occurs in the urine (as after an intravenous pyelogram), the specific gravity will be very high, but the solute concentration (osmolarity) will not be unusual. Thus osmolarity is the better measure of urinary concentration, since it more accurately reflects renal function. For purposes of approximation, a rough conversion between urinary specific gravity and urine osmolarity may be made using Table 2-4.

Table 2-4
Comparison of Urine Osmolarity
and Specific Gravity*

Specific Gravity	Osmolarity
1.001	50 mOsm/liter
1.010	300 mOsm/liter
1.020	600 mOsm/liter
1.030	1000 mOsm/liter
1.040	1400 mOsm/liter

* These values represent approximate equalities between urine specific gravity and osmolarity. The variation under usual circumstances will approximate 10%–20% for osmolarity and ± 0.002 for specific gravity. Under unusual circumstances, such as excretion of radiopaque materials in urine following intravenous pyelograms, the specific gravity may be extremely high and the osmolarity within the usual range. Therefore osmolarity is the preferred measurement for evaluating renal concentrating function.

stances the volume of urine tends to determine the fluid intake, whereas in a state of health the fluid intake tends to determine urine volume.

The relationships among solute load, solute concentration, and urine volume can be exemplified as follows: An adult male on a regular diet creates 1200 mOsm of solute. If his kidneys can concentrate his urine to 1200 mOsm/liter (specific gravity 1.030), 1 liter of urine will contain his daily solute load. If his kidneys cannot concentrate his urine above 600 mOsm/liter, it will require 2 liters (2000 ml) to contain his daily solute load. If a person has chronic renal disease and is unable to concentrate urine above the osmolarity of glomerular filtrate (300 mOsm/liter), the volume of urine required to excrete the solute will be 4 liters (1200/300). With chronic renal disease, this person might well be placed on a low-protein diet, and his daily solute load would decrease correspondingly. Such a diet might result in an 800-mOsm solute load and at a concentration of 300 mOsm/liter (specific gravity 1.010); his urine volume could be reduced to 2.67 liters or 2670 ml (800/300). Conversely, if a patient with a solute load of 1200 mOsm has a high enough fluid intake so that he has a urine volume of 3000 ml, the urine osmolarity can then be estimated as 400 mOsm/liter (specific gravity 1.012), since 1200 mOsm/3.0 liters = 400 mOsm/liter. A general formula can be used to express these relationships:

$$\text{urine volume } (U_V) = \frac{\text{urine solute } (U_s)*}{\text{urine solute concentration } [U_s]\dagger}$$

From such a formulation, any one factor can be determined if the other two are known. As an example, if urine volume = 1500 ml and urine concentration = 750 mOsm/liter (specific gravity 1.020), urine solute (U_s) = $U_V \times [U_s]$ = 1.5 liters × 750 mOsm/liter = 1125 mOsm.

Changes in solute load occur because of changes in intake (particularly protein and ionic substances) and because of unusual constituents or unusual concentrations of constituents in glomerular filtrate. The most frequent example of the latter is the presence of glucose in glomerular filtrate at a concentration exceeding the ability of the renal tubule to reabsorb it. This occurs in diabetic hyperglycemia; the resultant high solute load increases urine volume, and the ensuing polyuria is termed solute diuresis. Other high urine solute loads can result from administration of ions that are poorly reabsorbed (e.g., SO_4^{--}), rapid infusion of highly concentrated urea or glucose, or reduction in tubular reabsorption of a substance that is normally reabsorbed (e.g., Na^+).

Under more usual circumstances, a good approximation of the fluid intake required to replace fluid lost as urine can be obtained by estimating the solute load (mOsm/kg) from the full-diet line in Figure 2-3 and then dividing that value by the assumed urinary concentration (in mOsm/liter):

$$\text{urine volume (ml/kg)} = \frac{\text{osmolar load (mOsm/kg)}}{\text{urine osmolarity (mOsm/liter)}} \times 1000$$

EXAMPLE.   What would be the urine volume of a 1-year-old child? From Figure 2-3 it is seen that a 1-year-old child on a full diet has a solute load of 37 mOsm/kg. Assuming a moderate concentrating ability (to 600 mOsm/liter) the urine volume would be

$$\text{urine volume (ml/kg)} = \frac{37}{600} \times 1000 \text{ ml} = 62 \text{ ml/kg/day}$$

Lines A and B in Figure 2-3 are scales for the urine volume (ml/kg) at two arbitrary urine solute concentrations: A for 600 mOsm/liter and B for 300 mOsm/liter. Similar scales could be constructed for any assumed urine solute concentration. Using such scales, the urine volume can be read directly after solute load and urine solute concentration are selected.

---

* Parentheses indicate quantity or the total amount present without regard to volume.
† Note again that brackets indicate concentration.

ESTIMATION OF RENAL WATER LOSS AS A
FUNCTION OF AGE

In order to arrive at an average figure that will serve as a starting point in fluid calculations for a hospitalized child requiring parenteral fluids, two assumptions are made:

1. Urine concentration will be between 300 and 600 mOsm/liter. This takes into account the frequent temporary reduction in renal function associated with many childhood illnesses.

2. Solute load will be between that of a well child on intravenous fluids and that of a fasting child. This level is selected because the usual child on parenteral fluids is not well and thus has a somewhat higher matabolic requirement than a healthy child. This line is shown as the dash line in Figure 2-3.

On this basis urine volumes of 33–66 ml/kg (or an average of 50 ml/kg for the infant under 6 months) and 16–33 ml/kg (or an average of 25 ml/kg for the 16-year-old) are obtained. Values for intermediate ages can be interpolated.

Table 2-5 is an expansion of Table 2-3, with the addition of values for renal water requirement. As has already been indicated, the values for renal water can vary over an extremely large range. An example should make this clearer.

EXAMPLE. A 3-month-old infant with nephrogenic diabetes insipidus is unable to concentrate his urine above 60 mOsm/liter and is on a cow's milk formula. What fluid volume will be required to meet his renal water loss alone? His solute load = 38 mOsm/kg (from Figure 2-3).

$$\text{urine volume} = \frac{\text{osmolarity}}{[U_s]} = \frac{38}{60} = 0.633 \text{ liter/kg} = 633 \text{ ml/kg}$$

If the child weighs 4 kg, his water requirement, just for urine volume, is $4 \times 633 = 2532$ ml.

Table 2-5
Maintenance Fluid Requirements: Renal*

	7 kg (5 months)	60 kg (16 years)
Kilocalories/kilogram	95	47
IWL (ml/kg)	40	20
Renal (ml/kg)	50	25

* Renal water requirements for infants and for 16-year-old children. these values are based on usual solute load and urine osmolarity of approximately 600 mOsm/liter or specific gravity of approximately 1.020. Values for intermediate ages may be obtained by interpolation.

If a low-solute formula is given instead of whole cow's milk, what will be the urine volume? The solute load from the diet will be about half of the previous value, or 19 mOsm/kg. (For the composition of various milk formulas, see the Appendix.)

$$U_V = \frac{19}{60} = 0.317 \text{ liter/kg} = 317 \text{ ml/kg}$$

This is a value that is still about six times the average requirement for an infant of this age, but it is considerably less than if the child were on whole milk; this can be very important from a clinical and practical management viewpoint.

Gastrointestinal Loss

Fluid is usually lost from the gastrointestinal tract as stool water, but losses by vomiting, gastrointestinal suction, colostomy drainage, etc., are also included in this category. The volume of fluid lost in normal stool is quite small, even though formed stool is about 80%–90% water. In the healthy infant, stool water can be assumed to be about 5 ml/kg/day, and the value for the healthy adult is about half of that (2.5 ml/kg/day).

During diarrhea, stool losses can become extremely large, and they require equally large intakes of fluid to compensate for them. As an example of an extreme situation, adults with cholera may have stool losses up to 1 liter/hour (about 5 gallons/day or 300 ml/kg/day). Comparable values have not been reported for infants, but stool losses of 100 ml/kg/day have been reported. However, the diarrhea that is generally seen as part of a nonspecific gastroenteritis in the United States usually results in stool water loss of about 35 ml/kg/day for infants and about half that for adults.

Fluid losses from vomiting are unpredictable and can only be estimated or determined by measurement in individual cases. Similarly, fluid removed by suction or drainage from the gastrointestinal tract cannot be determined by theory; it must be estimated or measured as it occurs.

The potential for fluid losses by suction or ileostomy can be appreciated from the fact that the gastrointestinal tract in an adult produces over 8 liters of fluid per day. In healthy individuals over 95% of this is reabsorbed, and less than 200 ml is lost in stool. The majority of this reabsorption takes place in the large bowel, which functions not only to reabsorb the fluid passing through the ileocecal valve but also to modify its electrolyte composition.

Determination of the quantity of fluid lost from the body by the gastrointestinal tract completes the estimations for the three normal routes of fluid loss. The values are shown in Table 2-6. Two things that are

Table 2-6
Maintenance Fluid Requirements: Gastrointestinal*

	7 kg (5 months)	60 kg (16 years)
Kilocalories/kilogram	95	47.5
IWL (ml/kg)	40	20
Renal (ml/kg)	50	25
Gastrointestinal (ml/kg)	5	2.5
Total fluids	95	47.5

* Values for gastrointestinal losses when there is no diarrhea or malabsorption. Under these circumstances the total maintenance fluids will average 95 ml/kg for the 7-kg infant and 47.5 ml/kg for the 16-year-old person. Intermediate values may be obtained by interpolation.

apparent from Table 2-6 result from some of the arbitrary values selected for the "sick" patient: (1) Total fluid losses (in ml/kg) are equal to total kilocalories (in kcal/kg). (2) Values for total fluid loss and for each of the constituents in the 16-year-old person are half as high as values for the 6-month-old infant.

MAINTENANCE REQUIREMENTS

Definition

By determining quantitative values for each of the routes of fluid loss, one can determine total maintenance fluids. Maintenance fluid is defined as that quantity of intake that will provide the fluid necessary to match fluid losses. Furthermore, maintenance fluid for the usual patient can be calculated by the same rule that was used to calculate caloric requirements.

Estimation of Body Fluid Losses

VOLUME

The formula $95 - (3 \times$ age in years$)$ = maintenance fluid (in ml/kg) will be appropriate under the following conditions: (1) from about 1 month to 16 years of age; (2) when there is no abnormality in metabolic rate, solute load, renal function, or gastrointestinal function. Calculation of maintenance fluids when these conditions do not hold is covered in the next section on composition.

EXAMPLE. What are the maintenance fluid requirements for an 8-year-old child weighing 26 kg? Using the standard formula, 95 − (3 × age) = 95 − (3 × 8) = 95 − 24 = 71 ml/kg; 71 × 26 = 1846, or 1850 ml/day.

COMPOSITION

In addition to providing the body with the fluid necessary to compensate for fluid losses, one must replace the inorganic ions that are lost along with the fluid if body fluid composition is to be maintained. IWL (the fluid evaporating from skin and pulmonary mucous membranes) contains no appreciable quantity of salt,* and therefore the fluid provided as replacement for this loss should not contain any ionic material.

Sweat does contain ionic substances, primarily Na^+ and Cl^-, with some K^+ as well. In the average person the concentrations of these ions in sweat are relatively low, and only when very large quantities of sweat are lost is salt replacement as well as volume replacement needed. In general, Na^+ and Cl^- concentrations are about 20%–30% of those in ECF; thus one-fourth to one-third of sweat losses may be replaced with an isotonic† salt solution and the other three-fourths to two-thirds may be replaced with a 5% dextrose solution.‡ A notable exception occurs in the sweat electrolyte concentrations of patients who have cystic fibrosis. Their sweat salt concentration is two-thirds to three-fourths that of plasma, and in such cases sweat losses need to be replaced by solutions that are two-thirds to three-fourths isotonic salt, with the remainder being 5% dextrose in water.

The process used to determine the ionic component of renal water loss is somewhat more complex. Urine contains a variety of inorganic ions, and most of them are present because of excess intake that is not needed by the body; yet urine that is totally free of such ions does not exist. Therefore there is some minimal quantity of inorganic ions that represents an obligatory loss in urine. For Na^+, Cl^-, and K^+ this amounts to approximately 1 mEq/kg body weight per day for an infant and about half that for an adult. The amounts for the other ions are negligible for clinical considerations.

---

* The term *salt*, as used herein, is a general term signifying any cation–anion compound; it does not specifically mean NaCl.

† The term *isotonic* will be used to refer to a solution that has an osmolarity similar to that of plasma: e.g., 0.9% NaCl (0.9 g/100 ml = 9000 mg/liter; molecular weight of NaCl = 58; 9000/58 = 155 mM NaCl; since NaCl is completely dissociated to Na^+ and Cl^-, 155 mM NaCl = 310 mOsm/liter); 5% dextrose in water (5 g/100 ml = 50,000 mg/liter; molecular weight of glucose = 180; 50,000/180 = 280 mOsm/liter). Since 310 and 280 mOsm/liter are similar to the value for plasma, 0.9% NaCl and 5% dextrose in water are considered isotonic solutions.

‡ Since they are isotonic with plasma, 5% dextrose solutions are generally used as a substitute for water when giving fluids parenterally. However, the dextrose can be metabolized, and thus it provides no solute load for renal excretion.

Table 2-7
Table of Maintenance Fluid Requirements*

| | 7 kg (5 months) | | | | 60 kg (16 years) | | | |
	H_2O†	Na^+	K^+	Cl^-	H_2O	Na^+	K^+	Cl^-
IWL	40	0	0	0	20	0	0	0
Renal	50	1	1	1	25	0.5	0.5	0.5
Gastrointestinal	5	1	1	1	2.5	0.5	0.5	0.5
Total	95	1–2	1–2	1–2	47.5	0.5–1	0.5–1	0.5–1

* Electrolyte requirements for maintenance in the infant and the 16-year-old person.
† H_2O given in ml/kg/day; Na^+, K^+, and Cl^- given in mEq/kg/day.

The gastrointestinal tract does not appear to have any regulatory function vis-à-vis the electrolyte composition of body fluids. Therefore the ionic constituents of stool must be replaced by corresponding intake to maintain body fluid homeostasis. Although the fluid reaching the ileocecal valve is comparable in composition to the ECF, the normally functioning large bowel exchanges some Na^+ for K^+ and some Cl^- for HCO_3^- and reduces the overall concentrations of these ions. Thus, normal stool has somewhat lower concentrations of Na^+ and Cl^- and a higher concentration of K^+ than does the ECF. As stools become more voluminous and more liquid, representing disturbed large bowel function, the inorganic ionic composition of stool approaches that of the ECF.

In infants with normal stools, losses of Na^+, K^+, and Cl^- are slightly less than 1 mEq/kg body weight per day for each ion. The loss of each of these ions is less than 0.5 mEq/kg body weight per day in the adult. With diarrhea, gastrointestinal suction, ileostomies, and fresh colostomies, the composition of the fluid approaches that of ECF so closely that replacement can be accomplished with solutions in which the inorganic constituents are at concentrations similar to those in plasma. Again, the ultimate example is seen in cholera, with stool sodium concentration averaging 137 mEq/liter. Comparing such values with those for a patient with a fresh ileostomy (Na^+ 129, K^+ 11, Cl^- 116 mEq/liter) indicates the similarity and suggests the marked degree to which large bowel function has been impaired in cholera.

The table of maintenance fluid requirements (Table 2-7) can be utilized if one knows the fluid volume and the ionic requirements to compensate for the three routes of output. These average requirements can be met by a single solution in the infant and older child, since the absolute ionic requirements decrease with age in proportion to the decrease in fluid volume requirements: 1.5 mEq of Na^+ per 95 ml = 0.75 mEq of Na^+ per 47.5 ml. Converting these ionic quantities to concentrations per liter yields a solution that has about 15 mEq/liter of Na^+, K^+, and Cl^-. To allow for possible individual variation, a range of values is more appropriate. The range for each of the ions Na^+, K^+, Cl^-, and HCO_3^-* is 10–20 mEq/liter.

Commercially available solutions for maintenance fluid administration tend to cluster at the higher end of this range, since at this level of concentration the kidney can more easily compensate for a slight excess of these ions than for a deficit. Therefore most commercial solutions for maintenance fluids have concentrations in the following ranges: Na^+ 20–25 mEq/liter, K^+ 15–20 mEq/liter, Cl^- 20–25 mEq/liter, HCO_3^- 15–20 mEq/liter, with a total cation (or anion) concentration of 40–50 mEq/liter.†

EXAMPLES

EXAMPLE 1.   What would be the fluid requirement for a 6-year-old 22-kg boy who is on intravenous feedings following a routine herniorrhapy? Since there is no reason to expect any alteration in metabolic rate, renal function, or gastrointestinal function, an average overall maintenance figure can be used. Using the general formula 95 − (3 × age), the value is 95 − (3 × 6) = 95 − 18 = 77 ml/kg. Since his weight is 22 kg, the total daily fluid requirement is 22 × 77 = 1694 ml (or 1700 ml) of a standard (commercial) maintenance fluid. (For composition of various parenteral fluids see Appendix.)

EXAMPLE 2.   If this child were febrile postoperatively and his temperature were 40°C (104°F), how would this affect his maintenance fluids? In this circumstance, metabolic rate is increased, and the IWL will be increased 10% for each 1°C rise in body temperature. Therefore, each element of maintenance fluid must be calculated separately. The first step is to determine the value for each component of maintenance needs in the absence of any abnormality. Beginning with the values in Table 2-6, one can interpolate by dividing the change in requirement from birth to 16 years of age by 16 to obtain the change per yer (Table 2-8). After the "normal" values have been obtained, these can be modified by estimating the effect of altered physiology on fluid needs.

There is a 30% (3°C × 10%) increase in IWL, which increases its value by 10 ml/kg (30% × 32.5 ml/kg = 10 ml/kg). Thus the appropriate value for IWL in this patient is 42.5 ml/kg. Then the total daily maintenance fluid is IWL 42.5 ml/kg + renal loss 41.0 ml/kg + gastrointestinal loss 4 ml/kg = 87.5 ml/kg. Then, 87.5 ml/kg × 22 kg = 1925 ml/day (an increase of 225 ml/day due to the fever).

---

* HCO_3^- is used to complete the cation–anion balance and to provide for acid–base equilibrium, which is discussed in Chapter 6. Lactate or other H^+ acceptors can also be used, but in this section the term HCO_3^- will be used for simplicity.

† The total osmolarity for each of these solutions is comparable to that of plasma, since they are prepared in either 2.5% or 5% dextrose; the osmolarity is thus 220–380 mOsm/liter: $glucose = (25,000/180) − (50,000/180) = 140–280$ mOsm/liter, and cations plus anions = 80–100 mOsm/liter.

Table 2-8
Fluid Requirements: Intermediate Age*

	5 Month	16 Years	6 Years
IWL	40 ml/kg	20 ml/kg	32.5†
Renal	50 ml/kg	25 ml/kg	41.0‡
Gastrointestinal	5 ml/kg	2.5 ml/kg	4.0§

  * Methodology involved in determining maintenance fluid requirements for a child intermediate between the infant and the 16-year-old.

  † The decrease in IWL is 20 ml/kg over 16 years; thus it is 20/16 or 1.25 ml/year. In 6 years this is a decrease of 7.5 ml; so the figure at age 6 is $40 - 7.5 = 32.5$ ml/kg.

  ‡ In the same way, renal water decreases 25/16, or roughly 1.5 ml/year, or 9 ml in 6 years, for a figure of $50 - 9 = 41$ ml/kg.

  § In the same way, gastrointestinal loss comes out about 4 ml or one-tenth of the renal figure.

In this example the additional 225 ml does not represent any additional "salt" loss, since the increase is entirely the result of increased IWL; thus this fluid could be slightly less "salty" or more "dilute" in terms of ionic concentration. There are three alternative methods for meeting these needs:

1. One may prepare a solution exactly equivalent to his estimated needs. This is quite laborious, and the situation is not sufficiently unusual to justify it.

2. One may provide the fluids as for normal maintenance and add 225 ml of 5% dextrose in water.

3. Since the kidney has a relatively large capacity to adjust to the "salt" load present in a maintenance solution, one may provide the entire 1925 ml as a standard maintenance solution, recognizing that this provides a small amount more Na^+, K^+, Cl^-, and HCO_3^- than is needed for this patient.

EXAMPLE 3. Assuming that the surgery in this patient was for urinary diversion in the presence of marked hydronephrosis with associated isosthenuria (a urine with an osmolarity that is similar to that of plasma because of inability to concentrate or dilute the urine), what would be his maintenance fluid requirement if he were not febrile? IWL = 32.5 ml/kg (see previous example); his solute load would be 13–16 mOsm/kg (from Figure 2-3). Assuming 15 mOsm/kg and a urine concentration of 300 mOsm/liter (specific gravity 1.010),

$$U_V = \frac{U_s}{[U_s]} = \frac{15}{0.300} = 50 \text{ ml/kg}$$

Each day, IWL = 32.5 ml/kg, renal loss = 50.0 ml/kg, and gastrointestinal loss = 4.0 ml/kg; therefore total loss = 86.5 ml/kg, and 86.5 ml/kg × 22 kg = 1903 ml/day.

In this situation it would be wiser to use the second of the three approaches listed in example 2, i.e., provide the 200 ml of fluid required in excess of the "average" as 5% dextrose in water, since the reduced renal function makes any unnecessary solute an extra handicap.

EXAMPLE 4. Alternatively, if the surgery had been an ileostomy, which later drained at 25 ml/hour, what would be his maintenance requirement? IWL = 32.5 ml/kg (see Example #2), renal loss = 41.0 ml/kg (see Example #2), and gastrointestinal loss = 25 ml/hour = 600 ml/day. His expected value had been 4 ml/kg × 22 kg = 88 ml/day. The new value exceeds the expected by 512 ml (600 − 88 ml). Thus his daily maintenance is the "average" 1700 + 512 ml for added gastrointestinal loss, or a total of 2200 ml/day. Since this additional volume is to replace drainage from a fresh ileostomy, the additional fluid should be similar to plasma in its ionic composition. Two alternatives are available for estimating the composition of total maintenance fluids.

1. Calculate a specific composition:

		mEq/liter				mEq			
	Volume	Na^+	K^+	Cl^-	HCO_3^-	(Na^+)	(K^+)	(Cl^-)	(HCO_3^-)
Average maintenance solution	1700 ml	25*	20	25	20	42.5†	34	42.5	34
Additional plasma like solution	500 ml	140	6	110	36	70.0	3	55.0	18
Total	2200 ml					112.5	37	97.5	52

* Values are concentrations (in mEq/liter) for these ions in a hypothetical maintenance solution.
† Values are in total milliequivalents, i.e., the amount present in 1700 ml if the concentrations are those shown in the preceding columns.

The final concentration of the ions can be determined by dividing the total milliequivalents by the total volume:

$$Na^+ = \frac{112.5}{2.2} = 51 \text{ mEq/liter}$$

$$K^+ = \frac{37}{2.2} = 17 \text{ mEq/liter}$$

$$Cl^- = \frac{97.5}{2.2} = 45 \text{ mEq/liter}$$

$$HCO_3^- = \frac{52}{2.2} = 24 \text{ mEq/liter}$$

There are commercial solutions approximating such composition, but if one is not available the hospital pharmacy can prepare a solution with this composition.

2. Since the maintenance fluid requirement is equivalent to 1700 ml of an average solution and an additional 500 ml of a plasmalike solution, the total maintenance fluids could consist of 1700 ml of regular maintenance plus 500 ml of 0.85% NaCl,* or lactated Ringer's solution (similar to 0.85% NaCl except that some of the Cl⁻ is replaced by lactate ions).

---

* The 0.85% NaCl is similar to 0.9% NaCl for clinical application. With 0.85% NaCl (8.5 g/liter), the molarity = 8.5/58 = 0.147 molar; 0.147 × 1000 = 147 mM NaCl. This means that the Na^+ and Cl^- concentrations are both 147 mEq/liter, and since NaCl is essentially completely ionized, the osmolarity is twice the molarity. Then, this is 294 mOsm/liter. Thus, 0.85% NaCl is closer to plasma in its osmolarity than 0.9% NaCl, but the difference is probably not significant clinically; thus the two solutions are interchangeable for most purposes.

3
Body Fluid Regulation

Regulation of body fluids involves maintenance of volume and composition of both the extracellular fluid (ECF) compartment and the intracellular fluid (ICF) compartment. Under normal circumstances the ECF volume is regulated to a remarkably fine degree in spite of wide daily variations in intake of water and solutes. Only the control of ECF volume will be discussed here, because in pathologic states variations in the volume of this compartment can occur rapidly and can be relatively large. Changes in ECF volume are usually reflected by similar, but more limited, changes in ICF volume. However, it is important to remember that while variations in total body water alone will be reflected in qualitatively similar changes in both the ECF volume and the ICF volume, a variation in solute concentration in one body fluid compartment (ECF or ICF) may have a different effect on the volume of the other fluid compartment. For example, addition of sodium chloride to the ECF that results in an increase in the concentration of sodium chloride* (and osmolarity) in this compartment will draw water from the ICF, thus reducing the volume of the ICF while increasing the volume of the ECF.

Regulation of the ECF volume requires control of both the volume of fluid and the concentration of sodium, i.e., the osmolarity of the ECF. In general, the intake and output of water are responsible for the maintenance of volume and composition of the body fluids. However, it is the renal regulation of sodium excretion that is the primary mechanism for control of fluid volume. Since water tends to follow sodium passively, retention of sodium by the kidney results in retention of water and isotonic expansion of ECF volume. Because excretion of both sodium and water is regulated primarily by the kidney, a brief review of renal function is appropriate.

RENAL FUNCTION

While it is not possible to discuss all aspects of renal function in detail, an attempt will be made to present an overview and summarize the available information concerning normal glomerular and tubular function. The interested reader should consult the appropriate references for more detailed discussion. Renal control of sodium and water excretion by the kidney will be emphasized. Control of potassium excretion will also be considered.

---

* With the exception of a few special situations, the osmolarity of the serum equals twice the Na^+ concentration: $2 \times [Na^+]$. This situation results from the fact that Na^+ and its associated anions make up the bulk of the osmotically active constituents of serum. Therefore the terms *sodium* and *osmolarity* will be used interchangeably.

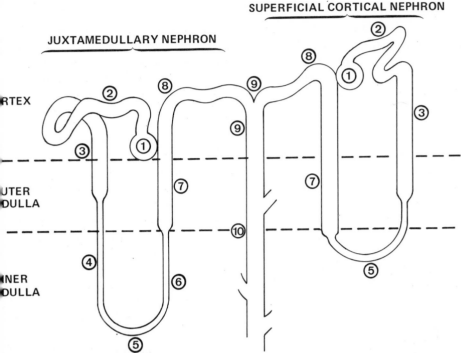

Fig. 3-1. Schematic diagram of the superficial cortical nephron and the juxtamedullary nephron illustrates the relationships of the following parts of the
nephron: (1) glomerulus, (2) proximal convoluted tubule, (3) proximal straight
tubule (pars recta), (4) thin descending loop of Henle, (5) loop of Henle, (6) thin
ascending limb of loop of Henle, (7) thick ascending limb of loop of Henle, (8)
distal convoluted tubule, (9) cortical collecting tubule, (10) medullary collecting
duct.

Nephrons

The nephron, the functional unit of the kidney, is diagrammed in
Figure 3-1. Two types of nephrons have been described. The superficial
cortical nephrons have short loops of Henle that descend only into the
outer medulla. The deep cortical nephrons, or juxtamedullary nephrons,
send long loops of Henle deep into the medulla. A second difference
between the two types of nephrons is that the efferent arterioles of the
juxtamedullary nephrons form vascular loops called vasa recta that run
parallel to the loops of Henle. These and other structural differences are
associated with some functional differences in the two populations of
nephrons.

Glomerular Filtration

As blood passes through the capillary loops of the glomerulus, an ultrafiltrate of plasma is formed by filtration into Bowman's space. The driving force for this process of filtration is related to the imbalance between transcapillary hydrostatic pressure and colloid osmotic pressure across the glomerular capillary membrane. This process can be expressed as follows:

$$q = K_f (P_{GC} - P_t) = (\pi_{GC} - \pi_t)$$

where q is the rate of fluid flow across the glomerular capillary membrane, K_f is the filtration coefficient (a factor that is proportional to the permeability of the capillary membrane and the total surface area of the capillary available for filtration), P_{GC} is the intraglomerular capillary hydrostatic pressure, P_t is the intratubular hydrostatic pressure in Bowman's space or proximal tubule, π_{GC} is the colloid osmotic pressure of the plasma in the glomerular capillaries (essentially proportional to the albumin concentration), and π_t is the colloid osmotic pressure of the tubular fluid (a factor that in practice may be assumed to be zero).

The most important factor in the fine regulation of glomerular filtration is the hydrostatic pressure within the glomerular capillaries, P_{GC}, which is under control of the vasomotor tone in the afferent and efferent glomerular arterioles. For example, vasodilatation of the afferent arteriole will result in an increase in P_{GC} and an increase in both renal blood flow and glomerular filtration. A decrease in the resistance in the efferent glomerular arteriole (vasodilatation) will result in a decrease in P_{GC} and a decrease in glomerular filtration, but an increase in renal blood flow. Furthermore, there is evidence that the rate of glomerular filtration and factors that control the filtration rate may be different in the superficial and juxtamedullary nephron populations. The physiologic importance of these observations is not clear.

Since the glomerular filtrate is an ultrafiltrate of plasma (contains no protein), the concentration of protein in the blood within the glomerular capillaries increases; thus π_{GC} increases until $\pi_{GC} = P_{GC} - P_t$, and then glomerular filtration stops. This situation has been demonstrated experimentally in animals, but its significance in man remains unknown. Furthermore, while variations in the filtration coefficient K_f could result in changes in glomerular filtration, at the present time there is little evidence to implicate changes in K_f in the abnormalities in glomerular filtration that are seen in various disease states.

In the adult with normal renal function, 150–175 liters of glomerular filtrate are formed each day (100–125 ml/min). This fluid is an ultrafiltrate of plasma, its ionic composition being similar to that of the plasma water and each liter containing 140–150 mEq of sodium. This process of filtration thus results in delivery of 25,000 mEq of sodium per day to the renal tubule. Since this latter quantity is 10 times the amount of sodium contained in the total body water, regulation of the composition of body fluids is critically dependent on reabsorption by the renal tubule of all but a small portion of the glomerular filtrate.

Proximal Tubular Function

During passage of the glomerular filtrate through the proximal tubule, approximately 70% of the filtered fluid and sodium is reabsorbed. The sodium, other solutes, and water are reabsorbed into the interstitial tissue and from there are returned to the body by way of the peritubular capillaries. (It is of interest that the intercellular space is the site for the active reabsorbing mechanism.) The proximal tubules cannot be considered to comprise a homogeneous unit, because portions of the proximal tubule differ both anatomically and functionally. In addition, recent evidence suggests that a given proximal nephron segment may function in different ways depending on whether it is derived from superficial cortical or juxtamedullary nephrons.

In the early portions of the proximal convoluted tubule, the major reabsorptive process for sodium is an active process (requiring energy). In this portion of the tubule, in addition to sodium, other solutes, including bicarbonate, glucose, and amino acids, are actively reabsorbed. The processes of reabsorption of these latter solutes are in part coupled to sodium, since their absence from the filtrate has been shown to result in a reduced rate of sodium transport by the proximal tubular cells. As solutes are reabsorbed from the tubular lumen, water follows as a consequence of the osmotic gradient that is generated.

In the late portions of the proximal convoluted tubule, conditions are changed, in part because the composition of the tubular fluid has been altered by transport processes in the earlier segments and possibly because of intrinsic differences in segments of the tubular epithelium. There is some evidence that in this late segment of proximal tubule, the reabsorption of sodium comes about by both active and passive processes, the latter being the result of movement of water (solvent drag) due to osmotic forces generated in earlier portions of the tubule.

In the straight portion of the proximal tubule (pars recta), sodium transport is similar to that of the late portion of the convoluted tubule, being both active and passive. However, the net transport of fluid and sodium is less than in the convoluted portion of the tubule. In addition, the coupling between sodium and glucose and amino acid transport is not present in the pars recta. Finally, current evidence indicates that it is within the pars recta that secretion of organic acids from the plasma into the tubular fluid takes place.

All of these processes within the proximal tubule result in the reabsorption of an isotonic fluid. Thus the 30% of the fluid remaining at the end of the proximal tubule, which is then delivered into the loop of Henle, is essentially isotonic with the plasma.

There are many complex factors that alter the absorption of fluid, sodium, and other solutes from the proximal tubule. While it is not possible to discuss these factors in detail, it must be kept in mind that changes in blood pressure, renal blood flow, glomerular filtration rate, and plasma protein concentration may all be important in the control of proximal tubular reabsorption.

Loop of Henle

Passage of the glomerular filtrate through the loop of Henle results in further reabsorption of solutes and water and generation of the hypertonic medullary interstitium, which eventually leads to the formation of a concentrated urine if antidiuretic hormone (ADH) is present. Figure 3-2 shows the final result of the process of countercurrent multiplication by the loop of Henle. While the exact mechanisms involved in this process remain debatable (they are discussed in detail elsewhere), the end result is clear: the concentration of solutes (sodium chloride and urea) in the medullary interstitium increases from the outer to the inner medulla at the tips of the papillae (Fig. 3-2). This high osmolarity in the medullary interstitium is the driving force for reabsorption of water from the collecting ducts (see below).

While the gradient represented in Figure 3-2 is shown as the total solute concentration (in mOsm/liter), it is important to note that this solute is made up of both sodium chloride and urea. In fact, urea makes up a major portion of this solute, and concentration of urea in the medulla is required in order that the urine may eventually be concentrated. This important function of urea is clearly demonstrated in the newborn. Prior to feeding, the ability of the newborn to concentrate urine is limited to approximately 700 mOsm/liter. When protein is added to the diet, the ability to concentrate urine rapidly increases. This finding suggests that lack of urea (generated from protein metabolism) limits the medullary gradient.

As fluid moves through the thin segments of the loop of Henle, both water and sodium are reabsorbed. This process is probably passive in some species. By the time the fluid enters the thick ascending limb of the loop, it not only is reduced in volume but also is hypotonic because of reabsorption of more sodium chloride than water in the thin ascending

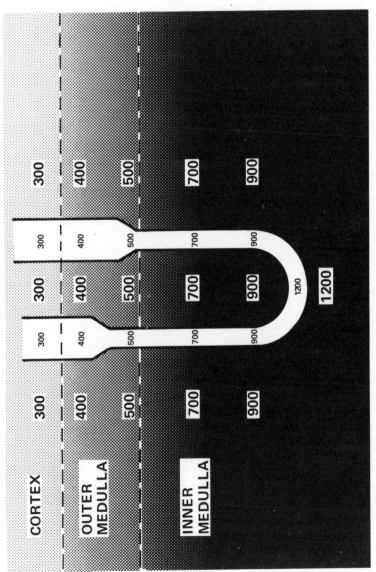

Fig. 3-2. Countercurrent multiplication in the loop of Henle. Osmotic pressure (in mOsm/liter) is shown in the renal interstitium of the medulla. The high osmotic concentration is made up of sodium and chloride ions and urea.

limb. The thick ascending limb is impermeable to water, but it can actively reabsorb chloride. As chloride is removed from the tubular fluid, sodium follows passively, and the tubular fluid becomes even more dilute. Thus the fluid entering the distal tubule may have an osmolarity approaching 50 mOsm/liter. This fluid is basically the dilute urine that is excreted in the absence of ADH. The thick ascending limb of the loop of Henle has been referred to as the diluting segment of the renal tubule.

An additional comment about the countercurrent mechanism is in order. The hypertonic medullary interstitium is formed by a system known as countercurrent multiplication, which involves the long loops of Henle of the juxtamedullary nephrons. The vascular supply (vasa recta) in this area of the kidney also forms loops that run parallel to the loops of Henle. These vascular loops form a countercurrent exchange system that prevents the solute (both sodium chloride and urea) present in the hypertonic medullary interstitium from being washed out in the blood and leaving the medulla. In spite of the countercurrent exchange in the vasa recta, under certain conditions increased medullary blood flow may result in depletion of interstitial solutes (wash out), with resultant decrease in ability to concentrate urine.

Distal Convoluted Tubule

The distal convoluted tubule begins at approximately the level of the macula densa* and extends a variable distance until the cortical collecting tubule begins. The basis for the division between the distal convoluted tubule and the cortical collecting tubule is both anatomic and functional.

Tubular fluid entering the distal convoluted tubule is hypotonic because of active chloride reabsorption in the thick ascending limb of the loop of Henle, which is impermeable to water. Sodium reabsorption in the distal convoluted tubule is active, although the rate of reabsorption is less than in the proximal tubule. The distal convoluted tubule is also impermeable to water, which means that the fluid becomes increasingly hyposmotic in this area. ADH probably has no effect on water permeability in this segment, and aldosterone probably does not affect sodium transport in the distal convoluted tubule, although the situation remains unclear.

Cortical Collecting Tubule

The segment of the nephron known as the cortical collecting tubule extends from the distal convoluted tubule to the outer medulla. Sodium is actively reabsorbed in the cortical collecting tubule. Since this segment of

---

* The macula densa is that portion of the distal convoluted tubule that lies in opposition to the juxtaglomerular apparatus. This aggregate of cells has a primary role in renin secretion and thus in the control of Na^+ reabsorption.

the tubule is sensitive to ADH, the final concentration of solute in the fluid depends on the degree of water reabsorption. In the absence of ADH, the tubule is impermeable to water, and the fluid remains hyposmotic. When ADH is present, water can diffuse into the more concentrated (but isosmotic) cortical interstitial space, and the fluid leaving the cortical collecting duct will be isotonic. Aldosterone also acts in this segment to increase sodium reabsorption and potassium excretion.

Collecting Ducts

The collecting ducts are formed by the confluence of cortical collecting tubules. Active reabsorption of sodium also takes place in this nephron segment. Recent evidence suggests that sodium reabsorption in this segment of the renal tubule is a major factor in the control of urinary excretion of sodium under a variety of conditions. Reabsorption of sodium in the collecting duct, like that in the cortical collecting tubules, is responsive to aldosterone. In addition, while there are some data to suggest that ADH affects sodium reabsorption in the collecting duct, the exact nature of this effect is not clear.

ADH has another major function in the collecting duct: control of water permeability. In the presence of ADH, the collecting duct is highly permeable to water. As the tubular fluid passes into the area of the hypertonic medullary interstitium, water is extracted by the osmotic forces, and the solute concentration in the urine rises. Maximum solute concentration is reached when the tubular fluid and medullary interstitium are in equilibrium.

Removal of ADH results in decreased water permeability of the collecting duct epithelium. However, even in the absence of ADH the collecting duct is still permeable to water, and reabsorption continues, although at a much reduced rate. The lack of ADH results in an increase in urine flow rate, as well as excretion of large volumes of dilute urine. It should be noted that since the collecting ducts reabsorb sodium, during water diuresis the collecting duct, like earlier segments of the renal tubule (thick ascending limb, distal convoluted and cortical collecting tubules), contributes to the formation of dilute urine.

Other Aspects of Renal Function:
Potassium and Other Solutes

In addition to controlling the concentration and volume of urine (processes dependent on regulation of sodium chloride reabsorption), the kidney has three other major roles in the maintenance of body fluid homeostasis: reabsorption of solutes other than sodium chloride, excretion of excess or waste solute, and regulation of acid–base equilibrium. Since essentially all of the solutes in the plasma (with the exception of plasma proteins) are filtered at the glomerulus, total solute equivalent to that contained in the total ECF is filtered every 2.5 hours in the adult and every 1.5 hours in the infant. Thus, some mechanism is necessary to return these filtered solutes to the body. When intake or metabolism results in concentration of potentially toxic substances in the ECF, they must also be removed. The renal handling of sodium has already been reviewed; chloride, potassium, and the divalent cations calcium and magnesium will be briefly considered. Hydrogen, bicarbonate, and phosphate will be discussed in reference to acid–base phenomena. In addition, a brief discussion of the reabsorption of glucose and amino acids and the secretion of organic acids will be presented.

As has previously been demonstrated, active reabsorption of either sodium or chloride results in passive movement of the other ion in order to maintain electroneutrality. However, under certain conditions, such as vomiting with hypochloremic metabolic alkalosis, loss of chloride from the body (as hydrochloric acid) results in bicarbonate being reabsorbed as a major balancing anion. This situation contributes to continuation of the high level of serum bicarbonate.

Potassium is the major intracellular cation, and it plays an important role in such basic physiologic processes as neuromuscular function and acid–base balance. Relatively small changes in serum potassium may have striking physiologic consequences, i.e., a decrease of serum potassium to 1.5 mEq/liter results in flaccid paralysis of skeletal muscles. Since major aspects of the regulation of potassium balance will be considered under acid–base disturbances, only a brief review of renal regulation will be undertaken here.

In the proximal tubule 70% of filtered potassium is reabsorbed. Further reabsorption of potassium in the thick ascending limb of the loop of Henle reduces the amount of potassium to approximately 10% of that filtered (90% has been reabsorbed). In the distal convoluted tubule, in the cortical collecting ducts, and possibly in the medullary collecting ducts, the situation becomes more variable. When intake of potassium exceeds the requirements for metabolic function, there is secretion of potassium into the tubular fluid. On the other hand, when potassium intake is very low, additional reabsorption takes place. Therefore, depending on the intake of potassium, the amount excreted in the urine can vary from 1% or 2% of that filtered to more than 100%. Mineralocorticoids (aldosterone) affect potassium secretion in the distal nephron segments but not in the proximal tubule. Lack of these adrenocortical hormones results in potassium retention and hyperkalemia. Other factors that modify potassium excretion include sodium balance, acid–base balance, and diuretics.

The renal handling of calcium and magnesium is complex and is related to a variety of factors, including parathyroid function and vitamin D metabolism, not all of which are completely understood. Both calcium and magnesium exist in plasma, partly in a free ionized form and partly bound to serum protein. It is the free calcium or magnesium that is filterable. In general, 99% of filtered calcium is reabsorbed. While factors affecting renal calcium handling are complex, reabsorption of calcium generally tends to follow that of sodium in the various nephron segments. It appears from recent work that the major control of excretion of calcium takes place in distal segments of the nephron. Parathyroid hormone (PTH) appears to affect transport of calcium in the distal tubule: administration of PTH stimulates reabsorption of calcium and decreases calcium excretion. In addition to PTH, other hormones (calcitonin, growth hormone, and thyroid hormone) may directly or indirectly modify calcium excretion. Acid–base alterations and the state of intravascular volume may affect calcium excretion. The control of renal excretion of magnesium still requires further study. As with calcium, a variety of hormones, changes in acid–base status, and altered intravascular volume may modify magnesium handling by the kidney. Magnesium reabsorption by the kidney may be limited by a maximum rate of transport.

Glucose is filtered at the glomerulus and is essentially completely reabsorbed in the proximal tubule until the plasma concentration exceeds 180 mg/dl. As the plasma concentration of glucose increases, glucose appears in the urine, and urinary excretion of glucose increases linearly with plasma concentration.

Substances such as glucose are said to have a renal threshold: the active transport system in the proximal tubule appears to have an upper limit or maximum rate of transport (abbreviated t_m for transport maximum). Thus, as higher concentrations of glucose appear in the proximal tubular fluid, the ability of the tubule to reabsorb glucose is surpassed, and glucose is excreted in the urine. Many other substances also display transport maxima, including magnesium, phosphate, and amino acids. As previously mentioned, reabsorption of some substances such as glucose, amino acids, and bicarbonate may be linked to reabsorption of sodium in the proximal tubule.

Reabsorption of filtered substances like glucose and amino acids results in conservation of these substances. On the other hand, a number of compounds are actively secreted by the kidney, including a variety of drugs and endogenous compounds. Most of these substances are weak organic acids; the prototype compound for this system (organic acid transport system) is p-aminohippurate (PAH). This system, which is t_m-limited, is important because it is the route of elimination of potentially toxic substances of endogenous and exogenous origin.

GLOMERULAR FILTRATION AND THE CONCEPT OF CLEARANCE

General Principles

As discussed previously, formation of the glomerular filtrate is due to a number of forces acting on the fluid within glomerular capillaries. The glomerular filtration rate can be determined by use of a substance that has the following properties: (1) It reaches the urine by filtration alone, i.e., it is not secreted by the tubules. (2) It is not reabsorbed by the renal tubule. (3) It is not metabolized by the kidney. (4) It is nontoxic. While there are several such substances available, the prototype is inulin, a starchlike polymer of fructose. If inulin is infused intravenously at a constant rate, a constant plasma concentration will be reached in 1–2 hours. At that point the rate of filtration of inulin (F_{IN}) can be calculated:

$$F_{IN} \text{ (mg/min)} = \text{GFR (ml/min)} = P_{IN} \text{ (mg/ml)}$$

where GFR is glomerular filtration rate (an unknown) and P_{IN} is plasma concentration of inulin. If the urine is collected during a known time period, the rate of excretion of inulin (E_{IN}) can be calculated:

$$E_{IN} \text{ (mg/min)} = V \text{ (ml/min)} \times U_{IN} \text{ (mg/ml)}$$

where V is urine flow rate and U_{IN} is concentration of inulin in urine. Since, by definition, all of the inulin in the urine was obtained by filtration,

$$F_{IN} \text{ (mg/min)} = E_{IN} \text{ (mg/min)}$$
$$\text{GFR (ml/min)} \times P_{IN} \text{ (mg/ml)} = V \text{ (ml/min)} \times U_{IN} \text{ (mg/ml)}$$

and rearranging

$$\text{GFR (ml(min)} = \frac{V \times U_{IN}}{P_{IN}}$$

Since all the values on the right-hand side of the equation can be determined, the GFR can be calculated. However, the quantity $(V \times U_{IN})/P_{IN}$ is also called "clearance of inulin," C_{IN}. This value C_{IN} is defined as that volume of plasma from which all the inulin is removed by the kidney in a given period of time (in this case 1 min). Several points concerning this technique for measurement of clearance should be noted: (1) It is a general technique that can be applied to any substance:

$$C_x = \frac{V \times U_x}{P_x}$$

the volume of plasma from which all of the given substance x is removed (cleared) in a given period of time. (2) The plasma is being cleared of the substance, which then is excreted in the urine. (3) The units of clearance (volume/unit time, i.e., ml/min, liters/day, etc.) refer to the volume of plasma from which the substance has been cleared during the given time.

While inulin may be used to determine the GFR in man, in practice creatinine,* an endogenous product of muscle metabolism, is usually used.

Clinical Determination of GFR

The use of the endogenous creatinine clearance as an estimate of GFR is practical for two reasons. First, as already discussed, creatinine is excreted in the urine primarily via glomerular filtration (a small fraction being secreted by the tubule). Second, creatinine is formed by the metabolism of creatinine in muscle, and the amount of creatinine excreted in the urine is proportional to muscle mass and is independent of renal function. Thus if renal function is constant, the plasma concentration of creatinine is also relatively constant from day to day.

With knowledge of the plasma creatinine concentration and the rate of urinary excretion of creatinine (as calculated by $U_{creat} \times V$), the clearance of creatine can be calculated: $C_{creat} = (U_{creat} \times V)/P_{creat}$.

The critical measurement in this formula is the urine flow rate V. In general, errors in determination of V can be reduced (but not eliminated) by using long collection times, e.g., 24 hours. The larger the volume of urine collected, the smaller the percentage error resulting from loss of urine or error in measurement of urine volume. Determination of 24-hour creatinine clearance is preferred to determinations over shorter collection periods. Creatinine clearance is usually expressed in milliliters per minute, even though the urine is collected over longer time periods.

EXAMPLE. An 8-year-old boy has a serum creatinine of 1 mg/dl. In

---

* In man, creatinine is secreted by the renal tubule, and the GFR estimated from creatinine is slightly greater than when inulin is used. However, in the actual determination of endogenous creatinine clearance, the chemical methods used measure not only creatinine but also some "noncreatinine chromogens." Since these noncreatinine substances have higher concentrations in plasma than in urine, the value for the clearance of creatinine is artificially reduced. This error tends to offset the error introduced by active tubular secretion of creatinine. Thus the endogenous creatinine clearance in man is a reasonable estimate of GFR.

24 hours he excretes 800 ml of urine with a creatinine concentration of 125 mg/dl.*

$$C_{creat} = \frac{800 \text{ ml/24 hours} \times 125 \text{ mg/dl}}{1 \text{ mg/dl}} = 100,000 \text{ ml/24 hours}$$

$$\frac{100,000 \text{ ml/24 hours}}{1440 \text{ min/24 hours}} = 69 \text{ ml/min}$$

After calculation of creatinine clearance as an estimate of GFR, the values are generally normalized to a surface area of 1.73 m². If the example patient has a surface area of 0.93 m², his corrected creatinine clearance is

$$69 \text{ ml/min} \times \frac{1.73}{0.93} = 129 \text{ ml/min/1.73 m}^2$$

Figure 3-3 shows creatinine clearance (in ml/min) plotted against age (in years), with the corresponding average surface area for age shown below. From 2 years to 13 years of age there is a linear increase of GFR with age, as expressed by the formula GFR = 30 + (5 × age in years). This formula permits rapid estimation of the normal creatinine clearance for children 2–13 years of age. Several points should be noted. First, below 2 years of age the creatinine clearance is less than would be predicted by the formula. Second, the values used for surface area are based on average size for age; for more precise evaluation of GFR a surface area nomogram or table (see Appendix) that takes both height and weight into consideration should be used. Third, above 13 years of age the values again deviate from the line, as most children enter puberty and growth rate increases. The surface-area nomogram is important for this group because of the wide variation in growth rate from patient to patient. Fourth, variability in determination of creatinine clearance is not shown in Figure 3-3. By present methods, the range of values for children ages 2–13 years varies approximately ± 25 ml/min/1.73 m². Thus the normal range of values of creatinine clearance for children 2–13 years of age is 95–145 ml/min/1.73 m², with a mean value of 120 ml/min/1.73 m². Fifth, determination of creatinine clearance is a steady-state measurement. It requires a constant rate of excretion of creatinine ($U_{creat} \times V$). During conditions in which renal function is changing rapidly (as in acute renal failure) or when renal function is greatly impaired (as in chronic renal failure), creatinine clearance is much less reliable. Finally, the difficulty in collecting urine

---

* Note that the units used for plasma and urine concentrations of creatinine must be the same. The units used (mg/dl or mg/ml) are not important, since they cancel in the equation.

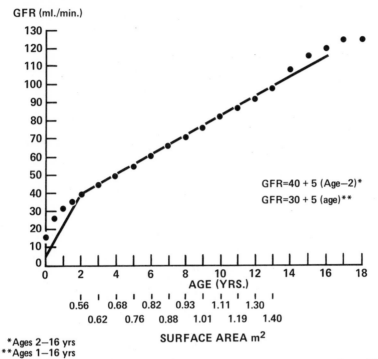

GFR (ml./min.)

GFR=40 + 5 (Age−2)*
GFR=30 + 5 (age)**

AGE (YRS.)

0.56   0.68   0.82   0.93   1.11   1.30
   0.62   0.76   0.88   1.01   1.19   1.40

SURFACE AREA m²

*Ages 2–16 yrs
**Ages 1–16 yrs

Fig. 3-3.   GFR as a function of age or surface area. From 2 to 16 years of age GFR increases essentially linearly and can be described by either of two equations: GFR = 40 + [5 × (age − 2)]; GFR = 30 + (5 × age). Below the age of 2 years there is marked reduction in GFR because of lack of maturation of the kidney.

from small children makes accurate estimation of GFR even more difficult.

Inspection of the formula for clearance demonstrates that since creatinine excretion ($U_{creat} \times V$) is constant and is unrelated to renal function, plasma creatinine is proportional to creatinine clearance ($C_{creat} \sim 1/P_{creat}$), i.e., as creatinine clearance decreases, plasma creatinine increases, and vice versa.* Thus plasma creatinine is an estimate of renal function. Normal values for plasma creatinine in children of several ages are given in Table 3-1. It must be kept in mind that the value for plasma creatinine will depend on the method used to determine creatinine and on the amount of noncreatinine chromogens present in the plasma. However, in spite of all limitations, endogenous creatinine clearance and plasma

* It appears that in chronic renal failure there is some enteric circulation of creatinine. As a result, the serum creatinine level may not rise quite as rapidly as predicted by the fall in GFR. However, this effect is presumably small and may be ignored when one is trying to make a clinical estimate of change in renal function.

Table 3-1
Plasma Creatinine as a
Function of Age*†

Age (years)	Mean Value ± 2 SD (mg/dl)
Birth	0.75 ± 0.24
1	0.32 ± 0.14
3	0.34 ± 0.12
5	0.40 ± 0.14
10	0.52 ± 0.18
Adult female	0.77 ± 0.24
Adult male	0.97 ± 0.25

* Adapted from: Rubin MI, Barratt TM: Pediatric Nephrology. Baltimore, MD, Williams & Wilkins, 1975; Lieberman E: Clinical Pediatric Nephrology. Philadelphia, PA, Lippincott, 1976.

† The gradual fall in plasma creatinine values from birth to 3 years of age and then the gradual rise to adult values are shown. The plasma creatinine value is a function of muscle mass and GFR. The values are higher in infancy because of the relative reduction in GFR. They increase in later childhood and adult life because of the relative increase in muscle mass. The difference between the female and male adult values is also a reflection of the difference in muscle mass.

creatinine remain the bases for rapid and simple clinical estimates of renal glomerular function.†

Urea Clearance and Blood Urea as Estimates of Renal Function

While urinary excretion of urea is mainly derived from urea that is filtered, the clearance of urea is in part dependent on urine flow rate. Tubular reabsorption of urea decreases as urine flow increases. Therefore urea clearance is not a good estimate of glomerular filtration. In addition, excretion of urea is a reflection of protein intake in the diet, and excretion from day to day is considerably more variable than that of creatinine.

† Schwartz and associates recently reported that GFR (ml/min/1.73 m^2) can be estimated by the formula GFR = $0.55 \times$ length (cm)/P_{creat} (mg/dl). Their correlation was quite good, and such a relationship may be a useful tool for monitoring renal function in children.

While urea excretion is valuable for estimation of protein intake (see below), clearance of urea is now little used as a measure of renal function. On the other hand, blood urea nitrogen (BUN) is a useful tool in screening for renal disease, keeping in mind the effects of protein intake.

Urea and Protein Intake

Another useful relationship inherent in the clearance concept is that the numerator $(U \times V)$ of the equation is the amount of substance excreted in the urine per unit time and is equal to the amount ingested or produced by metabolism (minus that amount excreted by other routes, such as feces) when the body is in a balanced state. Since 80% of excreted nitrogen is eliminated as urea, the amount of urea excreted per day can be used to estimate protein intake in a stable state, or it can be used to estimate protein catabolism when there is no intake. If renal function is constant, plasma urea will vary with intake, since $C_{urea} = (U_{urea} \times V)/P_{urea} = $ intake$/P_{urea}$. Several examples of the use of the clearances of creatinine and urea will aid in interpreting such data.

EXAMPLE 1.   A 4-year-old girl who weighed only 12 kg and who was 90 cm tall was being investigated because of her small size. Her mother stated that she ate a high-protein diet containing about 1400 kcal. She drank a pint of milk a day, but was said to eat large quantities of cheese, eggs, and meat. The physical examination revealed a small thin child with no other physical evidence of disease. As part of the evaluation, creatine clearance and urea N_2 excretion were determined.

Plasma urea N_2 concentration =   7.1 mg/dl
Plasma creatinine concentration =   0.5 mg/dl
Urine volume (24 hours) = 855   ml
Urine urea N_2 concentration = 280   mg/dl
Urine creatinine concentration =   32.8 mg/dl

$$C_{creat} = \frac{\frac{855}{1440} \times 32.8}{0.5} = 39 \text{ ml/min}$$

From the surface-area nomogram her surface area was found to be 0.54 m² (note that because of her small size she deviated considerably from the surface-area values given in Figure 3-3). Her GFR corrected for surface area was $(39 \times 1.73)/0.54 = 125$ ml/min/1.73 m², a value well within the normal range.

The quantity of urea N_2 excreted in urine is equal to U_{urea} (mg/ml)* $\times V$

---

* It is now important to convert U_{urea} from mg/dl to mg/ml: U_{urea} (mg/dl)/100 = U_{urea} (mg/ml).

(ml/24 hours): 2.80 mg/ml × 855 ml/24 hours = 2395 mg/24 hours. This value represents about 80% of nitrogen output; so total nitrogen output = (100/80) × 2400 = 3000 mg/day. Furthermore, protein is on the average 16.7% nitrogen, or protein intake is six times nitrogen intake. Assuming she was in a steady state, her 3000-mg output of nitrogen per day should be balanced by a 3000-mg intake. If her input of nitrogen was 3000 mg, her intake of protein was six times that value, or 18 g.* This represents 1.5 g/kg body weight, which is quite a low figure for a child of her age, and it suggests that the mother's evaluation of her diet was quite faulty. (Recommended protein intake at 4 years of age is approximately 2.5 g/kg.)

EXAMPLE 2.   An 8-year-old boy was being evaluated because of poor growth. He was 21 kg and 119 cm, values less than the 3rd percentile for his age. At 4 years of age he had been at the 25th percentile for height and weight. He was not a big eater, but his mother thought his diet was adequate. Among other studies, a 24-hour urea excretion and creatinine clearance were obtained:

$$
\begin{aligned}
\text{Serum creatine} &= 1.1 \quad \text{mg/dl} \\
\text{BUN} &= 16 \quad \text{mg/dl} \\
\text{Urine volume (24 hours)} &= 1440 \quad \text{ml} \\
\text{Urine creatinine concentration} &= 44 \quad \text{mg/dl} \\
\text{Urine urea } N_2 \text{ concentration} &= 384 \quad \text{mg/dl}
\end{aligned}
$$

From the surface-area nomogram his surface area was found to be 0.83 m^2. His GFR corrected for surface area was 40 × (1.73/0.83) = 83 ml/min/1.73 m^2. His creatinine clearance was approximately two-thirds the expected normal mean value of 120 ml/min and was well outside the range of normal. It should be noted that his BUN was within the normal range for most laboratories, and thus his decrease in function would have been overlooked had BUN been used as the sole screening procedure. On the other hand, his serum creatinine, which was normal by the usual adult standards used in most laboratories, was elevated when compared for age and surface area. Subsequent evaluation revealed that the patient had bilateral hydronephrosis secondary to ureteral reflux.

The patient's protein intake can also be estimated as previously described: 3.84 mg/min × 1440 ml/24 hours = 5530 mg urea/24 hours; 5530/0.8 = 6913 mg N$_2$. Input 7 g N$_2$ × 6 = 42 g protein/24 hours, or 2 g protein per kilogram of body weight. Although this value is low, it is adequate for reasonable nutrition at his age.

One year following corrective surgery his serum creatinine was 0.9 mg/dl. However, his height and weight had increased, and his surface area

---

* Protein intake would be greater than this value by the amount being retained for growth. For a 4-year-old child, weight gain rarely averages more than 7 g/day, and of this, only 1–1.5 g will be protein.

was 0.88 m². When determination of his creatinine clearance was repeated, his urine output was 960 ml/24 hours, and U_{creat} was 74 mg/dl.

$$C_{creat} = \frac{74 \times \dfrac{960}{1440}}{0.9} = 55 \text{ ml/min}$$

$$55 \times \frac{1.73}{0.88} = 108 \text{ ml/min/}1.73 \text{ m}^2$$

This increase in creatinine clearance of about 38% (from 40 to 55 ml/min) was associated with an 18% decrease in serum creatinine (from 1.1 to 0.9 mg/dl). An increase in surface area resulted in increased excretion of creatinine (from 0.44 to 0.49 mg/min). Creatinine clearance was still probably subnormal; serum creatinine remained above normal value for age. However, it is important to note that because of the wide range of normal values due to uncertainties in clearance determination, it cannot be said that the value of 108 ml/min/1.73 m² is decreased.

EXAMPLE 3.   A 10-year-old girl was followed for chronic renal disease over a period of 1 year. Her plasma creatinine increased from 2.5 to 5.0 mg/dl, and her BUN increased from 28 to 85 mg/dl. When her plasma creatinine was 2.5 mg/dl, C_{creat} was 35 ml/min uncorrected for surface area. During the year she grew less than most 10-year-olds. However, her appetite was good, and her mother reported that she did not follow the protein-restricted diet that was prescribed. What occurred in her renal function? At age 9 years,

$$C_{creat} = \frac{U_{creat} \times V}{P_{creat}} = \frac{U_{creat} \times V}{2.5 \text{ mg/dl}} = 35 \text{ ml/min}$$
$$U_{creat} \times V = 2.5 \times 35 = 87.5$$

It can reasonably be assumed that her creatinine excretion per unit time remained unchanged at age 10 years, since she was about the same size. Thus,

$$C_{creat} = \frac{87.5}{5.0} = 17.5 \text{ ml/min}$$

Her GFR decreased by 50%, while her plasma creatinine doubled.

If production of creatinine does not change, a decrease in C_{creat} must result in a rise in P_{creat}. This situation derives from the original equation: $P_{creat} \times \text{GFR} = U_{creat} \times V$. If $U_{creat} \times V$ is a constant reflecting formation of creatinine, then as GFR (or C_{creat}) falls, P_{creat} must increase.

While the same general principle holds for urea, BUN is very sensitive to protein intake. In the present situation, BUN increased by almost threefold, whild serum creatinine only doubled. This situation most likely represents a disproportionate increase in intake of protein. Indeed, when the patient was finally placed on a diet with 1.5 g of protein per kilogram per day, her BUN fell to 45 mg/dl.

EXAMPLE 4. A 7-year-old boy with bilateral ureteral reflux and urinary tract infection had a 24-hour creatinine clearance of

$$C_{creat} = \frac{77 \times \dfrac{720}{1440}}{0.6} = 64 \text{ ml/min}$$

$$C_{creat} = 64 = \frac{1.73}{0.87} = 127 \text{ ml/min/1.73 m}^2$$

One year later, following surgery, creatinine clearance was again obtained:

$$C_{creat} = \frac{83 \times \dfrac{486}{1440}}{0.7} = 40 \text{ ml/min}$$

Because he had grown normally, his surface area was then 0.93 m².

$$C_{creat} = 40 \times \frac{1.73}{0.93} = 74 \text{ ml/min/1.73 m}^2$$

Inspection of the data demonstrated that the seeming decrease in creatinine clearance (37%) was out of proportion to the increase in plasma creatinine (17%), which can be explained on the basis of growth. The apparent creatinine excretion $[U_{creat} \text{(mg/ml)} \times V \text{(ml/day)}]$ decreased from 554 to 403 mg/day. Such a change would require considerable loss of muscle mass. Further questioning of the mother revealed that some of the urine was lost during collection, and when the procedure was repeated the creatinine clearance was found to be normal. This situation illustrates that under steady-state conditions a decrease in creatinine clearance is not due to a fall in creatinine excretion but to an increase in plasma creatinine.

In summary, serum creatinine and creatinine clearance are convenient methods for clinical estimation of renal function. It must be kept in mind that there is considerable error in the estimation of serum creatinine and urine volume. In considering changes in creatinine clearance, the variability of the specific method and laboratory must be considered. Also, the age- and growth-related changes in renal function and thus in serum creatinine must be kept in mind.

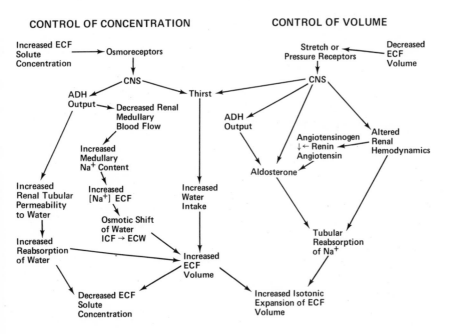

Fig. 3-4. Control of body fluid concentration and volume. Increases in solute concentration stimulate the osmoreceptors, which in turn produce thirst and an increased output of ADH. The end result of both of these stimulations is to increase the volume of the ECF. As a result of this change in volume, the ECF solute concentration will decrease. A reduction in ECF volume, as shown in the right-hand side of the figure, stimulates thirst, ADH output, and aldosterone. The primary response to aldosterone release is reabsorption by the renal tubule of increased amounts of sodium. This will increase the concentration of sodium in the ECF, but if it is accompanied by concomitant increase in volume through the thirst mechanism or secondarily through the ADH mechanism shown on the left, it will result in isotonic expansion of the ECF. In summary, the osmoreceptors primarily affect ECF volume, and the volume receptors primarily affect solute concentration.

CONTROL OF BODY FLUID COMPOSITION AND VOLUME

Maintenance of the concentration and volume of the ECF and ICF compartments requires that intake and output of water and sodium be equal. The most common imbalance occurs when output exceeds intake, with the result that the volume of body fluids decreases. The reverse situation is much less common and is frequently iatrogenic. A gain or loss of water without a similar change in sodium will result in modification of body fluid composition (hyponatremia or hypernatremia or osmolarity). While the mechanisms that control body fluid composition and volume will be discussed separately, several experimental and clinical situations have demonstrated that the control mechanisms are not independent. The processes involved are summarized in Figure 3-4.

Body Fluid Composition

Body fluid composition is regulated by factors that affect intake of water (e.g., thirst*) and factors that affect renal water loss (antidiuretic hormone and the function of the renal tubule).

If water is withheld or if excess sodium chloride is given to a person, the osmolarity of the ECF will increase. Water will then move from the ICF into the ECF to equalize the osmotic concentrations. This cellular dehydration is sensed within the hypothalamus, and the sensation of thirst is stimulated. In addition to its being caused by cellular dehydration, thirst may also be stimulated by decreases in ECF volume (specifically, the intravascular volume). Thus thirst is a prominent clinical feature of hemorrhage. Other factors that reduce ECF volume, such as sodium restriction or loss (e.g., sodium depletion due to diuretics) or sequestration of ECF, will stimulate thirst. Recent evidence suggests that angiotensin II is a potent stimulator of thirst and that the renin-angiotensin system is important in the control of this sensation.

If the osmolarity of the ECF is increased, the cellular dehydration is sensed by osmoreceptors that stimulate thirst, and other such receptors located in a different area of the hypothalamus are stimulated, with resultant release of ADH. Stimuli from these latter osmoreceptors pass to specialized neurons that synthesize ADH. The ADH thus formed is transported to the posterior pituitary where it is released into the circulation. The original signal from the osmoreceptor stimulates both synthesis and release of ADH. Factors other than osmolarity that also stimulate synthesis and release of ADH include various types of stress and pain, decreases in blood volume, a variety of drugs, and possibly changes in arterial Po_2.

Once ADH is released, its major site of action is the renal tubule.† The hormone reaches the cortical collecting tubules and collecting ducts

---

* Another factor is salt appetite, a phenomenon that is only poorly understood. While it is clear that changes in salt appetite are important in some species, it is difficult to demonstrate a role in man.

† Although ADH also has vasopressor activity, it is unclear whether this hormone is important in the regulation of blood pressure.

and produces an increase in the permeability of the tubular epithelium to water. Water then can diffuse back into the hypertonic medullary interstitium. The result of this diffusion of water out of the tubule is an increase in concentration of the urine. In addition to its effect on water permeability, ADH probably also increases the permeability of the medullary collecting ducts to urea and sodium. While the importance of changes in sodium permeability is not clear, changes in urea permeability result in an increase in reabsorption of urea. This process contributes to the high urea content of the medullary interstitium. Finally, ADH may have an effect on medullary blood flow, decreasing flow in the vasa recta. However, while such a process would help keep the sodium content of the medulla high, this role for ADH has not been proved.

If the opposite situation occurs, and the ECF becomes hypotonic, the osmoreceptors will be depressed and ADH production and secretion will be decreased. Since the half-life of ADH in the circulation is measured in minutes, the ADH levels will fall rapidly, water permeability in the renal tubule will decrease, and dilute urine will be excreted. The resulting loss of water in excess of sodium increases the osmolarity of the ECF. Stimuli (in addition to hypotonicity) that inhibit ADH release include alcohol, as well as situations that result in expansion of the ECF.

Body Fluid Volume

Whereas control of solute concentration in body fluids is achieved by rather straightforward control of thirst (intake) and water excretion (output), control of volume is achieved largely by regulation of sodium excretion. The mechanisms involved in control of sodium excretion are quite complex and are still under study. It is worth reemphasizing that volume control and composition control are interrelated. It should also be kept in mind that the concept of volume control is related to the capacity of a compartment to hold fluid. In general, control of the ECF volume is related to the capacity of the vascular compartment to hold fluid. When the vascular volume becomes either overfull or underfull, there is modulation via the kidney.

This capacity to monitor the fullness of the circulation is in part related to the presence of volume receptors, probably located at several sites, including the heart, the arterial and venous circulations, and the kidney. Increases or decreases in the volume of fluid in the circulation act as signals to these receptors. If fluid volume increases, as when dietary sodium intake is increased, an increase in renal sodium excretion follows. When the volume decreases, sodium excretion also decreases. It should be noted that the volume may be increased or decreased by methods other than intake of sodium. A large arteriovenous fistula is sensed as a volume decrease, and sodium is retained. When the fistula is closed, there is an increase in sodium excretion. Other situations, such as congestive heart failure, lead to similar changes in sodium excretion.

The net result of changes in the volume of the ECF is stimulation of several mechanisms that tend to restore fluid balance. A decrease in volume stimulates ADH production and secretion, the sensation of thirst, possibly an increase in salt appetite, and retention of sodium by the kidney. When the volume is overexpanded, the reverse mechanisms come into play. The first three mechanisms have been reviewed. The fourth, renal control of sodium excretion, will be discussed next.

In recent years the mechanisms involved in control of sodium excretion by the kidney have come under intensive study. While several of these factors will be reviewed briefly, their physiologic significance remains to be determined.

CHANGES IN RENAL PERFUSION PRESSURE

Changes in the hydrostatic pressure perfusing the kidney are known to modify renal sodium reabsorption, but they are unrelated to changes in GFR. Several specific mechanisms have been proposed, including effects of perfusion pressure on the filtered load of sodium, on the pressure in the glomerular and peritubular capillaries, and on the renin-angiotensin-aldosterone system.

CHANGES IN PLASMA ONCOTIC PRESSURE

When the ECF is increased with isotonic saline, the protein concentration of the plasma falls. Loss of fluid that contains no protein will raise the plasma protein concentration. Results of several studies have suggested that the rate of sodium reabsorption by the proximal tubule may be affected by the concentration of protein (oncotic pressure) of blood in the peritubular capillaries. Thus an increase in oncotic pressure would favor reabsorption of sodium, and a decrease would inhibit reabsorption. Changes in GFR or renal blood flow independent of one another might also affect the oncotic pressure in the peritubular capillaries and thus tubular reabsorption.

CHANGES IN SYMPATHETIC TONE

Stimulation of volume receptors can change the tone of the sympathetic innervation to the kidney. Changes in sympathetic tone may act to change renal sodium reabsorption via the renin-angiotensin-aldosterone system by altering the secretion of renin. Also, sympathetic control over the renal vascular resistance may alter the relationship between glomerular filtration and renal plasma flow, thus altering peritubular hydrostatic or oncotic pressure.

HORMONES

It has been suggested by several investigators that hormones produced within the kidney or elsewhere in the circulation may control sodium excretion by the kidney (natriuretic hormones). Validation of this mechanism awaits additional study, but data do suggest that hormonal factors other than aldosterone may play a role.

The effects of several possible mechanisms are shown in Figure 3-4. It is not possible at present to rank these factors in importance. Furthermore, it is clear that the isolated kidney without nervous or hormonal input can vary sodium excretion. Also, recent studies suggest that while changes in ECF volume change proximal tubular sodium reabsorption, it is within the collecting duct that the final level of sodium in the urine is controlled. It should be noted that changes in GFR have not been discussed as mechanisms for control of sodium excretion by the kidney. While there is evidence to suggest that there is a balance between sodium excretion and GFR, filtration does not appear to be a major factor in adjustments involved in control of ECF volume. For example, ECF volume expansion leads to an increase in urinary sodium excretion, despite maneuvers that result in decreases in glomerular filtration.

In summary, several factors have been implicated in the mechanisms by which the kidney responds to changes in ECF volume. The exact mechanism or mechanisms that control the final rate of sodium excretion and that can explain all the clinical and experimental observations remain to be determined.

Interaction between Volume Control and Concentration Control

It is worth reemphasizing that the control mechanisms for ECF volume and concentration cannot be completely separated. For example, contraction of the ECF volume (hypovolemia) is a much more potent stimulus for ADH secretion than an increase in ECF concentration (hypernatremia). Several clinical states where this interaction is important will now be considered.

In the clinical setting there are four states that can be considered to be pure variations in the state of hydration: gain or loss of sodium and gain or loss of water. The shifts in ECF and ICF volume and composition secondary to these states are considered in Part II. In practice, such changes almost never occur alone. For example, water containing no sodium is almost never lost from the body.* Rather, a hypotonic fluid is lost, as in diarrhea. The resulting changes in ECF volume and composi-

---

* Losses via the lung are the major exceptions.

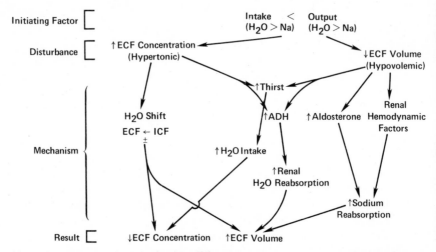

Fig. 3-5. Hypertonic dehydration. When intake is less than output, dehydration will result. When water loss exceeds sodium loss, the dehydration will be hypertonic in character. The mechanisms that the come into play are illustrated in this figure. The result of these mechanisms is a decrease in the solute concentration in the ECF and an increase in the ECF volume.

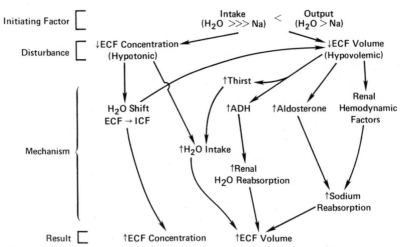

Fig. 3-6. Hypotonic dehydration. When the intake (although less than the output) results in a net sodium loss greater than the water loss, the result will be a decrease in ECF solute concentration and a decrease in ECF volume. The same mechanisms illustrated in Figure 3-5 will be involved, but the directions of changes will differ, so that the result is an increase in solute concentration and an increase in volume.

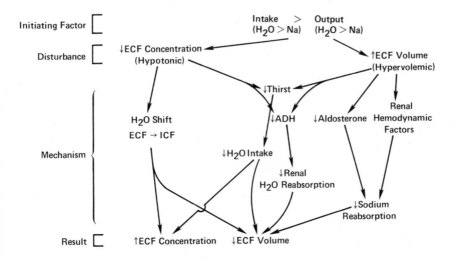

Fig. 3-7. Hypotonic overhydration. When intake exceeds output, and the net water increase is greater than the net sodium increase, the solute concentration in the ECF will fall when the volume of the ECF increases. The same mechanisms as in the previous two figures are again called into play, but in altered directions, so that the result is a reduction in volume and an increase in concentration within the ECF.

tion bring into play compensatory mechanisms that entirely or partly maintain homeostasis. Several specific examples will now be considered.

ISOTONIC OR HYPERTONIC DEHYDRATION

Loss of hypotonic fluid in excess of intake (Fig. 3-5) results in isotonic or hypertonic dehydration, depending on the volume of fluid lost, the amount of sodium ingested, and the efficiency of the compensatory mechanisms. Loss of hypotonic fluid will initially decrease volume and increase ECF solute concentration. An intake of water and a shift of ICF to ECF tend to overcome this increase. In the most common clinical situation, the net result is isotonic dehydration. Thus, even though losses are hypotonic, the net result when all mechanisms come into play is a decrease in ECF volume without a change in composition. When losses are large and more hypotonic than intake, the serum sodium concentration may rise, with resulting hypertonic dehydration. This may also happen because too much sodium is present in oral fluids. While retention of sodium and water by the kidney helps compensate for ECF losses, dehydration will occur as long as output exceeds intake.

HYPOTONIC DEHYDRATION

Hypotonic dehydration results from loss of hypotonic or isotonic fluid in excess of intake when intake is very dilute (Fig. 3-6): intake ($H_2O >>> Na$) < output ($H_2O > Na$). In this situation the sodium being taken in is much less than that being lost. A volume depletion occurs, but the net loss of sodium is greater than the loss of water, and a decrease in the solute concentration in the ECF occurs. This situation may come about when fluid with relatively more sodium is lost, but it can also occur when attempts to restore volume are made with very solute-poor fluids. The decreased ECF concentration results in a shift of water from the ECF to the ICF (Fig. 3-6). The shift partially corrects the low ECF concentration, but it contributes further to reduction in ECF volume. While both thirst and ADH mechanisms are important for maintenance of ECF volume, they may contribute to the hypotonic state. In this situation the regulating mechanisms for volume override those for concentration.

HIGH INTAKE OF HYPOTONIC FLUID

There are high-intake situations in which intake of hypotonic fluid exceeds output (Fig. 3-7): intake ($H_2O > Na$) > output ($H_2O > Na$); or intake ($H_2O > Na$) > output ($H_2O \sim Na$). These states are unusual, but they do occur. In the face of normal renal function it is difficult for them to produce serious consequences, since excess water is rapidly excreted and serum sodium concentration is maintained (Fig. 3-7). However, in states where renal or cardiovascular function is compromised, excessive intake of hypotonic fluid may result in serious dilution of the ECF volume and water intoxication.

HIGH INTAKE OF ISOTONIC OR HYPERTONIC FLUID

There are high-intake situations in which intake of isotonic or hypertonic fluid exceeds output (Fig. 3-8): intake ($H_2O \sim Na$) > output ($H_2O >> Na$). This situation is also uncommon; it leads to overexpansion of ECF volume, and it has the potential to increase serum sodium concentration. However, again in the face of adequate cardiovascular and renal mechanisms, the sodium is excreted. However, very rapid intake of such fluids may lead to cardiac decompensation, especially if cardiac function is already borderline.

GENERALIZED EDEMA

Table 3-2 gives a list of conditions in which generalized edema may occur. Many of these problems are not important in children. However, heart failure, nephrotic syndrome, renal failure, and cirrhosis are factors associated with edema in children. While there are some important differ-

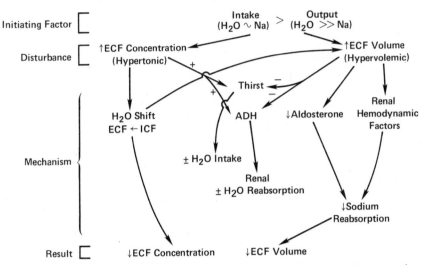

Fig. 3-8.   Hypertonic overhydration. When intake exceeds output, but retention of sodium is greater than retention of water, the concentration of solute will rise, as will the ECF volume. In this situation the contradictory stimuli on the mechanisms previously illustrated will result in a reduction in ECF concentration and a fall in ECF volume.

Table 3-2
Causes of Generalized
Edema*

Heart failure
Nephrotic syndrome
Renal failure
Liver cirrhosis
Obstruction of thoracic vena cava
Pregnancy
Toxemia of pregnancy
Endocrine–metabolic
Miscellaneous

* This is a partial listing of the causes of generalized edema that may occur in childhood and adolescence.

ences in these conditions, they all have in common renal retention of sodium at a time when ECF volume is increased, i.e., intake > output. The mechanisms by which the kidney retains sodium are complex and are still under investigation. However, they probably involve all the mechanisms previously discussed, including the renin-angiotensin-aldosterone system, changes in renal hemodynamics, and nervous and hormonal influences. It is still not clear whether retention of sodium by the kidney is primary or secondary to the processes of edema formation.

PART II

General Clinical Conditions

4
Volume Disorders

Volume disorders include those with net decreases in the volume of body water (dehydration), those with net increases in the volume of body water (overhydration), and those with movement of water within the body, with no net change in the total volume of body water (translocation).

DEHYDRATION

The term *dehydration* refers to a reduction in the volume of the body fluids. In the most common situations this reduction is distributed throughout the total body water in such a way that blood volume, ECF, and ICF are all diminished. However, the degree to which each is diminished depends on the rate of loss, the quantity of loss, and the composition of the loss.

Dehydration can be caused by primary reduction in intake of fluids that cannot be balanced by sufficient reduction in output, by an increase in output that cannot be offset by a concomitant increase in intake, or by a combination of reduced intake and increased output. Usually there are clear-cut distinctions between these mechanisms, and appropriate therapy can be administered. However, there are occasions when the sequence of precipitating events is ambiguous and the therapeutic approach may be unclear. In such circumstances a cautious therapeutic trial may serve as a diagnostic test.

Isotonic Dehydration

Dehydration can also be classified according to the proportions of water and solute that have been lost. When the net deficit of water is greater than the net deficit of solute, the body fluids will become more concentrated, or hypertonic. When loss of solute exceeds loss of water, the body fluids become more dilute, or hypotonic; when loss of solute and loss of water are proportional, the body fluids retain their usual concentration and are isotonic. In the first stage of most forms of dehydration, the body fluids remain isotonic, since the kidney is able to compensate for any disparity between water and solute loss by producing urine of the opposite composition. It is only at the second stage of dehydration, when the kidney no longer has the capacity to make this adjustment or when other factors have intervened to prevent further renal compensation, that the hypertonic or hypotonic state ensues.*

DECREASED INTAKE

The most common example of decreased intake as a cause of dehydration is voluntary or involuntary cessation of drinking. Involuntary lack of intake may occur as a result of severe anorexia, coma, or fluid restriction for surgery. In any case, the resulting events are similar.

One of the most important characteristics of the infant or small child (in contrast to the older child or adult) with regard to fluid balance is illustrated by the situation of limited intake. This was discussed by Gamble as one of the disadvantages of being small. Assuming, for simplicity, that both the infant and the adolescent have ECFs equivalent to 25% of body weight; then the ECF of a 6-kg infant is 1500 ml, and that of a 60-kg adolescent is 15,000 ml. The normal intake sufficient to match the usual output of the infant is 95 ml/kg, and that for the adolescent is 47.5 ml/kg. Thus for the infant the daily intake would be 570 ml (6 kg × 95 ml/kg), and for the adolescent it would be 2400 ml (60 kg × 40 ml/kg). In the case of the infant, his intake or average output represents a volume greater than one-third of his ECF (i.e., 570/1500), whereas for the adolescent his intake or output represents about one-sixth of his ECF (i.e., 2400/15,000). This is shown diagrammatically in Figure 4-1. It should be apparent that if intake ceases and output is not modified, the infant will lose his total ECF in less than 3 days, but the adolescent will not reach this state for 6 days. Actually, of course, output decreases when input falls; and as has been mentioned, losses are shared by the ECF. However, the illustration shows why fluid restriction creates problems in infants so much more rapidly than in older children and adults.

Cessation of intake for any reason initiates a sequence of events that partially compensates for this disturbance in fluid equilibrium. The reason that a disequilibrium occurs when intake stops is that output cannot stop. Insensible water loss (IWL) continues almost unchanged, and this loss is water that is almost solute-free. Continuing loss of solute-free water in the

---

* An exception is the chronically malnourished child who may have hypotonic body fluids to begin with, in which case the dehydration may further increase the hypotonicity.

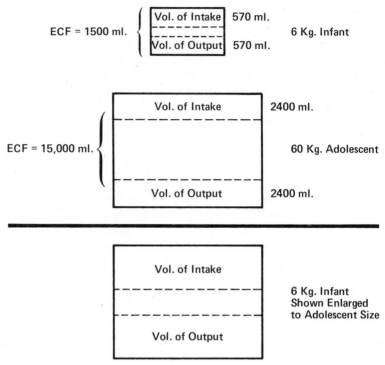

Fig. 4-1.   Magnitude of intake and output relative to volume of ECF. The rapidity with which an infant can become dehydrated may be seen by comparing the volume of output (or intake) to extracellular volume for the infant and for the adolescent or adult. It is apparent that the daily fluid output of the infant exceeds one-third of his ECF. In contrast, the daily fluid output of the adolescent is less than one-sixth of his ECF. Thus, relative to his size, the daily fluid output of the infant is more than double that of the adolescent. This concept is shown in the bottom portion of the figure, where the scale of the infant's ECF is enlarged to make it equivalent to that of the adolescent. It should be apparent that in the absence of intake, the infant will dehydrate approximately twice as rapidly as the adolescent or the adult.

absence of intake must result in higher solute concentration (hypertonicity) of a reduced volume of body fluids. However, compensation by the kidney and internal water shifts ameliorate the process for some time and maintain relative isotonicity of body fluids.

The renal response occurs as a result of stimulation of the volume receptors, reduction of GFR, increased aldosterone activity, and elaboration of ADH. The outcome of these reactions is urine of reduced volume and increased concentration, which can reach 1400 mOsm/liter (specific gravity ~ 1.040). It is important to recognize that children of all ages are capable of this response, but infants who are ill in addition to being dehydrated are not able to concentrate their urine as effectively as when they are not ill. Older children and adults are able to concentrate their urine independent of the presence of intercurrent illness. Another result of the response to dehydration occurs because of the fall in GFR: the plasma levels of substances that are largely dependent on glomerular filtration for their excretion will rise. These substances include urea, creatinine, phosphate, uric acid, etc. The greater the role of the tubule in the active excretion of one of these substances, the less its plasma concentration will be affected by the decrease in GFR. Creatinine and urea, with no active transport in the tubule, can be expected to rise with any fall in GFR. However, urea, which passively diffuses back through the tubule, may rise more than creatinine as GFR falls, because more passive back-diffusion can take place with the reduced rate of urine flow in the tubule. The frequent finding of elevated urea nitrogen in dehydration, in the absence of overt renal disease, led to use of the term prerenal azotemia. However, such azotemia is clearly renal, even if it is only transient and ultimately the result of dehydration.

Normally, less than 25% of filtered phosphate appears in the urine, and since reabsorption is active and can vary from 75% to 95% of filtered phosphate, a marked reduction in GFR is necessary before serum phosphate elevation will occur. The reabsorptive function for uric acid is still more flexible, and thus the serum level of uric acid will not rise until after serum inorganic phosphate has begun to rise.

In addition to the renal compensation for the decrease in intake, water shifts from the ICF to the ECF compartment. This occurs as a result of two separate phenomena: an increase in the osmolarity of the ECF and a transfer of solute from the ICF to the ECF.

Loss of water without solute from the ECF (primarily as IWL) raises the osmolarity of the ECF. The difference in osmotic pressure created by this ECF water loss results in water moving from within the cells to the ECF until the osmolarities are equal. This is shown diagrammatically in Figure 4-2, diagrams a–d. Diagram a is a conventional method of representing body water, with volume on the abscissa and concentration (solute as mOsm/liter or cation as mEq/liter) on the ordinate. The left half of the diagram represents ECF and the right half represents ICF. The area on each side represents the quantity of solute in milliosmoles or the quantity of cation in milliequivalents. In the situation of simple water loss from the ECF, the solute content remains unchanged. In diagram b the volume of the ECF has been reduced by 50 ml/kg, and diagram c shows the resulting increase in concentration of solute to 400 mOsm/liter (cation to 200 mEq/liter). In diagram d, water shifts into the ECF from the ICF as a result of the osmotic gradient until a new equilibrium is established. The new

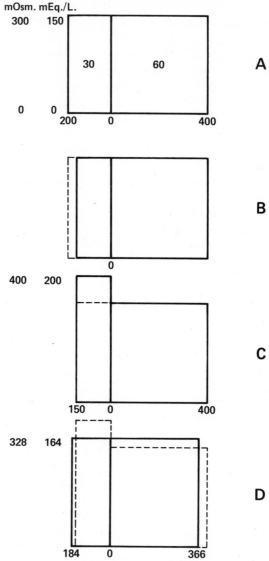

Fig. 4-2. Osmolar equilibration between ICF and ECF. Loss of fluid without solute from the ECF is illustrated in the progression from *a* to *g*. This results in an increase in the concentration of solute in the ECF, as shown in diagram *c*. The increased solute concentration in the ECF causes water to transfer from the ICF to the ECF, as shown in diagram *d*. The end result of water loss from the ECF is reduction in the volumes of ECF and ICF and increases in solute concentration in both compartments until equilibrium is again established.

equilibrium occurs when the loss of water from the ICF (with a resulting increase in ICF osmolarity) achieves sufficient expansion of the ECF so that the reduction in ECF osmolarity matches the new level of osmolarity in the ICF. The total amount of solute in each compartment remains the same, and the water loss is shared by the ECF and the ICF.

The second mechanism for movement of water from the ICF to the ECF in dehydration involves a transfer of solute, especially K^+ but also HPO_4^{--}. This occurs because cells are destroyed by the body for energy when caloric intake is inadequate and because K^+ is lost from intact cells as part of most catabolic processes. In the metabolic destruction of cells, the protein is converted to urea and other nitrogenous end products; the intracellular ions and the cell water become extracellular, because the cell no longer exists. The addition of K^+ and other intracellular ions to the ECF creates an additional burden on the kidney, which is acceptable initially; but later, as GFR falls further, K^+ (and to a lesser extent HPO_4^{--}) may accumulate in the ECF (and therefore in plasma) until toxic results occur.

The loss of K^+ from intact cells as part of the catabolic process is associated with loss of an osmotically equivalent amount of water to the extent that the K^+ is not replaced in the cell either by some extracellular cation (Na^+ and/or H^+) or by dissociation of previously undissociated cellular compounds. This transfer of K^+ may be influenced by aldosterone, which is increased as a result of the volume depletion. Under the influence of aldosterone, the excessive K^+ may be secreted by the renal tubular cells to facilitate reabsorption of Na^+ in the renal tubule.

The transfer of water from the cells, as a consequence of cell breakdown and K^+ loss from the cells, complements the transfer of water occurring in response to the osmotic pressure rise in the ECF. As was previously mentioned, the danger arises because the K^+ entering the ECF must be excreted, and when renal function falls, K^+ accumulation in the ECF may be lethal.

The net result of these processes for water transfer allows the ECF loss to be shared by the ICF. These reactions take place to varying degrees in all forms of dehydration; they are accentuated in the hypertonic form and are less pronounced in hypotonic dehydration. The consequences of this variation are that the ECF and the vascular volume are better maintained in hypertonic dehydration; they are less well supported in hypotonic dehydration, with a greater tendency to early cardiovascular collapse.

It is primarily the danger of hypovolemia and shock that makes dehydration a medical emergency. In order to assess the degree of dehydration and therefore the likelihood of cardiovascular failure, three levels of dehydration are generally distinguished: mild, moderate, and severe. The three descriptive terms are associated with three numerical values referring to acute weight loss: 5%, 10%, and 15%. These percentages refer to acute loss of body weight, which is assumed to represent primarily fluid lost from the total body water.

From a clinical viewpoint, a 5% weight loss is equivalent to a loss of 50 ml of body fluid per kilogram of body weight; a 10% weight loss represents a loss of 100 ml of body fluid per kilogram of body weight; a 15% weight loss reflects a loss of 150 ml of body fluid per kilogram of body weight.* A most important aspect of this classification is that it is essentially the same for infants and adults. This occurs because the percentages of water in the body are not markedly different over man's life span, and the factors leading to vascular collapse in body fluid depletion are primarily physical ones—essentially the functional vascular volume. When this vascular volume is depleted by some fraction, the response of the cardiovascular system will be consistent, regardless of the overall size of the individual. Thus the clinical criteria for recognizing these different degrees of dehydration will be comparable at all ages.†

Mild Dehydration.   Five percent dehydration (50 ml/kg) is usually considered to be the mildest level at which recognizable clinical findings of dehydration will appear. These findings include dryness of the mucous membranes, reduced turgor of skin and subcutaneous tissues, depressed anterior fontanelle (if it is patent), absence of tears, sunken eyeballs, reduced firmness of the globe of the eye, and thirst (unless anorexia is present). The urine volume is small, and the concentration is usually over 600 mOsm/liter (specific gravity > 1.020). With this degree of dehydration, renal function is usually reasonably adequate, and thus the body fluids will be isotonic: $[Na^+]_s = 140 \pm 10$ mEq/liter. Serum creatinine and BUN will be at the upper range of normal; $[K^+]_s$ and $[HPO_4^{--}]_s$ are also usually within the normal range. Metabolic acidosis, if present at all, will be mild and reasonably compensated: $[H^+]_s = 40$–60 nEq/liter (pH 7.40–7.22). Compensatory movement of water from the ICF to the ECF will have been adequate, so that shock will be neither present nor imminent. In any one person there is often some variability as to the presence or absence of specific findings, but marked deviation of any finding should lead to evaluation for some unsuspected complicating factor or process.

---

* Since these values are based on body weight, and since body water is 60%–70% of body weight, the 5%, 10%, and 15% figures represent 8%, 15%, and 23% losses when interpreted as loss of fluid per kilogram of body water (rather than per kilogram of body weight).

† Although use of actual weight would be a better method of assessing the extent of dehydration, predehydration weight is rarely available, and so clinical diagnosis is the procedure most commonly employed. If weights are available, obviously they should be used.

Moderate Dehydration. Ten percent dehydration (100 ml/kg), or moderate dehydration, is associated with an obviously ill-appearing child. In general, this degree of body fluid loss is potentially hazardous, and hospitalization is usually warranted. At this level of fluid depletion, compensatory mechanisms are at their limits, and early evidence of their failure is often present. The findings of dry mucous membranes, poor tissue turgor, depressed fontanelle, sunken eyes, reduced globe tension, absence of tearing and thirst are all present and are readily apparent.* Urine volume may be so reduced (oliguria) that temporary anuria may be suspected. Urine concentration is usually greater than 800 mOsm/liter (specific gravity > 1.025), except in sick infants. Renal function is sufficiently reduced that creatinine and urea are elevated, and K^+ and HPO_4^{--} concentrations may be at the upper range of normal or somewhat elevated. In addition, the ability to compensate for a primary loss of hypotonic fluid may be compromised, and $[Na^+]_s$ may be normal or increased. Metabolic acidosis is the most likely form of acid–base disturbance, and $[H^+]$ may be 50–120 nEq/liter (pH 7.30–6.92). At this point the compensatory shift of ICF to ECF is about at its limit, so that hypotension and shock are imminent.

Severe Dehydration. Fifteen percent dehydration (150 ml/kg) is about the limit that the human body can tolerate as an acute loss. A person with 15% dehydration appears extremely ill and is extremely ill. He is usually in shock, has a depressed sensorium, and is oliguric or anuric, as the physiologic compensating systems have been exceeded. The physical signs of dehydration are marked, blood pressure is low, the pulse is rapid and weak, and cardiac sounds are distant or faint. With the impairment of renal function, creatinine and urea nitrogen are elevated; K^+ and HPO_4^{--} are also usually high. The elevated serum K^+ may be sufficiently increased to produce electrocardiographic changes, best seen in limb lead II (high and pointed T waves, then absent P waves, and finally widening of the QRS complex, so that the ECG begins to look like a sine wave; Fig. 4-3). Metabolic acidosis is usually severe, with $[H^+] = 80–160$ nEq/liter (pH 7.1–6.8). There is appreciable mortality associated with dehydration of this severity, and very few persons survive dehydration in excess of this amount.

INCREASED OUTPUT

Increased output as a cause of dehydration can result from an increase in any one of the three routes of output or any combination of these three.

---

* See sections on hypertonic and hypotonic dehydration for exceptions.

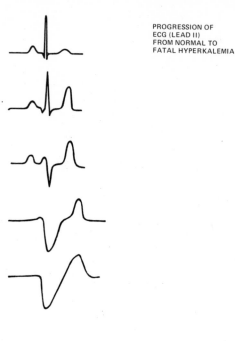

PROGRESSION OF
ECG (LEAD II)
FROM NORMAL TO
FATAL HYPERKALEMIA

Fig. 4-3.   Progression of electrocardiogram (EKG) changes from health to death as a result of hyperkalemia. The changes are schematically illustrated for limb lead II. First there is an increase in the amplitude of the T wave and widening of the QRS complex. Next there is a reduction in the R wave and an increase in the S wave. This is followed by absence of the P wave and then by a sine wave appearance. Finally, there is no electrical activity when the serum potassium has been elevated to a value of 10–12 mEq/liter. The exact serum values of $[K^+]_s$ associated with each of these changes cannot be defined because of the modifying effects produced by the concentrations of other extracellular ions and intracellular potassium.

Insensible Water Loss and Sweating.   Although the IWL can more than double under appropriate circumstances, such losses are usually adequately compensated by increased intake and/or a decrease in urine volume, with an increase in urinary solute concentration. To the extent that dehydration might occur as a result of increased IWL, the results would be similar to those seen with the dehydration described under decreased intake.

Although sweating is technically not a form of IWL, it is considered under this heading because it is a loss from the skin, and like IWL it has the function of dissipation of heat (Table 4-1). Sweat losses, in contrast to IWL, do contain low but significant concentrations of Na^+, K^+, and Cl^-.

Table 4-1
Sweat Losses*

	Infant (ml/kg/day)	Adult (ml/kg/day)	Surface Area Basis (ml/m²/day)
Mild sweating	0–20	0–10	0–400
Moderate sweating	20–100	10–50	400–2000
Severe sweating†	100+	50+	2000+

* These are approximate values for sweat losses in infants and adults. Because the ranges are great, accurate values are possible only by careful determination.

† Rates of sweating in excess of 1000 ml/hour have been measured in adults over short periods of time (< 6 hours).

With slight to moderate sweating the loss of ions is not a major problem, but when sweating is moderate to severe for an appreciable period of time, loss of Na^+ and particularly K^+ can be important. Thus the factors that determine the degree to which sweating must be considered are the concentration of ions in the sweat, the rate of sweat loss, and the duration. In addition, the rate of sweat loss, besides determining the volume of sweat produced per minute, also modifies the concentration of ions in sweat. The greater the rate of sweating, the higher the ionic concentration will be. In cystic fibrosis the ionic concentrations are at least twice normal values, and persons with asthma may have values intermediate between those of persons with cystic fibrosis and those of healthy persons. Because of the higher ionic concentrations in sweat from people with cystic fibrosis and people with asthma when sweating is profuse, salt losses in these persons can be serious.

The physiologic response to sweating has been studied under conditions of severe sweating, as in the desert or in athletic contests occurring in hot weather. The sequence of events is shown in Figure 4-4.* The sweat that is lost is relatively hypotonic, and so the remaining ECF begins to become hypertonic, but at smaller volume. The usual response to this includes loss of additional salt and water in the urine, but with relatively more salt than water being lost by the renal route. The high concentration of Na^+ in the urine restores isotonicity to the ECF, but at the expense of still further volume depletion. Often at this stage in the process some sort of treatment may be given, but either water alone or salt alone would be inappropriate. Water alone would tend to restore volume but would create

* The scales for the heights of the columns for water and Na^+ are adjusted so that when the columns show equal heights for water and Na^+, the relationship is at the ratio of 150 mEq of Na^+ to 1 liter of water; this represents an isotonic fluid. When the water column is taller than the Na^+ column, the fluid is hypotonic. When the water column is shorter than the Na^+ column, the fluid is hypertonic.

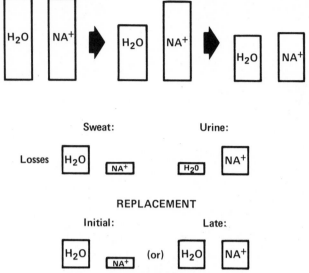

Fig. 4-4.   Adjustment to sweating. In the process of sweating, water is lost in excess of sodium. If no correction is made, the renal response is to excrete urine containing more sodium than water, so that ultimately the individual is depleted of both water and sodium. If replacement of sweat losses is undertaken early enough (essentially, as they occur), one can use a dilute salt solution such as those now available commercially. If replacement is to take place late, after renal compensation has occurred, then the fluid replacement must be both water and salt in essentially isotonic proportions.

acute hypotonicity. Salt alone would restore the body content of Na^+ but would not restore volume and would create hypertonicity. Obviously, if renal compensation is relatively efficient, the body fluids should be isotonic but of low volume; the ideal fluid treatment would be to provide fluids as some type of isotonic salt solution. As has been demonstrated in recent years in athletic contests, the best approach is preventive. This can be accomplished by providing a hypotonic fluid (with composition comparable to that of sweat) early in the process while the skin losses are occurring, so that renal compensation will never need to occur; thus body fluid volume and concentration will remain stable.

Renal Water.   In the presence of good renal function and a reasonable solute load, the volume of urine is determined by the amount of water available for urine formation—essentially the ECF excess. As available water becomes progressively more limited, or if there is no water available, the volume of urine decreases until the concentrating capacity of the kidney is approached. At that point further reduction in urine volume is dependent on reduction in solute load. If the solute load is excessive for

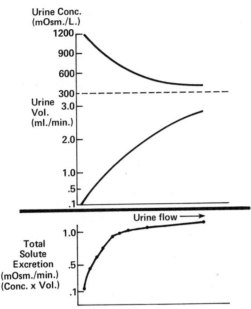

Fig. 4-5. Changes in urine in solute diuresis. The results of solute diuresis are a decrease in urine concentration, an increase in the volume of urine produced per minute, and an increasing total solute excretion. Although it is not shown in this diagram, if the urine is more dilute than plasma when a solute diuresis begins, urine concentration will rise, approaching 300 mOsm/liter asymptotically as urine flow increases and solute excretion increases.

available water or if the available water is inadequate for a usual solute load, reduction in ECF volume (dehydration) occurs.

Solute load.   One of the most common situations in which excess solute load occurs is in the presence of diabetes mellitus. When blood sugar exceeds about 180 mg/dl, the capacity of the tubule to reabsorb the filtered glucose is exceeded. At that point glucose will appear in the final urine in increasing amounts as the blood sugar rises further. Initially the increase in solute will require excretion of additional water and/or elaboration of urine with greater concentration of solute. However, as the amount of glucose being filtered continues to increase, the volume of water leaving the proximal tubule will increase, as the fluid in this portion of the nephron is always isotonic. The increased volume of fluid that will then reach the loop of Henle and beyond will dilate the tubule slightly and will also flow through the tubule more rapidly. The consequence of both of these actions is impairment of the reabsorptive process for both water and sodium. Impairment of reabsorption of water and Na^+ produces urine of greater volume, with concentration more like that of a plasma ultrafiltrate. Even though volume rises and concentration falls, the product volume $\times$

concentration increases, so that the response (as typified by glucosuria) is called a solute diuresis. The increased renal output of solute and water leads to loss of more Na^+ than would ordinarily be present in the urine in healthy states. This is shown diagrammatically in Figure 4-5.* The losses of water and Na^+ tend to produce an isotonic type of dehydration. The important characteristic of dehydration produced by solute diuresis is that urine volume remains large even when the other symptoms of dehydration may be very marked. It is quite late in this type of dehydration process that the ECF volume becomes so low that the GFR falls sufficiently for urine volume to become small. Another result of the persistence of high urine output is that creatinine and urea nitrogen levels in the blood do not increase as early in the dehydration process as they do in the absence of solute diuresis. An example of solute diuresis due to hyperglycemia follows.

EXAMPLE. A 15-year-old boy was admitted with a blood sugar of 900 mg/dl. He had had marked polyuria and polydipsia. Blood sugar = 900 mg/dl = 9 mg/ml. GFR = 110 ml/min. Glucose filtration = 110 ml/min × 9 mg/ml = 990 mg/min. The maximum rate of glucose reabsorption ($T_{m\ glucose}$) = 375 mg/min. If he filters 990 mg/min and can reabsorb only 375 mg/min, he will have to excrete 990 − 375 = 615 mg/min. If he excretes glucose at 615 mg/min, this can be converted to milliosmoles/minute by dividing 615 mg/min by the molecular weight of glucose (180); thus 615 mg/min ÷ 180 = 3.4 mOsm/min.

Maximum urinary concentration is 1400 mOsm/liter, or 1.4 mOsm/ml. If the kidney could excrete glucose at that concentration, urine flow would have to be 2.4 ml/min (i.e., 3.4/1.4). This rate of urine flow exceeds that at which maximum concentration can occur, and the other urinary solutes (Na^+, K^+, HPO_4^{--}, Cl^-, urea, etc.) have not even been considered. (These other solutes would increase the flow still more.) Under such circumstances the urine concentration approaches 300 mOsm/liter (that of glomerular filtrate). At 300 mOsm/liter, or 0.3 mOsm/ml, urine flow would exceed 11 ml/min (i.e., 3.4/0.3), which is a marked solute diuresis.

Inability to concentrate urine: renal insufficiency. Inability to concentrate urine above the osmolarity of plasma (but with an ordinary solute load, such as may occur in chronic renal disease) will approximately double the output figures given in Table 2-6. That is, urine volume will be approximately 100 ml/kg/day in the infant and 50 ml/kg/day in the adult. Although these are large volumes, they can usually be met by a comparable increase in intake. However, if for any reason intake becomes limited or other output also increases, as with fever or sweating or

---

* In Figure 4-5, the term *solute* refers to the total of all solute present in the urine. In most circumstances, excretion of the specific solute Na^+ is similar to that of total solute.

diarrhea, then fluid balance can be in jeopardy, and dehydration can easily ensue. Na^+ excretion is usually not impaired; so if dehydration occurs, it is usually isotonic. (Occasionally, chronic renal disease is associated with difficulty in reabsorption of Na^+; in such cases, dehydration can be hypotonic in character.)

Inability to concentrate urine: diabetes insipidus. Although diabetes insipidus generally leads to hypertonic dehydration, it is discussed in this section because it is one of the basic causes of increased urine output. A more extreme form of increased urine output occurs in diabetes insipidus, due either to deficient ADH secretion or to the nephrogenic form in which the renal tubules are unresponsive to ADH. In either case, urine concentration in untreated cases rarely exceeds 100 mOsm/liter and is often in the range 50–75 mOsm/liter (specific gravity < 1.003).* With an ordinary solute output of 40 mOsm/100 kcal metabolized, the solute load for an infant is about 40 mOsm/kg, and that for an adult is about 20 mOsm/kg. If urinary concentration cannot exceed 80 mOsm/liter, the infant must excrete 500 ml/kg to get rid of his solute load, and the adult must excrete 250 ml/kg to accomplish this same end. It is difficult to achieve an oral intake of fluid to match this volume of output; thus dehydration is almost inevitable. This type of dehydration tends to be hypertonic in nature, with $[Na^+]_s$ levels of 155–195 mEq/liter. Hypertonic dehydration occurs because the urine contains much more water than solute, and the effect of ADH on Na^+ reabsorption in the nephrogenic form of diabetes insipidus may not be impaired.† The treatment of such a situation involves increasing the intake of fluid as much as possible, reducing the solute load to the minimum compatible with health, and providing whatever medication is appropriate to increase renal concentrating power (Pitressin in ADH deficiency disease and thiazides in nephrogenic diabetes insipidus). With this combined approach it is possible to reduce an infant's solute load to 20 mOsm/kg and increase his concentrating ability to 120 mOsm/liter (specific gravity ~ 1.004). His urine volume would then be (20/120) × 1000 = 167 ml/kg/day; this is still a very large number, but it is one-third of the previous figure, and one that it is possible to match with intake.‡

---

* An exception can occur when dehydration is severe and GFR has fallen markedly. Then reabsorption of water can increase, and osmolarities of 300–500 mOsm/liter (specific gravity 1.010–1.018) have been repoted under these circumstances.

† There is no experimental evidence for this, but some of the highest $[Na^+]$ are noted in nephrogenic diabetes insipidus. ADH levels are usually elevated, and even though the distal tubule and collecting duct do not respond by becoming permeable to water, there is no specific reason to believe that the ADH stimulus to Na^+ reabsorption should be altered.

‡ Intake would have to be about 210 ml/kg: 40 ml/kg/day for IWL, 167 ml/kg/day for urine volume, and 5 ml/kg/day for stool loss.

Gastrointestinal Water. The solute content of most gastrointestinal fluid is comparable in composition to ECF. Gastric fluid is high in [H^+], [K^+], and [Cl^-], and pancreatic secretions are high in [HCO_3^-], but the remainder of the fluid passing through the ileocecal valve is similar to ECF. However, once this fluid reaches the large bowel, Na^+ begins to be exchanged for K^+ and Cl^- for HCO_3^-. In addition, as has been mentioned, over 90% of the total volume of fluid is reabsorbed, with a somewhat greater amount of solute being reabsorbed than water. The result of these actions is a stool containing hypotonic fluid of small volume.

Diarrhea. Diarrhea is the most frequent basis for an increase in gastrointestinal output. Losses of body fluid as stool water are normally very small, but with impairment of the reabsorptive process in the large bowel, the volume of stool water can reach 20 liters/day, as in adults with cholera. Infantile diarrhea and the forms of diarrhea in adults that are seen in the United States do not cause fluid losses of this magnitude; nevertheless, the losses they cause are quite sufficient to produce severe dehydration when intake cannot keep pace. The fluid and electrolyte transport processes of the large bowel deteriorate during diarrhea, with the result that reabsorption diminishes, and thus the volume of stool increases, the concentration of solute increases, and the expected electrolyte composition is altered. Nevertheless, except in persons with cholera, the stool water remains hypotonic.

The volume of water lost with the common forms of diarrhea is generally in the range of 30–40 ml/kg/day in the infant and 15–20 ml/kg/day in the adult. This degree of loss should be relatively easy to compensate by an increase in intake and/or a decrease in urine volume, with an increase in urinary concentration. However, several factors may militate against this compensation:

1. Anorexia is frequently part of the disease process, and it can easily lead to reduction of intake below the usual maintenance levels.

2. Vomiting is also common, and in addition to restricting intake, it becomes a source of increased output.

3. The concentrating function of the infant kidney is definitely decreased in response to dehydration when the infant is ill, in contrast to when he is well.

4. Frequently, when intake is increased, stool output increases still further.

Therefore diarrhea results in dehydration not only because it increases output but also because the process is almost always accompanied by decreased input.

Figure 4-6 illustrates the sequence of events in diarrhea and how the outcome depends on the type of oral intake provided during the process. The figure presents the situation in infancy, because in infants the intake

SEQUENCE IN DIARRHEA OF INFANCY—A
NO INTAKE

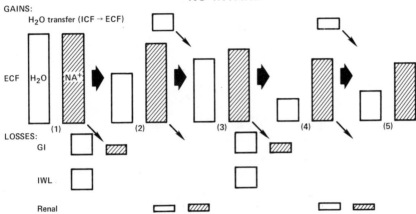

Fig. 4-6A.   Diarrhea in infancy without intake of fluids. This and Figures 4-6B through 4-6E are constructed to illustrate the hypothetical progression in diarrhea of the changes in ECF volume and sodium concentration and the changes that occur in fluid losses in the presence of different intakes of fluid and salt. In the situation shown here, there is no fluid intake; the gastrointestinal and IWL (illustrated by the clear areas) are greater than the sodium loss (illustrated by the shaded areas). In stage 2 of the process, the ECF has become hypertonic and hypovolemic. The result of this is transfer of water from the ICF to the ECF and marked reduction in urine volume associated with an increase in urine sodium concentration. As a result of these mechanisms, the ECF volume is increased slightly and the sodium concentration is decreased by stage 3. If diarrhea persists, the process will result in more marked loss of extracellular volume and increasing hypernatremia. At this point, the volume of water that can be transferred from the intracellular fluid is reduced; the kidney is no longer able to concentrate the urine because of reduced function. The end result (stage 5) is hypovolemic, hypernatremic dehydration.

tends to be limited by anorexia or vomiting and the renal compensation is poor,* with the result that the process is more exaggerated than in adults. Approximately the same sequence of events can occur in older children and adults if the diarrhea is severe enough and prolonged enough and if intake is limited.

In section A of Figure 4-6, the reactions that occur in the absence of any fluid intake are illustrated. The volume and Na^+ content of the ECF are shown at five stages (1–5); the scales are such that when the heights of

* Even though urine concentration may be 400–800 mOsm/liter, which in itself is less than in older children or adults under similar circumstances, urinary [Na^+] rarely exceeds plasma levels, even in hypertonic dehydration in infants; thus the hypotonic gastrointestinal losses and IWL are not well compensated by renal function.

SEQUENCE IN DIARRHEA OF INFANCY—B
SMALL WATER INTAKE

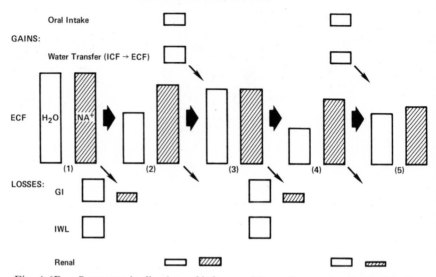

Fig. 4-6B.   Sequence in diarrhea of infancy with small water intake. In this illustration the same changes will take place as were shown in Figure 4-6A. However,
the presence of a small intake of water will act to ameliorate the process, so that by
stage 5 the degree of hypovolemia will be less and the degree of hypernatremia will
also be less.

the two columns (for H_2O and Na^+) are equal, the fluid is isotonic, as it is
in stage 1 prior to onset of diarrhea. The events occurring between stages
1 and 2 and between stages 2 and 3 happen simultaneously, so that stage 2
does not actually ever exist, but this intermediate stage is shown to
simplify discussion.* The loss with diarrheal stool is hypotonic, but it
does contain Na^+. IWL is water only. The result will be markedly hypertonic dehydration, as illustrated in the hypothetical stage 2, except that
the kidney does excrete some Na^+ along with water, and there is a sizable
transfer of water from the ICF to the ECF. The result of this process,
stage 3, is a slightly hypertonic dehydration that might not have been
hypertonic at all if the kidney had excreted urine with a somewhat higher
$[Na^+]$. However, as the diarrhea continues, stage 3 to stage 4, the compensatory capabilities represented by the kidney become limited by a
falling GFR, and the transfer of water from ICF to ECF is diminished by
rising ICF osmolarity. These reduced compensations, as shown between

* The same thing is true between stages 3 and 4 and between stages 4 and 5. Thus stage
4 also never actually exists.

SEQUENCE IN DIARRHEA OF INFANCY—C
SMALL HYPOTONIC INTAKE

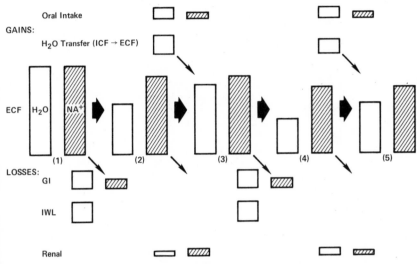

Fig. 4-6C.   Sequence in diarrhea of infancy with small hypotonic fluid intake. In a situation where the volume of fluid taken orally is less than the insensible loss, the sodium content of the oral fluids tends to be retained, and the degree of hypernatremia is greater than it is in Figure 4-6B; the degree of hypovolemia is essentially unchanged.

stages 4 and 5, result in an ECF that is markedly reduced in volume and clearly hypertonic in concentration, as shown in stage 5.

Sequence B illustrates how this process is modified by a small intake of water (about 50 ml/kg in this example). Isotonicity of the ECF is maintained more easily in the early stage 3, and the degree of hypertonicity is much less by stage 5, when there is some intake of water.

Sequence C illustrates the impropriety of providing solutions containing any Na^+ when the oral intake is small. Although the results (stage 5) are better than with no intake at all, and the volume of the ECF is the same as with a comparable intake of water, the degree of hypertonicity is greater than when water of equal volume is given (as in sequence B). This would suggest, as has been demonstrated empirically, that when intake of fluid is less than IWL, such fluid should be given as water or as water with carbohydrate and should not contain Na^+. If sweating (sensible water loss) is profuse, some Na^+ will have to be given with the water.

Sequence D illustrates the situation when the infant accepts larger volumes of fluid (the example is 150 ml/kg) but still not enough to maintain ECF volume. In this sequence, with no Na^+ intake and a continuing Na^+ loss, primarily in stool, the ECF volume diminishes, but not as much as

SEQUENCE IN DIARRHEA OF INFANCY—D
LARGE WATER INTAKE

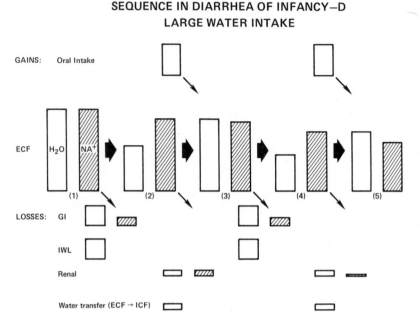

Fig. 4-6D. Sequence in diarrhea of infancy with large water intake. In a situation where there is large water intake without solute, dehydration may continue to occur, but the continuing loss of sodium results in hyponatremia and transfer of water from the ECF to the ICF. The end result is intracellular overhydration, extracellular dehydration, and hyponatremia.

the ECF Na^+. The result, which may include a net transfer of some water into cells, is a hypotonic dehydration that is not as severe a volume depletion as in the previous sequences but that may create other problems in management.

Sequence E represents the response to a more appropriate approach to therapy. The volume of intake used in this example is still not adequate to compensate for the losses; thus some dehydration still occurs.* By providing water or glucose-water up to an amount equivalent to the IWL and then providing a hypotonic salt solution or its equivalent to the extent the infant will accept it, isotonicity of body fluids will be maintained, even though some decrease in volume may occur.

Vomiting.   Vomiting may occur as a single source of excess gastrointestinal output, or it may be only part of the losses sustained in gastroenteritis. Vomiting of gastric secretions usually produces metabolic alkalosis with dehydration; however, vomiting of small-bowel fluid pro-

---

* If the volume were somewhat greater, body fluids could be maintained quite adequately in terms of volume and concentration.

SEQUENCE IN DIARRHEA OF INFANCY—E
"BALANCED" INTAKE

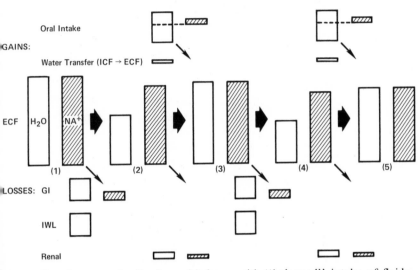

Fig. 4-6E. Sequence in diarrhea of infancy with "balanced" intake of fluids. This sequence illustrates what occurs when the oral intake provides water in an amount equivalent to the insensible loss and a hypotonic salt solution in addition to this water. This is the ideal method of providing oral fluids for an infant with diarrhea. As can be seen, there is a minimal degree of dehydration. The result is isotonic body fluids and a minimum degree of intracellular dehydration in association with the extracellular dehydration. Renal function is preserved, and the severity of the fluid problem is greatly reduced.

duces a response similar to that seen with loss of small-bowel fluid from an ileostomy, etc.

Pyloric stenosis is the classic problem associated with "pure gastric vomiting" that is seen during childhood. The pattern of response is similar when vomiting of gastric fluids occurs at other ages and for other reasons.

Gastric secretions are composed predominantly of Na^+, H^+, and Cl^-, with a moderate amount of K^+ as well. The total osmolarity is similar to that of ECF. An interesting series of events arises as a consequence of these losses. Initially the loss of Na^+, H^+, and Cl^- produces a mild metabolic alkalosis and dehydration. The kidney responds by secreting a small volume of concentrated urine that contains HCO_3^- and is alkaline. The loss of buffer base (HCO_3^-) occurs as an attempt to balance the loss of H^+ from the gastric mucosa. The cation accompanying the HCO_3^- in the urine may be Na^+ at first, but the combination of gastrointestinal and renal Na^+ loss quickly sets in motion the Na^+ reabsorptive process, which begins by exchanging K^+ for Na^+ in the renal tubule. For a period of time the urine contains large amounts of K^+ and HCO_3^-. This excretion of K^+

facilitates the transfer of K^+ and H_2O from the ICF to the ECF, thus helping to maintain ECF volume. The K^+ excretion continues for a period of time until sufficient K^+ has been lost to create a significant K^+ deficiency state. As the K^+ shortage begins to have its effects, the body's loss of Na^+ is so great that the kidney must continue to reabsorb as much Na^+ as it can; and if there is insufficient K^+ to exchange for all the reabsorbable Na^+, then H^+ must be used to exchange for Na^+. Thus as the dehydration becomes moderate (10% loss of body weight) the urine becomes acid, and the ECF then becomes still more alkaline. Finally, as K^+ deficiency increases (for even after the urine has become acid with the H^+–Na^+ exchange, the K^+–Na^+ exchange still continues), the renal concentrating mechanism begins to fail, leading to urine that is less concentrated; dehydration accelerates, GFR falls, and azotemia appears. The relatively large loss of Na^+Cl^-, along with the water loss, leads to a dehydration that is usually isotonic in nature. From a therapeutic point of view, it is clear that the need is to reexpand the ECF and provide additional K^+.

Other gastrointestinal losses.   Loss of small-bowel fluid by suction or ileostomy results in loss of fluid very similar in composition to the ECF. Such losses tend to produce a dehydration that is isotonic, usually with a tendency toward metabolic acidosis.

MIXED INTAKE AND OUTPUT DISORDERS

As has already been discussed in the section on diarrhea, many cases of dehydration result from both decreased intake and increased output. It is also apparent from that discussion that the character of the intake (whether it is limited or not) is of great significance in determining not only the degree of dehydration but also the type: isotonic, hypertonic, or hypotonic. Ideally, when losses are hypotonic, which they usually are, intake should be hypotonic; when fluid intake is markedly limited, it should be water or a renal solute-free solution such as glucose-water. Table 4-2 lists fluids frequently used in the care of ambulatory dehydrated patients; it also provides the Na^+, K^+, and Cl^- concentrations, as well as the caloric values and solute loads of these fluids.

Hypertonic Dehydration

ETIOLOGY

The mechanisms by which hypertonic dehydration usually occur have been described in the section on isotonic dehydration. In summary the fluid losses that usually occur and that lead to dehydration are hypotonic, and if the kidney is unable to elaborate urine that is appropriately hypertonic and/or if hypotonic intake is not sufficient, the body fluids will become hypertonic.

Table 4-2
Composition of Oral Fluids*

Fluid	Na⁺	K⁺	Cl⁻	Solute (mOsm/ liter)	Calories (kcal/ liter)
		(mEq/liter)			
Water	0	0	0	0	0
"Sugar water" (5%)†	0	0	0	0	200
Lytren	25	25	30	135	280
Pedialyte	30	20	30	115	280
Coca-Cola	0.5	13	0	27	435
Pepsi Cola	7	1	0	15	480
Ginger ale	3	1	1	10	380
Seven-Up	7.5	0.5	0	15	420
Orange juice	2	48	2	100	410
Gatorade	.23	2.5		50	167
Boiled skimmed milk‡	27	43	31	350	410
One-half boiled skimmed milk§	13	21	15	175	205

* This table presents the electrolyte, solute, and caloric content of commonly used fluids given to infants who are unable to take their usual food intake.

† Prepared at home by using 3 tablespoons/quart of water.

‡ Assuming no evaporation. In practice, boiling creates an evaporative loss, producing higher values than those shown.

§ This term refers to equal amounts of water and skimmed milk.

An additional problem that has increased the incidence and severity of hypertonic dehydration is inadvertent use of high-solute feedings in the treatment of diarrhea. These consist of improperly diluted commercial and prescription salt and carbohydrate solutions for home treatment of gastroenteritis. These solutions are meant to have [Na⁺] of 15–35 mEq/liter and [K⁺] of 10–25 mEq/liter. However, they are often prepared at three to five times that strength when tablespoons (15 ml) are used instead of teaspoons (5 ml) for measuring and when the patient subscribes to the theory that if a little is good, a lot is better.

When a small volume of intake (less than that required to offset the IWL) is all that is consumed by a patient with diarrhea, *any* level of Na⁺ or solute load content at all will be more likely to result in a hypertonic state than if water alone is consumed. Commercial "salt" solutions and skimmed milk are particularly notorious in this regard in patients under 2 years of age.*

* Very few instances of hypertonic dehydration have occurred in children older than 2 years under these circumstances; presumably they take large enough volumes (their IWL is somewhat smaller) and/or their kidneys function more efficiently in terms of Na⁺ removal and water conservation.

In the absence of gastroenteritis, high salt intake, or restricted water intake, hypertonic dehydration may occur in patients with untreated diabetes insipidus (especially the nephrogenic type) or occasionally with a case of head trauma, CNS mass lesion, or CNS inflammatory process. In cases of CNS lesions that do not produce diabetes insipidus, it has been postulated that the damage may be in the thirst mechanism or in the osmoreceptor areas. In such a patient the body would still be able to concentrate or dilute the urine, and ADH could be released, but either the patient would show no inclination to drink fluids when hypertonic or the solute concentration at which the regulatory center responds would be elevated.

One additional form of hypertonicity that should be mentioned is hypertonicity due to excessively high concentrations of glucose or other nonionic solutes. Hyperosmotic, nonketotic diabetic coma belongs in this category. In such an instance the $[Na^+]$ may be normal or low, but the total osmotic pressure (solute concentration) of the plasma is markedly elevated. (A blood sugar of 1200 mg/dl is equivalent to a solute concentration of 67 mOsm/liter. The impact would be similar to a $[Na^+]$ of 172 mEq/liter.)

PHYSIOLOGY

Whatever the etiologic basis, the responses of the body fluids to hypertonic ECF are similar. As illustrated in Figure 4-2 in the diagram representing response to loss of water from the ECF, there is transfer of water from the ICF to the ECF until the osmolarities are again equal—but both are elevated.

An example of changes leading to hypertonicity in diarrhea is given in Figure 4-7. The important aspects of this example are that with a water loss of 1000 ml, there was only a 30-mEq loss of univalent cation (Na^+ 15 mEq, K^+ 15 mEq) and there was a net gain (intake > output) of Cl^-. This example is consistent with many cases studied under similar circumstances. The gain in Cl^- is associated with both a relative preservation of the ECF volume and a metabolic acidosis (note that the increase in $[Cl^-]$ exceeds the increase in $[Na^+]$).

SYMPTOMATOLOGY

The relative preservation of the ECF volume occurs at the expense of a relatively greater loss of ICF volume than in isotonic dehydration. There are three highly significant consequences of this difference from isotonic dehydration in the apportionment of the fluid loss between ECF and ICF:

1. For a total body fluid loss of 100 ml/kg, less will have come from the ECF; so the clinical signs and symptoms with moderate dehydration will be less pronounced. This will be equally true of any other level of dehydration. In other words, the signs and symptoms of dehydration that

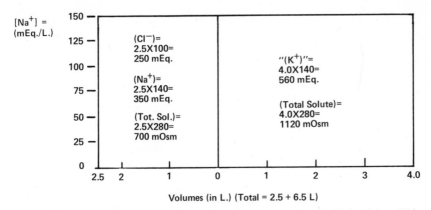

Fig. 4-7A. Body fluid changes in hypertonic dehydration: initial values. This figure illustrates the fluid volume and ionic status of a 10-month-old boy weighing 10 kg. Assuming normal distribution of body water, the initial $[Na^+]$ = 140 mEq/liter; $[Cl^-]$ = 100 mEq/liter. There is a normal ECF of 2.5 liters, an ICF of 4.0 liters, and an osmolarity in body water equivalent to twice the sodium concentration, or 2×140 = 280 mOsm/liter. The quantity of these electrolytes is illustrated in the figure.

reflect ECF volume (and most of them do) will be milder than they should be for the degree of total body water loss; expressed another way, the actual extent of dehydration will be greater than that suggested by the loss of skin turgor, dryness of mucous membranes, etc. Doughiness of subcutaneous tissue has frequently been reported as a sign of hypertonic dehydration, but it is highly variable in frequency and onset; thus little reliance can be placed on an absence of the finding.

2. Shock due to reduction in cardiovascular volume will be less likely to occur, because there is relatively better maintenance of ECF volume.

3. The increased loss of cellular fluid will have its major impact in the skull. Here, as brain volume shrinks due to loss of cellular fluid, the skull remains fixed; so there is great tension on the bridging vessels between the skull and the brain cortex. Thus signs of brain hemorrhage (specifically subarachnoid), CNS depression, and other CNS disorders are more marked in the hypertonic form of dehydration than in any other type. Unusual somnolence, stupor or coma, and convulsive seizures have all been noted in association with this state, and abnormal electroencephalograms and elevated spinal fluid protein have also been reported.

DIAGNOSIS

Diagnosis of hypertonic dehydration requires two items: evidence for dehydration (which is usually based on physical findings) and elevation of serum osmolarity (either due to a serum $[Na^+]$ greater than 150 mEq/liter or due to an increase in a nonionic solute such as glucose). An elevation of

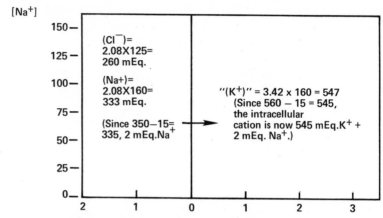

Fig. 4-7B. Body fluid changes in hypertonic dehydration: after diarrhea. After 3 days of diarrhea during which careful measurements and analyses of intake and output were made, the child's weight was 9 kg; $[Cl^-]$ = 125 mEq/liter, $[Na^+]$ = 160 mEq/liter. From the balance studies it was ascertained that there was a net gain to the body of 10 mEq of $[Cl^-]$ and a net loss from the body of 15 mEq of $[Na^+]$ and 15 mEq of $[K^+]$. Assuming that all of the chloride is extracellular, the new ECF volume = new total Cl^-/new $[Cl^-]$ = (250 + 10)/125 = 260/125 = 2.08 liter. The new ICF volume equals new total body water minus new ECF volume = (6.5 liters − 1 liter) − 2.08 liters = 5.5 − 2.08 = 3.42 liters. Having calculated the new volumes, one can then determine what has happened to sodium. In this example, the sodium contained in the new ECF = 2.08 × 160 = 333 mEq, but since there was a total Na^+ of 350 mEq initially and 15 mEq were lost, the total body sodium is now 335 mEq; therefore 2 mEq were transferred to the ICF. These 2 mEq of sodium added to the 545 mEq of potassium would provide 547 mEq of cation in the ICF, and this would then satisfy the volume times concentration calculation for the ECF. It is from studies such as this that information has been obtained on the transfer of cation between ECF and ICF in various states of abnormal hydration.

blood glucose by itself is insufficient evidence for establishing hypertonicity, as the serum $[Na^+]$ may be decreased to compensate for the glucosemia.

EXAMPLE 1. Blood sugar (BS) = 1200 mg/dl = 12,000 mg/liter; $[Na^+]$ = 110 mEq/liter; molecular weight of BS = 180; osmolarity = 12,000/180 = 67 mOsm/liter. Serum osmolarity = (2 × $[Na^+]$) + increment due to nonionic solute* = 220 + 67 = 287 mOsm/liter, which is in the normal range.†

EXAMPLE 2. BS = 900 mg/dl = 9000 mg/liter; osmolarity = 9000/180

---

* Normal glucose concentration of 90–120 mg/dl = 900–1200 mg/liter = (900/180)–(1200/180) = 5–6.7 mOsm/liter.

† Normal serum osmolarity = 260–300 mOsm/liter.

= 50 mOsm/liter; $[Na^+]$ = 135 mEq/liter. Serum osmolarity = (2×135) + 50 = 270 + 50 = 320 mOsm/liter, which represents an increase above the normal range and would be considered indicative of hypertonicity.

TREATMENT

Fundamentally, treatment involves replacing more fluid than solute in repair of the dehydration loss. Generally, the water loss is very large and the solute loss is minimal. However, there are reasons, as yet incompletely explained, for avoiding an essentially water-only replacement. Presumably the events leading to the hypertonic state required several days to evolve, and in that period some adjustment to the reduced cell volume took place, especially in the CNS.‡ If very hypotonic solutions are infused therapeutically, the ECF will rapidly become more dilute than the cells (even though both could actually still be hypertonic). Then a fairly rapid movement of water into cells will occur, and the internal functioning of the cells could be deranged. For example, when very hypotonic solutions have been used to treat the hypertonic dehydration occurring in infantile diarrhea, convulsive seizures have frequently been noted. Therefore there are two basic approaches: the rather slow infusion of markedly hypotonic solutions or the more rapid infusion of only moderately hypotonic solutions. Although the former process seems to be rational in terms of correction of the abnormal concentration, it is the latter process that is most commonly employed, because the volume replacement has priority. Using either the moderately hypotonic fluid ($[Na^+]$ + $[K^+]$ = 50–75 mEq/liter) rapidly or the very hypotonic fluid ($[Na^+]$ + $[K^+]$ = 10–40 mEq/liter) slowly, there will be a reduction in the osmolarity of the body fluids. Since there has been no comparative trial using the two approaches, it is not possible to know which is more advantageous.

Hypotonic Dehydration

ETIOLOGY

In this section three hypotonic states will be discussed, although only one of them (acute symptomatic hypotonicity) has the characteristics of being symptomatic as well as requiring specific therapy. The other two are hyponatremia without hypotonicity and asymptomatic hypotonicity. All three of these states can occur in the presence of dehydration, but they can also be seen with adequate hydration as well as with overhydration.

‡ For example, there may have been a compensatory increase in the volume of cerebrospinal fluid to fill the void created by the shrinking cells.

Hyponatremia Without Hypotonicity. Hyponatremia can be defined by a serum $[Na^+] < 130$ mEq/liter, and it can occur in association with high levels of nonionic solutes such as urea or glucose. If serum osmolarity is to be estimated by doubling the $[Na^+]$, there must be laboratory confirmation that urea and glucose are not elevated; this will validate the reasonableness of the osmolarity estimation. If urea and/or glucose are elevated, their concentrations (in mOsm/liter) must be added to twice the $[Na^+]$ to obtain an adequate prediction of serum osmolarity.

EXAMPLE 1. $[Na^+] = 115$ mEq/liter; $[BUN] = 140$ mg/dl $= 1400$ mg/liter; molecular weight of $N_2 = 28;^*$ $1400/28 = 50$ mOsm/liter. Hyponatremia with normal osmolarity $= (2 \times 115) + 50 = 280$. Therefore this is not hypotonicity.

EXAMPLE 2. $[Na^+] = 115$ mEq/liter; $[BUN] = 70$ mg/dl $= 700$ mg/liter; $700/28 = 25$ mOsm/liter; $(2 \times [Na^+]) + [urea] = (2 \times 115) + 25 = 255$ mOsm/liter. This is hyponatremia with hypotonicity of body fluids.

EXAMPLE 3. $[Na^+] = 125$ mEq/liter; $[BUN] = 160$ mg/dl $= 1600$ mg/liter; $1600/28 = 57$ mOsm/liter. Serum osmolarity $= (2 \times 125) + 57 = 250 + 57 = 307$ mOsm/liter. This is hyponatremia with hypertonicity of body fluids (osmolarity > 300 mOsm/liter).

It is important to recognize that hyponatremia can occur with hypotonicity, isotonicity, or hypertonicity of body fluids; but hypotonicity is always accompanied by hyponatremia.

Asymptomatic Hypotonicity. Hypotonicity and hyponatremia have been observed in children and adults with a variety of chronic illnesses and with malnutrition, but without the signs and symptoms usually associated with hypotonicity. In addition to the fact that these patients appeared to tolerate their dilute body fluid status quite well, the hypotonicity appeared to be chronic rather than acute. Finally, following recovery from their chronic illnesses or malnutrition, the tonicity of their body fluids spontaneously returned to normal.

It would appear that for reasons still somewhat obscure, these individuals reestablished their osmotic regulatory system at a new low level when they developed their underlying illnesses or malnutrition. This concept is supported by the observation that if such patients are given added salt loads, the additional salt is excreted, and the $[Na^+]$ returns to its previous low level. However, the actual excretion of the added salt may be a slow process, and in the interim an equivalent amount of water may be consumed and/or retained by the patient, producing serious overhydration and possibly cardiac failure. Therefore, salt therapy in asymptomatic

---

* The molecular weight of N_2 is used because each molecule of urea contains two nitrogen atoms, each of which has a weight of 14. Furthermore, it is the urea nitrogen value that is determined when a BUN is requested.

hypotonicity is usually contraindicated. The chronic illness in which this type of hypotonicity has been reported most frequently is tuberculosis, including tubercular meningitis, miliary tuberculosis, and the pulmonary form. However, in recent years the syndrome of asymptomatic hypotonicity (also termed asymptomatic hyponatremia)* has been seen in a variety of other chronic conditions. It would appear that the impaired metabolism of these patients in some way depletes their cellular solutes, producing first an intracellular hypotonic state, followed by readjustment of the ECF to the same solute level. However, the mechanisms are far from clear. It must also be recognized that patients with asymptomatic hypotonicity can also develop a superimposed acute symptomatic hypotonicity; in fact, they may be somewhat more susceptible than normal individuals to such events.

Acute Symptomatic Hypotonicity.   Both hyponatremia without hypotonicity and asymptomatic hypotonicity must be distinguished from acute symptomatic hypotonicity, since there are important reasons to provide additional salt to the acute symptomatic patient and there are contraindications to such treatment in the nonsymptomatic states. Acute symptomatic hypotonicity can be seen with dehydration, with normal hydration, and with overhydration. The syndrome as seen with overhydration is discussed in the section on overhydration.

As has already been discussed, hypotonic dehydration occurs primarily when intake is more hypotonic than output. Usually this occurs only when the intake is water or carbohydrate and water and when the volume of intake exceeds the free water of the output (free water is the volume of a fluid in excess of the amount that would make the solute concentration isotonic).

EXAMPLE 1.   In a 15-kg infant the following output values were found:

Source	Volume	Solute Concentration	Total Solute
IWL	600 ml	0	0
Urine loss	700 ml	500 mOsm/liter	350 mOsm
Stool loss	400 ml	200 mOsm/liter	80 mOsm
Total	1700 ml		430 mOsm

For 430 mOsm to exist as a solution with a concentration of 300 mOsm/liter (that of body water) would require $(430/300) \times 1000 = 1433$ ml. Thus 1433 ml of the output would contain all the solute of the output at

---

* As was previously discussed, hyponatremia can occur without hypotonicity; so the term asymptomatic hyponatremia is somewhat ambiguous.

a concentration similar to that of body water. The remaining output is 1700 − 1433 = 267 ml. This is the free water of the output.

When the free water of the intake exceeds 267 ml there will be a tendency for the body fluids to become more dilute. But before this will happen to any appreciable extent, the kidney will generally begin to produce more dilute urine. However, after whatever renal compensation does occur, if the intake of free water exceeds the output of free water, the body fluids will become hypotonic.

EXAMPLE 2.   An 8-kg infant in one 24-hour period had an intake of 16 ounces of skimmed milk, with a urine output of 10 ounces (specific gravity 1.015) and a stool output of 8 ounces. Weight loss was 400 g. Given this information about this child, a number of assumptions can be made that will enable the physician to perform several calculations that in turn will provide a better understanding of the situation.

One form of output that is unknown is the IWL. The change in weight in 1 day is primarily due to changes in water balance. Therefore, intake − output = weight change, and output = IWL + renal loss + gastrointestinal loss. Thus intake − IWL − renal loss − gastrointestinal loss = weight change. Rearranging terms and converting ounces to milliliters (ounces × 30).

$$
\begin{aligned}
\text{IWL} &= \text{intake} - \text{renal loss} - \text{gastrointestinal loss} - \text{weight change} \\
&= 480 \quad\;\; - 300 \qquad\quad - 240 \qquad\qquad\qquad - (-400)^* \\
&= 480 \quad\;\; - 300 \qquad\quad - 240 \qquad\qquad\qquad + 400 \\
&= 340 \text{ ml} \\
&= \frac{340 \text{ ml}}{8 \text{ kg}} = 42.5 \text{ ml/kg/day}
\end{aligned}
$$

The next area to be examined is the balance in water and solute. Intake[†] = 480 ml with solute concentration = 350 mOsm/liter and total solute = (480/1000) × 350 = 168 mOsm. The free water in the intake will be that amount in excess of the amount required to contain 168 mOsm at a concentration of 300 mOsm/liter. The volume required for the solute is (168/300) × 1000 = 560 ml, but this is greater than the intake; so the volume for the free water in the intake is negative: −80 ml.

---

* Weight change is a loss, and so it is entered as a negative number.

† Skimmed milk contains $[Na^+]$ = 27 mEq/liter, $[K^+]$ = 43 mEq/liter, and 3.5% protein. $[Na^+] + [K^+]$ = 70 mEq/liter. Therefore the osmolarity due to ions = 2 × 70 = 140 mOsm/liter. One gram of protein = 167 mg of N_2, and 167 ÷ 28 = 6 mOsm of N_2. The milk contains 3.5 g of protein in 100 ml, or 35 g/liter; 35 × 6 = 210 mOsm of N_2 per liter; 210 + 140 = 350 mOsm/liter.

Output:

	Volume	Solute Concentration	Total Solute
IWL	340 ml	0	0
Renal loss	300 ml	450 mOsm/liter*	135 mOsm
Gastrointestinal loss	240 ml	150 mOsm/liter†	36 mOsm
Total	880 ml		171 mOsm

* A specific gravity of 1.015 corresponds roughly to an osmolarity of 450 mOsm/liter.
† Assuming stool to be about half isotonic to plasma = 150 mOsm/liter.

The free water of the output (that amount in excess of the amount required to make the 171 mOsm of solute isotonic) will be 880 − [(171/300) × 1000] = 880 − 570 = 310 ml.

The balance of free water, as with the balance of any substance, is obtained by subtracting the output from the input. Balance of free water = free water in the intake (−80 ml) − free water in the output (310 ml). Intake − output = (−80) − 310 = −390 ml, which is a negative balance of free water.

With solute intake (168 mOsm) about equal to output (171 mOsm), it is apparent that this infant has suffered primarily a loss of free water (−390 ml). The result must be hypertonic dehydration, and serum [Na$^+$] would have risen from 140 mEq/liter to 152 mEq/liter.*

EXAMPLE 3. Now, assuming the same output figures, except for a 480-ml intake of pure water (therefore it is all free water), what would be the effect? Free water balance = 480 − 310 = +170 ml. Solute balance = 0 − 171 = −171 mOsm. The solute lost from the body was accompanied by an appropriate volume of fluid: (171/300 × 1000 = 570 ml. The body has in effect lost 570 ml of isotonic fluid and gained 170 ml of free water; this should lead to a decrease in osmolarity.

The new volume of isotonic body water will be 4.8 liters − 0.570 liter = 4.33 liters; 4.33 × 300 = 1299 mOsm, but the addition of 170 ml of free water will make the actual volume 4.4 liters, still containing 1299 mOsm. The resulting final osmolarity is 1299/4.4 = 295 mOsm/liter, still a normal value, but less than before. The [Na$^+$] would only change from 140 mEq/liter to 138 mEq/liter.

EXAMPLE 4. Again using the same data, but with greater volumes of

* Assume initially a normal body water of 60% of body weight; 0.60 × 8 kg = 4.8 liters. Assume an initial [Na$^+$] of 140 mEq/liter in the ECF and a [K$^+$] of 140 mEq/liter in the ICF. Then the Na$^+$ + K$^+$ of the body = 140 × 4.8 = 672 mEq. Since solute content does not change appreciably (providing BUN does not rise), the new [Na$^+$]$_{ECF}$ or [K$^+$]$_{ICF}$ will be 672 mEq ÷ 4.41 = 152 mEq/liter.

intake and output, the results could be as follows: Intake of 5% carbohydrate = 600 ml. Output: IWL = 340 ml; renal loss = 400 ml at 450 mOsm/liter = 180 mOsm; stool loss = 300 ml at 180 mOsm/liter = 54 mOsm; total loss = 1040 ml and 234 mOsm. Weight change = 600 − 1040 = −440 ml (or g). The free water of the output = 1040 − [(234/300) × 1000] = 1040 − 780 = 260 ml. The free water balance = intake − output = 600 − 260 = 340 ml. The change in isotonic body fluids, since there is no solute intake (again assuming no change in BUN), will be a loss equivalent to the solute loss, or (234/300) × 1000 = 780 ml.

Now we have a final solute content of body water = (4.8 liters − 0.78 liter) × 300 = 1206 mOsm. And the volume of body water = 4.8 − 0.78 + 0.34 = 4.36 liters. The resulting concentration is 1206/4.36 = 275 mOsm/liter,* which would correspond to a $[Na^+]_s$ of 128 mEq/liter. This figure lies in the range of hypotonicity, and since there has been a net loss of 340 ml of body water, or 55 ml/kg (or g/kg), there is a 5.5% weight loss, which represents a mild dehydration. If the intake and output were still further increased in this manner, or if they were continued as they stand for several days, which is the usual situation, it is apparent that the dehydration and the hypotonicity would continue to become more severe.

Thus the most common cause of acute symptomatic hypotonic dehydration is a net loss of solute greater than the net loss of water. Such a mechanism gives rise to a hypotonic dehydration that has the potential to be, or actually is, hypotonic from its onset.

By contrast, the second type of acute symptomatic hypotonic state begins with an isotonic volume depletion and becomes hypotonic as part of the attempt to repair volume. Under most circumstances, regardless of the proportion of salt to water in the intake or the output, the body is able to adjust one or the other so that the final state of dehydration occurs with a balanced net loss of salt and water. At this stage it is similar to any other isotonic dehydration, whether due to absence of intake, abnormal sweating, or diarrhea. Either the volume depletion results in thirst or the physician recognizes the state of dehydration and decides to administer fluids. Hypotonicity can develop when the fluid the patient selects or is allowed access to, or the fluid the physician selects, is essentially solute-free water.† The consumption of such fluid, orally or parenterally, will begin to expand the volumes of the body fluids, but only at the cost of diluting them. Whether the symptomatic aspect of the acute hypotonicity occurs

---

* Note that in these examples a solute concentration of 300 mOsm/liter has been used for the osmolarity of body water. This is a theoretical value and not the measured one. If a norm of 300 is used, the normal range is 280–320 mOsm/liter. The results will come out essentially the same whichever value is chosen.

† Solute-free in the sense that it contains only solutes that will be totally metabolized and will leave no solute requiring excretion, e.g., 5% glucose in water.

while the patient is being rehydrated but is still somewhat dehydrated or after adequate hydration has occurred will depend on the degree of dehydration and the rate and volume of replacement. In either case the physiologic responses and the symptomatology will be similar. This form of acute symptomatic hypotonicity, which arises from administration of what is essentially water to a patient who is isotonically dehydrated (occasionally the patient may actually be hypertonically dehydrated initially), is termed water intoxication.

PHYSIOLOGY

Since the only type of hypotonicity that requires treatment is the acute symptomatic form, this discussion of physiology is limited to that type of hypotonicity. The physiology of acute symptomatic hypotonic dehydration and of water intoxication can be illustrated using volume-concentration diagrams. Such a diagram for the preceding example 4 is shown in Figure 4-8. It is assumed that the patient initially has normal values. The intake (600 ml of 5% carbohydrate) and the output (1040 ml containing 243 mOsm of solute at a concentration of 234 mOsm/liter) are shown. The resultant state is given at the bottom of the figure. The dash lines indicate the original volume and osmolarity. The volume change (600 − 1040 = −440 ml) has not been taken equally from the ECF and ICF (as in isotonic dehydration), nor has it been taken more from the ICF (as in hypertonic dehydration); it has been taken entirely from the ECF. The volume loss of the ECF is much greater than that of the ICF, because the only way the ICF can contribute water to the ECF is by K^+ transfer and cell breakdown. In isotonic dehydration and in hypertonic dehydration, water is transferred from the ICF to the ECF because of the greater osmolarity in the ECF. However, in hypotonic dehydration the ECF has a lower osmolarity than the cells; so water moves from the ECF to the ICF, further depleting the ECF and more or less canceling the effect of the water moving in the opposite direction due to cell breakdown and cellular K^+ loss.

The changes seen in water intoxication can be illustrated by a previously published study of a 5½-year-old girl with nephrotic syndrome and an episode of apparent gastroenteritis. She became dehydrated, with a 2-kg weight loss from an original weight of 24.4 kg. She became very thirsty and drank sufficient water to return her weight to 24.4 kg, but in the process she became acutely and symptomatically hypotonic and was admitted and treated with hypertonic saline. The amount of salt required was about equivalent to the amount that would have rendered her 2-liter consumption of water isotonic. The diagrams representing her findings are shown in Figure 4-9. In the top drawing she was isotonically dehydrated. By comparing this drawing with the bottom one, it can be seen that she

Osmolarity

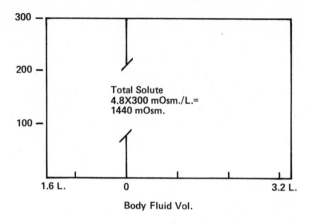

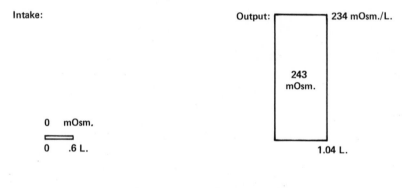

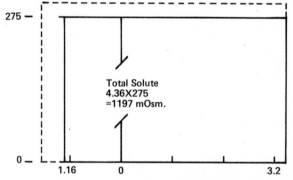

Fig. 4-8. Acute symptomatic hypotonic dehydration. Hypotonic dehydration may occur when output is nearly isotonic but intake is solute-free. In the upper part of the figure normal body fluid volume and solute concentration are shown. In the midportion, an output of 1.045 liters containing 243 mOsm and an intake of 0.6 liter with no solute are illustrated. The result is reduction of total body water by 0.44 liter (1.04 − 0.6) and a drop in solute concentration from 300 to 275 mOsm/ liter. In this and subsequent figures, the dash lines indicate the previous volume and concentration.

122

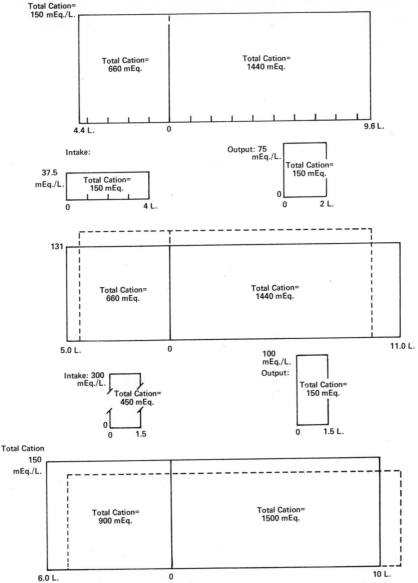

Fig. 4-9. Dehydration repair producing hyponatremia. In this series of diagrams, a nephrotic child who was moderately dehydrated consumed a large volume of low-solute fluids and had an output of half the ingested volume, but with the same total quantity of solute. The result, as shown in the middle part of the diagram, is expansion of both ICF and ECF and reduction in solute concentration (in this case, equivalent to a sodium concentration of 131 mEq/liter). Repair of this state was accomplished by use of a hypertonic sodium chloride solution, and the result was a net intake of 300 mEq (450 mEq intake − 150 mEq of sodium output). The final distribution of body fluids and their concentrations are shown in the bottom diagram. (Adapted from Weil WB, Wallace WM: Fluid therapy in renal disease. Pediatr Clin North Am 6:130, 1959.)

lost both ECF and ICF. After she consumed enough hypotonic fluid to provide a net gain of 2 liters, but no increase in cation, her total body fluid was restored to its normal value, but her cation concentration was abnormally low (corresponding to a $[Na^+]$ of about 121 mEq/liter). Furthermore, even though this "water" was absorbed into the ECF, osmotic readjustment moved an excessive amount of it to the ICF. Thus her cells were somewhat overhydrated, while her ECF was still dehydrated, but her total body water was normal. With administration of hypertonic solutions to provide a net gain of 300 mEq of cation (the amount necessary to make the previous gain of 2 liters of water isotonic), her osmolarity returned to normal; her total body water did not change, but the excess water in the cells (ICF) was transferred for osmotic equality to the ECF. (A small amount of cation also entered the cells; so they did not lose all the water they had gained but retained enough to repair the original ICF dehydration.) The important point to be made by this example is that the ECF is relatively more depleted of fluid in acute hypotonic states than in equivalent isotonic or hypertonic states of hydration or dehydration.

SYMPTOMATOLOGY

The physiologic changes that occur are directly related to the symptomatology found in acute symptomatic hypotonic dehydration, or water intoxication. These signs and symptoms affect the same four systems that have been discussed previously: the subcutaneous tissues, the cardiovascular system, the kidneys, and the central nervous system. Many of the findings are related to the relatively greater depletion of the ECF at any level of hydration.

In the subcutaneous tissues this is reflected by more marked symptomatology than would be expected for the degree of dehydration judged to be present on the basis of weight loss or clinical assessment of the disease process leading to the dehydration. The findings that would be more pronounced include the decrease in skin turgor, the dryness of mucous membranes, the depression of the anterior fontanelle, and the sunken appearance of the eyes.

In the cardiovascular system the shock due to diminished vascular volume occurs with less total body water loss than in other forms of dehydration. With the relatively greater reduction in blood volume and the fall in GFR, plus the resulting increased activity of aldosterone to reabsorb Na^+ and ADH action (in spite of the hypotonicity, ADH activity will be present as a result of stimulation from the volume receptors), the urine volume will be markedly reduced. This will decrease the kidney's ability to compensate for the hypotonicity. In addition, marked hypotonicity by itself produces oliguria, even when body water volumes appear to be normal. This type of oliguria in response to hypotonicity is not well understood, but it disappears when body water osmolarity returns toward normal.

Changes in the CNS are the result of the intracellular hypotonicity, which appears to alter the conductivity of the cells and the relative or absolute increase in cell water that is especially pronounced in water intoxication (hypotonicity with relatively normal total body water). The end results frequently are convulsive seizures, which may be localized or generalized in type, and which may be accompanied by some elevation of the spinal fluid pressure. The potential for diagnostic confusion is of some importance.

DIAGNOSIS

The signs and symptoms that can lead the physician to suspect a hypotonic state depend on the presence or absence of associated dehydration. Severe, acute symptomatic hypotonic dehydration presents with intense signs of ECF depletion in the skin and mucous membranes, incipient or frank shock, marked oliguria, and possibly seizures. The patient appears very ill, and his color may be pale or mildly cyanotic. Nausea may also be a prominent symptom. In the presence of dehydration, the signs and symptoms primarily represent an exaggeration of the pattern of findings expected at any particular level of water loss. By contrast, when hydration is more or less adequate, the signs and symptoms of acute symptomatic hypotonicity are nausea, oliguria or anuria, a sense of marked prostration, and at times convulsive seizures. The onset is rather rapid (usually in hours), and frequently a history can be obtained of a rather large intake of salt-free or salt-poor fluid, orally or parenterally, in the very recent past.

From the laboratory, the single most useful determination when a diagnosis of hypotonicity is suspectd is the $[Na^+]_s$. Since the $[Na^+]_s$ is usually a mirror of the osmolarity, caution must be observed when there is a possibility that the low $[Na^+]_s$ (<130 mEq/liter) may be associated with an elevation of urea or glucose that will leave the resulting osmolarity in the normal range. If urea and glucose are near the normal limits, a patient with a low $[Na^+]_s$ must be carefully evaluated to determine whether there is evidence of chronic illness (suggesting the asymptomatic form), whether there have been any recent acute symptoms (suggesting the symptomatic form), and most important, whether the change in $[Na^+]_s$ is of recent origin.

The final diagnostic test is actually a therapeutic test: administration of an isotonic or hypertonic salt solution sufficient to halve the assumed deficit. If there is dramatic improvement in the signs and symptoms and urine output, it is likely that the problem was an acute symptomatic hypotonic state. On the other hand, if there is no change, or if the patient becomes worse, it is most likely that the patient originally had the asymptomic form of hypotonicity. Cautious use of salt may be indicated, but all other diagnostic possibilities should be examined first.

TREATMENT

Therapy for the asymptomatic from of hypotonicity requires attention to the underlying illness, especially the patient's nutritional status, whereas treatment of the symptomatic form of hypotonicity requires administration of salt with varying amounts of water, depending on the state of hydration of the patient. Therapy can be oral or parenteral or both, depending on the tolerance of the patient and the acuteness of the problem.

The salt given is usually Na^+Cl^-, even though the patient may have a deficit of K^+ and/or a metabolic acidosis requiring H^+ acceptor (HCO_3^-) as part of the intake. K^+ is rarely used, because it is too easy to produce transient hyperkalemia. HCO_3^- is often given in lieu of some of the Cl^- when the metabolic acidosis is severe.

The amount of salt administered in acute symptomatic hypotonicity is based on the amount required to raise the $[Na^+]_s$ to normal. As a general rule, half the required amount is administered, and then the patient is reevaluated before the remaining portion is given. If the diagnosis is correct, and if the treatment is calculated appropriately, the patient should show striking improvement after the first half of the therapeutic requirement of salt is given.

The amount of $Na^+ Cl^-$ necessary to correct the $[Na^+]_s$ is determined by multiplying the concentration deficit by the assumed volume of body water. The volume of the total body water is used in this situation because the fluids of the body are all in osmotic equilibrium. Thus if the serum is hypotonic, the rest of the ECF and also the ICF will be hypotonic to the same extent. Even if only Na^+Cl^- is used to correct the hypotonicity, sufficient solute-free water will be drawn from the ICF to the ECF by osmotic forces to increase ICF osmolarity, and thus the end result will be the same as if salt had been added to all the body fluids. This is illustrated in Figure 4-10. A child with 9 liters of body water and $[Na^+]_s = 115$ mEq/liter (osmolarity = 230 mOsm/liter), as shown in the top diagram, theoretically could be given 90 mEq of Na^+ and 180 mEq of K^+ (with appropriate anions) and no additional water. The result would be an isotonic body water with no fluid shift, as shown in the middle diagram. However, administration of concentrated potassium solutions is *not done,* because of the danger of producing transient, and fatal, hyperkalemia. Therefore, the same amount of cation is given, but all as Na^+, and the final solute concentration of the body water will be the same; but a large volume of water (1.24 liters) will have moved from the ICF to the ECF in the process. This is shown in the bottom diagram of Figure 4-10. An alternative way of determining the amount of Na^+ needed is to calculate that the old ECF of 3 liters has to be raised 30 mEq/liter, and the new 1.24 liters of water transferred from the ICF has to be raised from 0 to 145 mEq/liter. Thus the total needed is $(30 \times 3) + (145 \times 1.24) = 90 + 180 = 270$ mEq. This is the same figure that was obtained by multiplying the total body water by the change in concentration (9 liters $\times$ 30 mEq/liter) = 270 mEq.

However, it can also be seen from the bottom diagram of Figure 4-10 that complete correction of the solute concentration deficit using Na^+ results in a relatively large load of fluid being added to the ECF. In addition, the salt must be given in some fluid, and this will also go into the ECF. Thus, in order to avoid too great an increase in ECF, and thereby in blood volume, only half the calculated amount of salt is given at one time (and that time is usually a period of 4–12 hours). After reassessment, and if there is evidence of improvement, sometimes the remaining half of the calculated amount may be needed the next day.

The volume of fluid to be used will be minimal when correcting an acute hypotonic state in an adequately hydrated patient. The maximum concentration generally used is 3% Na^+Cl^-, which is just over three times the solute concentration of body fluids ($[Na^+] = 500$ mEq/liter = 0.5 mEq/ml). This assures that the least possible amount of water accompanies of Na^+Cl^-.

One of the reasons that this therapy is occasionally ineffective is that the patient is allowed access to water at a time when a hypertonic salt solution is being administered. Even though the patient's body fluids may be hypotonic at the time, the infusion of hypertonic saline stimulates thirst. If the patient drinks water at the time of salt administration, the body fluids can become expanded more than the amount planned for, and then the final concentration will be less than that calculated.

If the patient is only mildly affected and is able to take fluids orally, administration of oral salt tablets and restriction of oral fluids can serve the same purpose as parenteral therapy. When using an oral replacement, some degree of fluid restriction must be strictly followed if the correction in concentration is to be effective.

If the patient is dehydrated and hypotonic, the total fluid to be given is the sum of that required for repair and that required for maintenance. The total salt to be given is the sum of the amounts required for repair of volume, for repair of concentration, and for maintenance needs. The resultant concentration of salt in the total fluids can be calculated by dividing the total salt by the total volume.

EXAMPLE. A 12-kg infant with severe gastroenteritis is admitted to the hospital with what appears to be marked dehydration, oliguria, rapid pulse, and a blood pressure of 60/30 mm Hg. His serum $[Na^+]$ is 118

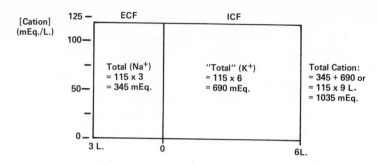

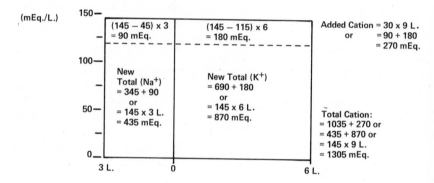

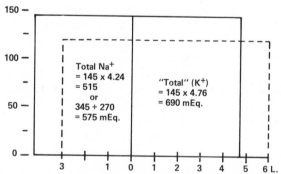

Fig. 4-10. Treatment of hyponatremia showing use of hypertonic sodium chloride to treat symptomatic hyponatremia in a person who is not dehydrated. The diagrams illustrate, from top to bottom, the shift of ICF to the extracellular compartment and demonstrate the need to calculate the total amount of electrolyte required on the basis of the total body water.

mEq/liter, his BUN is 20 mg/dl, and his blood sugar is 50 mg/dl. He is afebrile and appears to be at least 10% dehydrated. (Note that symptoms and signs may be pronounced with hypotonic dehydration.) His maintenance requirements are IWL = 40 ml/kg/day, renal loss = 50 ml/kg/day, gastrointestinal loss = 35 ml/kg/day, and total loss = 125 ml/kg/day. Repair in the first 24 hours: 60 ml/kg (the other 40 ml/kg will be given on the second day). Total fluid = 125 + 60 = 185 ml/kg/day; 185 × 12 kg = 2220 ml/day.

If, as in the usual isotonic dehydration, half of the fluid (60 ml/kg for repair and 35 ml/kg for gastrointestinal maintenance) were to be given as an isotonic salt solution,* the amount of salt to be given would be (2220/ 2) × 150 mEq/liter = 167 mEq of cation. In addition to this, there is a need to increase the cation concentration from 118 to at least 129 mEq/liter, as this would be half of the correction necessary to restore the $[Na^+]_s$ to 140 mEq/liter. To increase the $[Na^+]_s$ from 118 to 129 mEq/liter would require $(129 - 118) \times 8$ liters† = $11 \times 8 = 88$ mEq. This additional 88 mEq of cation would be added to the 167 mEq already known to be needed. The total (167 + 88) is 255 mEq. If this is to be administered in 2200 ml of fluid, the cation concentration will be 255 mEq/2.22 liters = 115 mEq/liter. Such a solution could be approximated by half-isotonic saline (Na^+ = 77 mEq/ liter) to which KCl is added up to the amount of 35 mEq/liter. The final cation concentration would then be 77 + 35 mEq/liter = 112 mEq/liter, which is very close to the calculated concentration. If H^+ acceptor is needed instead of some of the Cl^-, some other mixture can be developed, substituting 25 mEq/liter $NaHCO_3$ for 25 mEq/liter NaCl.

OVERHYDRATION

Edema, Overhydration, and Altered Vascular Volume

The terms *overhydration* and *edema* are not synonymous, although they are often used interchangeably. Overhydration refers to an absolute increase in total body water. Such an increase may be associated with relative reduction (or, occasionally, absolute reduction) in the water content of one component of body water, e.g., plasma volume, ECF, or ICF. Edema refers to excessive fluid in the ECF (particularly the nonvascular or interstitial portion of the ECF) manifest by swelling of the looser sub-

---

* This is equivalent to giving the total of 180 ml/kg as a half-isotonic salt solution; total cation concentration = 75 mEq/liter.

† The figure of 8 liters is based on the assumption that the total body water is 67% of body weight. For this infant (12 kg), total body water = 0.67 × 12 = 8 liters.

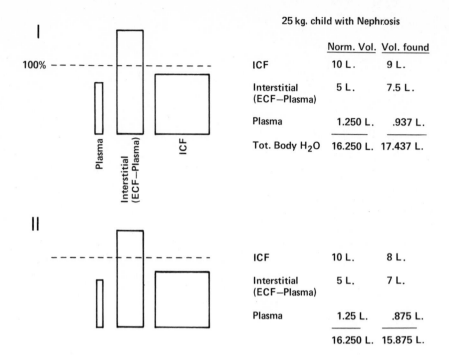

25 kg. child with Nephrosis

	Norm. Vol.	Vol. found
ICF	10 L.	9 L.
Interstitial (ECF–Plasma)	5 L.	7.5 L.
Plasma	1.250 L.	.937 L.
Tot. Body H$_2$O	16.250 L.	17.437 L.

ICF	10 L.	8 L.
Interstitial (ECF–Plasma)	5 L.	7 L.
Plasma	1.25 L.	.875 L.
	16.250 L.	15.875 L.

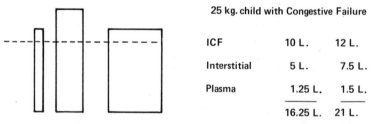

25 kg. child with Congestive Failure

ICF	10 L.	12 L.
Interstitial	5 L.	7.5 L.
Plasma	1.25 L.	1.5 L.
	16.25 L.	21 L.

Fig. 4-11. Edema with and without overhydration. The three illustrations of this problem are examples of edema with varying degrees of hydration in the plasma and ICF. The upper portion of the figure (I) represents the state of hydration of a child with massive edema and expansion of interstitial fluid, but with some reduction in the volume of the plasma and the ICF. This child's total body water is increased, but plasma volume and intracellular volume are below what one might expect for this particular child. Loss of fluid in this child could compromise plasma volume. The middle portion of the figure (II) represents a child with

cutaneous tissues, especially in dependent protions of the body, e.g., ankles, scrotum, labia, eyelids, etc. Localized edema can also occur in the pulmonary interstitium in left heart failure or in any specific location as a result of trauma, burn, or localized disease. Although massive edema is usually associated with total overhydration, this is not always the case. The confusion surrounding the relationship between edema and the states of hydration is illustrated by the child with nephrotic syndrome and very low serum protein concentration, markedly reducing the small osmotic gradient between the vascular system and the rest of the ECF. Such a child may have massive edema, reduced vascular volume, and normal, increased, or decreased ICF volume. Examples I and II in Figure 4-11 illustrate this situation. In example I there is mild overhydration of the total body water that is entirely accounted for by the expanded interstitial volume. The plasma volume is significantly reduced, and the ICF is slightly reduced. In example II there is reduction in volume in each of the areas (as compared to example I), a circumstance that might arise after the use of a potent diuretic. In this case there is still moderate edema (a manifestation of the expanded interstitial volume), but the plasma volume is critically reduced, and the ICF is also smaller. The total body water in this situation is actually less than normal; so the patient is mildly dehydrated overall but is in very serious danger of shock because of the severe volume depletion in the vascular system.

Example III could represent the volumes in a child with right-sided cardiac failure with normal serum protein concentration. In this example all the volumes are increased, and there is marked edema with severe total overhydration.

A fourth example (not shown) would be a child with an expanded vascular volume with normal or reduced interstitial and intracellular volumes. This is neither edema nor necessarily overhydration, although expansion of the vascular volume could be accompanied by edema and/or overhydration, as in example III. It should also be clearly understood that it is quite possible to have an expanded vascular volume in the presence of overall dehydration. Two circumstances may give rise to an independent increase in blood volume: (1) excessively rapid or excessively large in-

---

edema, but with reduction in plasma volume and ICF sufficient that total body water is actually decreased. This represents a dehydrated child with edema and a seriously compromised plasma volume. The bottom portion of the figure (III) represents an edematous child who has expansion of plasma volume, ICF, and interstitial volume. This child is severely overhydrated, and overhydration is present in all body water compartments. The first two examples represent problems that are commonly seen with reduced serum proteins, as in the nephrotic syndrome. The third example is more typical of the overhydration seen with congestive heart failure.

travenous infusions of any solution, since they go directly into the vascular system and a finite period of time is required for diffusion equilibrium to distribute the fluid to the other fluid volumes in the body; (2) an imbalance in the forces governing the distribution of fluid between the vascular and interstitial volumes (see the following section) in favor of transfer of water to the vascular side.

Etiology and Physiology

The distinctions between edema, overhydration, and expanded plasma volume carry over to their underlying pathophysiology. Overhydration depends primarily on expansion of the total of monovalent cations of the body—essentially Na^+. The formation of edema and/or the expansion of blood volume result primarily from disequilibrium in the forces first clearly delineated by Starling. These mechanisms are illustrated in Figure 4-12. The Starling forces are hydrostatic and osmotic. The solute concentration of the plasma is slightly greater than that of the interstitial fluid because of the presence of serum proteins (especially the albumin) in the vascular system. The effect of this is to draw water from the interstitial fluid into the plasma. This is countered by the hydrostatic forces, which differ on the arterial and venous ends of the capillary bed. On the arterial end the intravascular pressure is much greater than the hydrostatic pressure in the tissues, and the net hydrostatic pressure forcing water out of the vascular system is greater than the osmotic pressure drawing water in. Therefore there is a net movement of water from the blood vessels into the tissues. On the venous end of the capillary bed, the intravascular pressure is close to the tissue pressure and may be slightly more than tissue hydrostatic pressure (as in the legs) or slightly less (as in the areas above the heart). In either case the osmotic pressure drawing water into the vessels is greater than the net hydrostratic pressure so there is a net movement of water back into the vascular system on the venous end. Normally, the movement of water out of the vascular system on the arterial side is just balanced by the movement of water on the venous side.

Reduction in serum protein concentration (or increase in interstitial fluid protein) will reduce the osmotic difference between the vascular and interstitial fluids; this will result in an increased movement of water toward the interstitium and out of the vessels—hypoproteinemic edema. An increase in venous pressure will reduce the return of fluid to the vascular system and produce a net gain of fluid in the interstitial area—the edema of right-sided cardiac failure. Both of these processes will continue to enlarge the interstitial fluid volume until the increase results in a high enough tissue hydrostatic pressure to create a new balance of forces.

The forces of osmotic pressure and hydrostatic pressure are not the

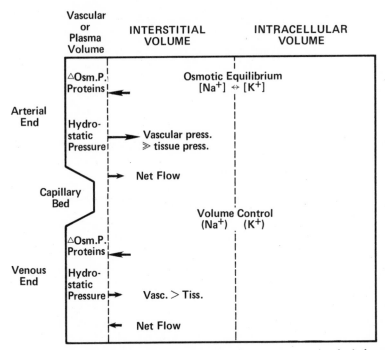

Fig. 4-12.   Fluid shifts and Starling forces. The diagram represents the balance of
forces acting on the fluid contained in the capillary bed. On the arterial end, the
balance of forces between the osmotic pressure due to serum proteins and the
hydrostatic pressure results in a net flow of fluid from the plasma volume to the
interstitial space. On the venous end, the net balance of these same forces results
in flow of fluid from the interstitial space back into the vascular volume.

only factors operating to determine the presence or absence of edema.
Lymphatic flow carries interstitial fluid back into the circulation, and thus
changes in lymph flow rates can affect the appearance or disappearance of
edema. A variety of circulatory and local tissue metabolic changes may
also modify the accumulation of interstitial fluid; in addition, a renal factor, possibly related to Na^+ reabsorption, seems to be important in the
phenomenon of edema formation. Thus, although an increase in interstitial
fluid arises as the end result of many factors, the balance between osmotic
pressure and hydrostatic pressure remains a highly significant aspect of
the process.

The areas where venous pressure is greatest and where tissue
pressure is least are the areas of greatest fluid accumulation. This explains
the propensity for edema formation in the lower legs and scrotal or vulvar
area when a person is upright and in the periorbital tissues and over the
sacrum when the person is recumbent.

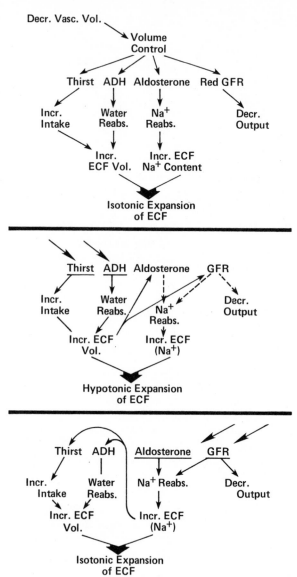

Fig. 4-13. Mechanisms for overhydration. Three basic mechanisms resulting in overhydration are illustrated. In the upper diagram the volume control mechanism is stimulated, usually through a decrease in vascular volume in the upper half of the body. In turn, four events occur: thirst is stimulated, ADH is increased, aldosterone is released, and effective GFR is reduced. The net result of these stimuli is to expand the ECF volume in an isotonic manner. If the volume control center responds because of local factors in its immediate environment, and if the person is not dehydrated, overhydration will occur. In the middle diagram the situation is illustrated in which only two of the four mechanisms involved in expansion of the ECF are stimulated: thirst and ADH stimulation. The result is

Simultaneously with the net transfer of fluid to the interstitial area, the reduction of the vascular volume will trigger the volume control mechanisms, altering renal vascular hemodynamics and elevating aldosterone activity and to some extent ADH activity, with increased reabsorption of Na^+ and water as the end reaction. Ultimately this can create true overhydration.

Overhydration requires an uncompensated increase in fluid intake or an uncompensated decrease in output or some combination of these processes. As with dehydration, combined alteration of intake and output is the most common underlying mechanism.

ISOTONIC AND HYPOTONIC OVERHYDRATION

In dehydration the net loss of hypotonic solution (both intake and total output usually being hypotonic) tends to lead toward development of hypertonicity once the compensating responses of the body have been overextended. In overhydration the net gain of hypotonic solution tends to lead toward development of hypotonicity when the body's compensating mechanisms have been surpassed. Here the comparison fails, however, because hypotonic dehydration, although the least common form of dehydration, does occur with a certain frequency, whereas hypertonic overhydration is extremely uncommon.

The physiologic responses leading to overhydration are summarized in Figure 4-13. In the upper diagram, diminished vascular volume, either throughout the body or confined to the areas of volume reception (primarily in the upper half of the body), is the initiating stimulus. Through the volume receptors the central control mechanism is activated, and four responses may be elicited: thirst, release of ADH, stimulation of aldosterone activity, and altered renal hemodynamic factors (labeled Red. GFR). The first two responses (thirst and ADH release) lead to intake of fluid and reabsorption of water, with subsequent expansion of ECF volume. This is balanced by the other two effects (aldosterone activity and changed renal function), which increase Na^+ reabsorption and provide the necessary solute to make the ECF expansion an isotonic one. Both increased intake and decreased output are involved in this general response pattern.

Alternatively, using this same model, if the intake is salt-free or very low in salt, even maximum Na^+ reabsorption will not increase the body's

---

hypotonic expansion of the ECF. If, as shown in the bottom diagram, activation of the other two mechanisms occurs, this tends to produce increased sodium reabsorption, which increases the concentration of sodium in the ECF. But this in turn stimulates the other two mechanisms, so that the ultimate result is an isotonic expansion of the ECF, as in the upper diagram.

salt content as much as volume can be increased, and the end result will be hypotonic expansion of the ECF, or hypotonic overhydration. This can be partially compensated by transfer of water into cells, but hypotonic expansion of the total body water must eventually occur.

The middle diagram in Figure 4-13 illustrates a second mechanism by which hypotonic overhydration can occur. In this example the primary stimulus can affect the thirst mechanism or ADH release or both. Such events can result from a variety of stimuli, e.g., pain, trauma, or anesthesia. The sequence of events will lead to primary water retention, volume expansion, and inhibition of those responses that might have produced increased Na^+ reabsorption. The final state will, of necessity, be hypotonic overhydration. Head trauma, meningitis, or cranial surgery may also stimulate ADH release and result in retention of water in excess of Na^+ producing hypotonic overhydration.

Alternatively, as diagrammed in the bottom scheme of Figure 4-13, stimuli leading to increased aldosterone activity and/or altered renal function can increase Na^+ reabsorption and decrease output, but the addition of more Na^+ to the ECF will in turn activate ADH release and thirst; thus water reabsorption and water intake will rise, and the final state will be isotonic overhydration.

HYPERTONIC OVERHYDRATION

Hypertonic overhydration results only under very unusual circumstances: the net gain in solute must exceed the net gain in water. This requires excretion of hypotonic urine and intake of a large volume of high-solute fluid. One of the situations in which this can occur is in the postoperative state. If a patient is given more fluid than required for maintenance, and this fluid is, for example, isotonic saline, and if the patient's renal function is depressed following surgery, the appropriate conditions will exist for development of hypertonic overhydration.

EXAMPLE. A 4-year-old boy weighing 20 kg underwent extensive abdominal surgery during which he had an episode of hypotension of moderate duration. He was adequately hydrated preoperatively, and postoperatively he had marked oliguria (urine output of about 5 ml/hour). On the basis of body weight, he appeared adequately hydrated, although as indicated in the section on translocation of fluid, he could have been "relatively" dehydrated because of fluid accumulating in the gastrointestinal tract. His temperature postoperatively was 40°C.

His fluid orders called for infusion of isotonic saline at 100 ml/hour. Actually the fluid ran somewhat faster, and at the end of 24 hours 3000 ml had been infused. The patient showed evidence of congestive failure and stupor. Assessment at that time yielded the following figures: Maintenance losses were IWL 34 ml/kg/day + 30% for fever = 900 ml; renal loss

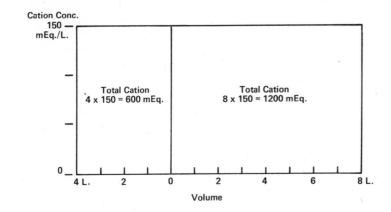

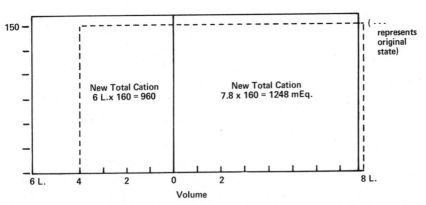

Fig. 4-14. Hypertonic overhydration. Using volume/concentration diagrams, the development of hypertonic overhydration is illustrated. This resulted from infusion of isotonic sodium chloride solution postoperatively in a child who was adequately hydrated. The child was oliguric as a result of stimulation of the ADH mechanism resulting from the stress of a surgical procedure (see text for details).

5 ml/hour = 120 ml; gastrointestinal loss (nasogastric suction) = 180 ml. Total maintenance loss = 1200 ml of fluid. Assuming that the urine and gastrointestinal suction losses were similar to isotonic salt solution with a cation concentration of 150 mEq/liter, the cation loss was (0.120 liter + 0.180 liter) × 150 mEq/liter = 45 mEq of cation.

The intake was 3000 ml of a solution with a cation concentration of 150 mEq/liter. Thus the intake of cation was 3 liters × 150 mEq/liter = 450 mEq. The net gain was 450 − 45 = 405 mEq of cation and 3000 − 1200 = 1800 ml of fluid.

If this boy had a normal body water initially, he had 60% of 20 kg or

12 liters of body water. At a cation* concentration of 150 mEq/liter, he had 12 × 150 = 1800 mEq of cation. After the infusion his body water was 12 liters + 1.8 liters = 13.8 liters, and his total cation content was 1800 mEq + 405 mEq = 2205 mEq. The new cation concentration was 2205 mEq/13.8 liters = 160 mEq/liter, an increase in cation concentration of 10 mEq/liter, which was reflected in a serum [Na^+] of 153 mEq/liter.

Thus this child sustained 15% overhydration and an increase in cation concentration producing hypertonic overhydration. Furthermore, not only will most of the administered fluid remain in the ECF, but additional water will be drawn from the ICF to the ECF to equalize the solute concentrations in the two volumes. This is shown diagrammatically in Figure 4-14.

Symptomatology and Diagnosis

The symptomatology associated with overhydration depends on the relative volumes of the plasma, the interstitial fluid, and the ICF, as well as the osmolarity of the body water. The one finding that is essential to the diagnosis of overhydration is weight gain. As in dehydration, this can be roughly quantitated as mild (5% weight gain), moderate (10% weight gain), or severe (15% weight gain). These figures are appropriate only when the additional fluid is more or less evenly distributed throughout the body water. When the excess fluid is primarily in the interstitial tissue, much larger volumes can be accumulated without critical adverse effects. Accumulation of large amounts of edema fluid, while cosmetically disfiguring and unpleasant, may be relatively benign physiologically while the patient is awake and more or less ambulatory during the day; however, as the patient becomes recumbent and metabolically less active at night, changes in venous pressure and cardiac function may allow much of this fluid to reenter the circulation, which can lead to episodes of nocturnal congestive failure with pulmonary edema.

Expansion of the interstitial fluid produces edema that tends to aggregate in the dependent and looser tissue areas. Compression of such areas with a finger may result in a depression that fills out slowly; this is termed pitting, and it first becomes manifest when there has been about a 5% gain in interstitial fluid volume. However, pitting does not routinely occur with edema; it also requires the presence of a specific physiochemical state in the tissues that is related to hyaluronidaselike activity. When the volume increase exceeds 15%, the overlying skin will become so thinned as to appear translucent; it may begin to split, so that some of the fluid from the subcutaneous tissue will ooze out. At this point the tissues

---

* Used in this manner, cation refers to the univalent cations—Na^+ and K^+.

appear to have increased susceptibility to bacterial invasion, and erysipelaslike infections may occur. In all cases of significant overhydration, the interstitial fluid volume will be increased.

As has been stated, plasma volume may be reduced, unchanged, or expanded in overhydration. Reduced plasma volume in overhydration results in the same group of findings that it causes in dehydration. These findings include the following: poor peripheral circulation, with coolness of fingers and toes and pallor or cyanosis of these areas; rapid, weak pulse; hypotension progressing toward shock; syncope from reduced cerebral circulation; sweating; reduced renal function from impaired renal perfusion; triggering of the volume control center in the CNS, with its sequelae of thirst, ADH release, increased aldosterone activity, and changes in renal function relative to Na^+ and water excretion.

Expansion of the vascular volume produces a plethoric facies, a slowed pulse rate, and some elevation in blood pressure. In man the GFR is only slightly increased under these circumstances. The most serious complication of increasing plasma volume arises from overloading in the circulation. As plasma volume expands, the venous and capillary vessels will accommodate most of the increased fluid. However, with increased venous filling, venous pressure rises, cardiac filling during diastole increases, and cardiac output must also rise. Changes in rate and stroke volume and cardiac dilatation compensate initially, but ultimately cardiac output no longer increases with dilatation; venous pressure and volume rise further. Frank cardiac failure is the final outcome.

Acute changes in intracellular volume that are compatible with survival appear to be of smaller magnitude than those seen in the other body fluid volumes. In addition, much less is known about the results of altered cellular hydration, with the possible exception of the changes occurring in the CNS. In the CNS the important aspect would seem to be the fact that the brain is almost completely enclosed in a solid container, the skull. Thus expansion of brain cell volume will produce increased intracranial pressure, with its own constellation of findings. However, there is scanty information on the quantitative relationships involved.

The diagnosis of overhydration is based on clinical observation of the findings just described for each of the body fluid volumes. Weight is one of the best quantitative assessments readily available. There are a variety of chemical substances that distribute in plasma, ECF, or total body water, and by use of combinations of these substances, the size of the various fluid volumes can be estimated. However, chemical determination of such volumes is still not widespread clinically. Measurement of the concentration of plasma Na^+ or Cl^- will not be at all useful unless extremely careful balance measurements of the intake and output of these substances are also performed; again, this is not a common clinical practice.

Treatment

Treatment of overhydration will depend more on whether the plasma volume is depleted, normal, or expanded than on the overall extent of change in the total body water.

EXPANDED VASCULAR VOLUME

When the plasma volume is expanded comparably to the remainder of the body fluids, there are three approaches to therapy: decrease intake, increase output, or improve the "pump." Limitation of intake can mean any degree of restriction on total fluid intake. This must include consideration of the water content of foods as well as liquids. Restriction of Na^+ intake is frequently utilized, but it has two important drawbacks: (1) Such restriction must be quite stringent to be effective, and this often leads to reduced caloric intake and undernutrition—at times when this can be important. (2) Sodium limitation does not always limit water intake or water retention, the result being the more complicated problem of hypotonic overhydration, with findings of an acute symptomatic hypotonic state, including oliguria, which reinforces the tendency to overhydration. Fluid restriction does not present these same problems, but it is difficult for the patient to maintain for any long period of time. However, fluid restriction can effectively reduce overhydration when intake is less than the maintenance needs that compensate ongoing losses. Even when fluid intake is zero, the reduction in overhydration can proceed only as fast as these ongoing losses are occurring. However, unless some fluid restriction is carried out, any other therapeutic measures may be ineffective.

Increasing the output is probably the most common approach to treatment, but unless simultaneous attention is paid to fluid intake, increases in output may gain little. Diuretic agents of many types and modes of action have been found useful. Some of the newer drugs that are extremely effective when plasma volumes are large are unfortunately still somewhat effective when plasma volumes are small. This can be fatal. Nevertheless, diuretics have an extremely important place in the therapy of overhydration. Most of their effectiveness involves interfering with reabsorption of Na^+, increasing its excretion, and providing a comparable volume of water to accompany the excreted Na^+ into the urine.

The third therapeutic approach involves a variety of interventions aimed at improving the circulation. In congestive failure, digitalization remains a primary maneuver. Other devices that can reduce venous return to the heart and thus improve the heart's efficiency include keeping the patient in a semiupright position, use of tourniquets on the extremities at just sufficient pressure to block venous flow, phlebotomy, and dialysis.

Extracorporeal dialysis can be a very effective technique for removing a protein-free solution from the circulation without losing valuable serum proteins or red blood cells. However, such a procedure is usually reserved for acute, critical situations.

With each of these measures, which are usually combined to one extent or another, the immediate impact is on the vascular volume. Constant reequilibration occurs with the interstitial volume, and to some extent with the intracellular volume as well, so that ultimately there is general alleviation of the overhydrated state.

EXAMPLE. An 8-year-old child with chronic cardiac insufficiency weighs 30 kg. His weight 3 months earlier had been 25 kg. He shows evidence of edema in the periorbital tissues, scrotum, and lower legs. He is having moderate respiratory difficulty. He has been fully digitalized for several months and has been on an intermittent program of diuretics and moderate salt restriction. Blood chemical values are within normal limits. One of the methods of treatment to be considered is limitation of fluids, and the question arises to what extent these should be limited. His fluid losses are as follows:

IWL: Since he is midway between the infant and the 16-year-old person, his IWL will be midway between 40 and 20 ml/kg, or 30 ml/kg. Since one can assume that his weight gain is fluid, the weight of 25 kg can be used to determine his total IWL: $30 \times 25 = 750$ ml/day.

Renal loss: He is eating poorly, but being provided a generous amount of carbohydrate; so his solute production can be considered at a low level, but not basal. From Figure 2-3 this can be estimated at 15 mOsm/kg, or a total of $15 \times 25 = 375$ mOsm/day. Assuming that he can concentrate his urine to 600 mOsm/liter (specific gravity 1.020), the urine volume required to excrete his solute load is $(375/600) \times 1000 = 625$ ml.

Gastrointestinal loss: He is not vomiting or having diarrhea; so his stool water content will be about 4 ml/kg (midway between 5 and 2.5 ml/kg), or 100 ml/day.

His total output should be $750 + 625 + 100 = 1475$ ml. Calculated per kilogram, it would be $30 + 25 + 4 = 59$ ml/kg ($59 \times 25 = 1475$ ml).

Assuming a diet of 1500 kcal (750 kcal from carbohydrate, 450 kcal from fat, and 300 kcal from protein) and assuming the food averages two-thirds water and one-third solids, his diet will weigh about 900 g, of which 600 g will be water. In addition, the water of oxidation, which averages about 0.1 ml/kcal and represents the water formed from oxidation of carbohydrates, fats, and proteins, will add another 150 ml (0.1×1500 kcal) to the intake. Thus, without any liquid to drink, the fluid balance will be intake − output = balance, or $(600 + 150) - 1475 = -725$ ml. If it is desired to have the patient lose 0.5 liter of fluid per day, intake of liquid can be set at 225 ml; then the balance will be -500 ml, or -0.5 liter.

Should his urine concentration rise to 1200 mOsm/liter (specific gravity 1.035),* his urine volume will be halved, or down to 312 ml. Then, if the patient had no liquid intake at all, his balance will be $(600 + 150) - (750 + 312 + 100) = 750 - 1162 = -412$ ml. Thus the patient could not even lose 0.5 liter of fluid per day under these circumstances.

DIMINISHED VASCULAR VOLUME

Most of the measures that can be employed in treatment of overhydration with expanded plasma volume are contraindicated when plasma volume is decreased in the presence of overhydration. Such measures are contraindicated because their primary or initial effects reduce plasma volume and their secondary effects reduce the volume of the remainder of body water. When plasma volume is already reduced, these therapeutic measures either will be ineffectual or will create a very real danger of vascular collapse.

Digitalization in the presence of cardiac failure with low plasma volume is a legitimate approach, but it may not be effectual in improving the circulation. Diuretics are almost always contraindicated, as are phlebotomy and dialysis for the purpose of removing fluid. Fluid restriction is usually contraindicated, but occasionally it can be tried if extreme caution is exercised.

The most efficacious therapeutic approach is to treat the cause of the reduced plasma volume. If the volume is low because of hypoproteinemia, as is often the case in children, the ideal approach is to increase the serum osmotic pressure with proteins or other large-molecule substances that cannot diffuse out of the vascular system. This should be done using as little fluid as is practical, since the increase in osmotic pressure of the serum will quickly draw water into the vascular system from interstitial volume. The major problem with this technique occurs in the nephrotic syndrome, as most of the administered protein (albumin) is excreted in the urine almost as fast as it is given. Nevertheless, it is sometimes possible to use this approach daily with very large amounts of protein and thereby make a little headway. In critical situations, massive albumin infusion followed by a single dose of a rapid-acting potent diuretic, with the procedure being repeated every day for several days, has been found to be moderately effective. In the majority of patients, however, reasonably liberal access to fluids is necessary to maintain a respectable plasma volume, and the overhydrated state is not attacked directly.

HYPOTONIC STATES

In the presence of low solute concentration (hypotonic overhydration), serum $[Na^+]$ will be low, but plasma volume may be small, normal, or large. In each of these circumstances, but particularly with reduced

* This is an unlikely occurrence, but it is used by way of illustration.

plasma volume, renal function may be impaired, so that oliguria is a common finding. Marked reduction in urine volume compounds the problem of overhydration because it is then very easy for intake to exceed output, which can lead to a continuing positive balance of water. Although administration of Na^+ is generally considered contraindicated in the presence of overhydration, its careful use when there is hyponatremia and hypotonicity of body fluids may be of remarkable benefit to the patient.

Sodium, usually administered as NaCl or as $NaHCO_3$ or as a mixture of the two, should be given with minimal amounts of fluid as a hypertonic solution when plasma volume is expanded and as an isotonic solution when plasma volume is contracted. The quantity of Na^+ used should not exceed half the amount necessary to correct the concentration defect in the total body water; in the presence of marked overhydration, it would be reasonable to begin with one-fourth of the total estimated need. The results of such an approach, if it is successful, should be an increase in urinary output and a mild to marked diuresis, with improvement in the patient's sensorium and general feeling of well-being. The major danger lies in the increase in plasma volume and the possibility that this could precipitate or increase congestive failure.

FLUID SHIFTS: TRANSLOCATION

There are occasions when total body fluids remain relatively constant but internal shifts of fluid occur from one volume to another. This shift produces symptomatology comparable to that exhibited with an absolute increase or decrease in a particular area.

Intraintestinal

One of the more frequent occurrences of translocation is seen after major abdominal surgery and/or in paralytic ileus. Under these circumstances, fluid moves initially from the plasma and then from the total ECF into the intestinal lumen. An alternative explanation for this phenomenon, with the same end result, is that when the secretions of the intestinal wall and the associated organs, such as the gallbladder and pancreas, continue to be formed but are not reabsorbed into the plasma, they accumulate in the bowel. In any case, the fluid that is translocated is isotonic and is comparable in composition to the ECF. The end result is production of all the signs and symptoms of isotonic dehydration, but with minimal change in weight and consequently essentially unchanged total body water. As far as the functioning of the various body systems is concerned, the fluid in the bowel does not participate; it acts as if it had been lost from the body. The difference is that with the recovery of bowel function, provided that the intraluminal fluid has not been removed by suction, the functionally "amputated" fluid can be returned to the plasma and ECF. When this occurs, a temporary overload can exist, especially if the ECF and plasma volumes have been restored to their normal amounts in the interim by parenteral therapy.

The quantitative aspects of fluid shifts of this type are difficult to ascertain. However, clinical evaluation of the degree of dehydration based on skin turgor, depression of the anterior fontanelle in infants, pulse rate, blood pressure, and urinary output is the best available technique for estimation. Whenever gastrointestinal suction is used, the volume of fluid removed by this technique also provides a good indication of the quantity of fluid trapped in the gut. In this case, however, once the fluid has been removed by suction, it no longer constitutes a problem of secondary relocation back to the plasma and ECF.

Therapy is based on these clinical observations. Fluid is provided initially as if the translocated fluid has been lost, whether it has actually been removed by suction or not.

EXAMPLE. A 2-year-old infant was hospitalized after 24 hours of vomiting, anorexia, and abdominal pain. He appeared mildly dehydrated on admission. He was immediately taken to surgery, where an intestinal obstruction was relieved, but only after extensive manipulation of the bowel.

During the 12-hour period following his admission and including surgery, he was given 360 ml of fluid (30 ml/hour) that was half-isotonic in its salt concentration. At the end of this 12 hours, the child appeared more dehydrated than he had on admission, and the fluid balance problem was reevaluated. His temperature was 39°C, which is what it had been since admission; his urine output for 12 hours had been 140 ml, and nasogastric suction had produced 100 ml of fluid. An estimated blood loss of 75 ml had been replaced during surgery. At the end of the 12-hour period his weight was 150 g less than his 12.0 kg on admission, but his serum chemical values were normal. His fluid status in the first 12 hours was as follows: IWL = 37 ml/kg (normal) + 8 ml/kg (20% for fever of 2°C) = 45 ml/kg/day = 540 ml/day = 270 ml/12 hours. Gastrointestinal suction loss = 100 ml + translocation (?). Renal loss = 140 ml. Total output for 12 hours = 270 + 100 + 140 + (?) = 510 ml + (?). Previous dehydration (5%) = 600 ml. Input = 360 ml. Current estimate of dehydration (8%) = 1000 ml. Net change in hydration, or "balance" = −400 ml (previous dehydration minus existing dehydration (600 − 1000). Intake − output = balance (obtained by estimates of dehydration): 360 − [270 + 100 + 140 + (?)] = −400 ml.

If the values are all approximately correct, the (?) for translocation should be 250 ml. This would also agree with weight change, since he lost 150 ml from his body (on the basis of weight loss), and if 250 ml were translocated and remained in the bowel, the total functional balance would be −400 ml (150 + 250).

At this point his fluid needs should be estimated for the next 36 hours. For the next 12 hours, his maintenance needs will be the following: IWL = 45 ml/kg/day = 540 ml/day = 270 ml/12 hours. Gastrointestinal suction (estimate based on last 12 hours) = 100 ml. Translocation is assumed to have ceased to accumulate. Renal maintenance should be 45 ml/kg = 540 ml/day or 270 ml/12 hours, but since functional output will be less than output at this time, the estimate for 12 hours is 200 ml. Repair of 8% dehydration: half of this (40 ml/kg) in 12 hours = 480 ml. Total for 12 hours = IWL + gastrointestinal + renal + repair = 270 + 100 + 200 + 480 = 1050 ml.

For the following 24 hours, his maintenance needs will be the following: IWL (assume normal temperature) = 37 ml/kg = 444 ml/day. Gastrointestinal (assume same rate of suction) = 200 ml/day. Renal (assume normal function) = 45 ml/kg = 540 ml/day. Total maintenance = 1184 ml/day. Repair of remaining dehydration (40 ml/kg) = 480 ml. Total fluids 1664 ml/day.

Composition of fluids: Gastrointestinal and repair fluids are those that should be replaced with isotonic salt solution; the remainder should be replaced with glucose in water. In the second 12 hours, salt solution = 100 + 480 = 580 ml; glucose solution = 270 + 200 = 470 ml. This is about half salt and half glucose; so the total fluid could be half-isotonic for salt ([cation] = 75 mEq/liter) or slightly greater. Since the patient is still not voiding well, and since serum $[K^+]$ is normal (although the patient probably has an overall K^+ deficit), the solution for this 12-hour period probably should not contain K^+. A reasonable type of composition could be $[Na^+]$ = 75 mEq/liter, $[Cl^-]$ = 50 mEq/liter, and $[HCO_3^-]$ = 25 mEq/liter.

In the next 24 hours, salt solution = 200 + 480 = 680 ml; glucose solution = 444 + 540 = 984 ml. This is slightly less than half-isotonic salt, but such a solution might balance the slight salt deficit of the previous 12 hours if half-isotonic salt was used then. However, to estimate the appropriate cation concentration more precisely, $[680/(680 + 984)] \times 150$ mEq/liter = $(680/1664) \times 150$ = 61 mEq/liter. At this time, renal function should be improving, and the potential K^+ deficit can be treated. Therefore, the ideal composition of fluid for this 24-hour period will be $[Na^+]$ = 35 mEq/liter, $[K^+]$ = 25 mEq/liter, $[Cl^-]$ = 40 mEq/liter, and $[HCO_3^-]$ = 20 mEq/liter.

It is very important to recognize that the fluids for this 24-hour period will not be ordered until the end of the preceding 12 hours, at which time the patient will be reevaluated to determine whether his progress has been as predicted and whether the losses have been as they were estimated. If either of these conditions is not met, the program for this 24-hour period must be reexamined. At the end of this period of treatment, assuming that losses, gains, and progress are all as anticipated, the fluids for the following day will consist entirely of maintenance fluids to balance the ongoing losses.

Ascites

Development of ascites is a second common form of translocation of fluid; it can produce marked reduction in plasma volume and functional dehydration of the body water. Ascites occurs as a result of low serum proteins and/or elevated portal venous pressure. In any case, the fluid accumulated in the peritoneal space is initially derived from plasma and is ultimately derived, to some degree, from the total body water. It is functionally inert, except for embarrassment to respiration because of elevation of the diaphragm; its presence creates a potential site for bacterial infection, and its volume, when very large, produces increased pressure on the inferior vena cava. This last effect may have two important consequences: (1) loss of additional fluid from the plasma as edema in the lower extremities as a result of the elevated peripheral venous pressure and (2) reabsorption of additional Na^+ by the renal tubules as a result of the increased renal venous pressure. Reabsorption of additional Na^+ leads to retention of additional water. The Na^+ and water retention, while increasing the tendency to ascites and edema formation, will also expand the vascular volume; this can be beneficial if hypovolemia existed previously.

One other potential danger that is inherent in the problem of ascites is that of removal of intraperitoneal fluid by paracentesis when this is done rapidly and/or in large volume. In a patient who already has decreased plasma volume, the formation of new ascitic fluid, which occurs quickly when intraabdominal pressure is low, may reduce plasma volume so much more that the patient may go into shock. This danger is not great when the initial plasma volume is normal or increased. In other respects the relative dehydration, if it exists, is managed as in the case of intraintestinal translocation of fluid.

Burns

Another common situation where there can be significant translocation of fluid involves the patient with extensive burns. The fluid lost into the burned area consists of an isotonic fluid like plasma, but the fluid translocated in burns also contains a significant quantity of plasma proteins that escape because of local damage to capillary walls. The protein concentration in such fluid may be about half its concentration in plasma. In addition, often there is destruction of significant numbers of red blood cells; so the rises in plasma protein and hemoglobin concentrations, which often reflect loss of fluid from the ECF in other forms of dehydration, will not be as large as might be anticipated in the burned patient.

The fluid tends to accumulate in the burned tissue within a very short time after the insult. A sizable amount will have been translocated in the first 4 hours, and the great majority will have been transferred by 24 hours. After 48 hours little additional fluid is lost into the damaged tissues. Beginning about the third or fourth day, the fluid will begin to move back into the circulation and be redistributed into the total body water. This must be considered when planning fluid therapy at that time, particularly if renal function is still depressed and the body is unable to excrete what may easily become surplus volume.

The amount of translocated fluid in burns is in the range of 5%–10% of body weight (50–100 ml/kg) when the burn covers 25%–50% of the body surface. Thus a significant degree of dehydration can result from this process.

In all cases of dehydration resulting from translocation of fluid, the thirst mechanism is activated. This is of greatest significance in burns because the process is so rapid. As a result, the patient tends to consume large quantities of water unless this is restricted. The large intake of water is not readily excreted, because not only is renal function depressed, but also the stimulus to water reabsorption is increased because of elevated levels of ADH. The ADH elevation arises from the action of the volume control center, and in burns it is also released as part of the response to trauma. A frequent end result of this process is hypotonicity of body fluids, as reflected by low $[Na^+]_s$.

5

Composition Disorders

Composition disorders of body fluids involve change in concentration of one or more of the solutes present in body water. Such changes in concentration may exist with or without concomitant changes in the volume of body fluids. Alteration in concentration of one or more solutes may also occur in the extracellular body water compartment or intracellular body water compartment independent of change in the other compartment. However, since current clinical practice does not include direct examination of intracellular water composition, only those intracellular changes that can be inferred from changes in plasma, serum, or ECF are discussed.

Two other considerations are important in interpreting the discussions in this section: the intracellular solute composition is usually unknown, and the actual volumes of the ICF and ECF are frequently unknown. Therefore, a change in concentration of a solute does not necessarily reflect a change in the quantity of that solute in the total body. The exceptions to this statement will be made explicit, and some of them are discussed in the chapter on volume disorders (Chapter 4).

The composition disturbances may be divided into two groups: those that involve the ionized solutes commonly referred to as the electrolytes and those that involve nonionized solutes such as urea and glucose. Some overlap is necessary, since a discussion of urea involves the concept of azotemia, which in turn involves both nonionized solute and electrolytes.

The plan in this chapter is to consider the effects of a change in concentration of each ion; under each change, four topics are presented: cause, implications, detection, and management.

IONIC DISORDERS

Alterations in concentrations of electrolytes, essentially those in the ECF, are discussed in terms of individual ions. However, it should be recognized that no single ion can be changed in concentration without affecting other ions, because a net charge, positive or negative, will result, and immediately some other ion or ions will have to change. For example, if there is an increase in $[Cl^-]$,* either $[HCO_3^-]$ or some other anion will have to decrease and/or $[Na^+]$ will have to increase.

All the cations and anions of the plasma are bound to some extent to the amphoteric serum proteins, and thus they are not free to participate in various ionic equilibrations. In the case of the major monovalent ions, about 15 mEq/liter of Na^+ and 10 mEq/liter of Cl^- are not ionized, but from a clinical perspective the only significance is to reduce the measured serum osmolarity to 280 mOsm/liter from the theoretical value of 300–310 mOsm/liter.

Sodium

Most of the disturbances of $[Na^+]$ are associated with volume changes and are included in Chapter 4. However, a brief recapitulation is appropriate in the context of this chapter.

---

* Concentration is indicated by brackets: $[Na^+]$; absolute amounts are indicated by parentheses: (Na^+).

INCREASE IN [NA⁺]

Cause. Although hypernatremia is most commonly associated with dehydration, this is not always so. When dehydration is part of the picture, elevated [Na⁺] results from net loss of water from the body in excess of net loss of Na⁺. This is accentuated when the intake of fluids consists of solutions containing Na⁺. If the total amount of fluid consumed is less than that necessary for the body's obligatory water loss (primarily insensible water), then any Na⁺ in such fluids is likely to be retained, adding to the likelihood of hypernatremia. This becomes particularly important if dehydration has developed to the point that renal function is impaired, thus limiting the kidney's ability to excrete the added Na⁺. When fluid intake is larger, the problem of hypernatremia may still arise if the Na⁺ content of the fluid is higher than the renal excretory system can handle.

The other group of conditions leading to hypernatremia involve the system utilized by the body for regulating the osmolarity of body fluids. This system, like most in the body, has three basic components: a sensing mechanism, a message mechanism, and an effector mechanism. In the osmolarity regulating system, the sensor is in the brain, probably in the hypothalamus; the ultimate message is the liberation of ADH from the posterior pituitary; the effector is the urine concentrating mechanism of the renal tubules. Abnormalities of function in any of these areas can result in hypernatremia.

At the level of the sensor, various CNS lesions have been implicated in the development of hypernatremia, i.e., brain tumors, cerebral hemorrhage, meningitis, trauma, subdural hematoma, and nonspecific brain damage. The message center can also be damaged by most of the same CNS lesions, and it is particularly prone to interference from a craniopharyngioma because of the location (adjacent to the pituitary gland) of that tumor. In some cases ADH production, storage, or release will fail, and yet there will be no identifiable lesion. In children, especially in infants, hypernatremia in the absence of obvious cause frequently indicates a congenital defect in the renal tubular concentrating mechanism. These children, predominantly males, are unresponsive to either exogenous or endogenous ADH, and they require high volumes of fluid with very low solute concentration to prevent the occurrence of hypernatremia. Other causes of failure to concentrate urine are rarely as profound as that seen with nephrogenic diabetes insipidus, and therefore they are far less likely to result in hypernatremia.

Implications. Hypernatremia is a term often used interchangeably with the terms hyperosmolarity and hypertonicity. The last two terms refer to increases in total solute concentration of body water (increased osmolarity). Because Na^+ is the predominant cation of the ECF, any significant increase in $[Na^+]$ cannot be offset by a decrease in the concentration of any other extracellular cation. Therefore the results of an elevation in $[Na^+]$ are an associated rise in some or all extracellular anion concentrations and, of necessity, an increase in extracellular osmolarity. The ability of water to cross the cell membrane in response to osmolar differences leads to a net shift of water from the cells to the ECF, thereby creating a hyperosmolar or hypertonic state throughout the body water. Thus the result of hypernatremia is hyperosmolarity, or hypertonicity, but the reverse is not necessarily true. Hyperosmolarity may result from an increase in the concentration of nonionized solute (urea or glucose), and hypernatremia is usually not present. Thus the terms are not synonymous under these circumstances.

As mentioned in the chapter on volume disorders, the principal effect of hypernatremia is the creation of marked intracellular dehydration. The organ most affected is the brain, because of its fixed container. If the acute loss of brain volume is severe enough, blood vessels bridging between the skull and the brain are disrupted and extracerebral hemorrhage occurs. Other changes, especially in cell function, are likely to occur, but they are less well documented.

Detection.   Both historical data and information gained by physical examination are useful as indications of hypernatremia, but determination of the serum value of $[Na^+]$ is essential for establishing the finding. The elements of history that may be significant are often in several constellations of clues. One includes marked diarrhea, vomiting, gastrointestinal suction and/or other fluid losses, reduced intake of fluid, and an intake of fluids containing any appreciable Na^+. This group characterizes the hypernatremia associated with gastroenteritis. Another set of symptoms includes failure to thrive, unexplained fevers, eagerness for water, and a family history of avid water drinkers; these are suggestive of the hypernatremia of nephrogenic diabetes insipidus. A third type of history involves head trauma, headaches, polyuria, history of encephalitis or meningitis, and other neurologic complaints; these are related to the group of etiologies centered on the sensor-messenger complex: the hypothalamic–posterior-pituitary axis.

The physical findings due to the hypernatremia include fever, dehydration, and depression. The dehydration is less evident than the historical data would suggest, because there is some sparing of extracellular volume at the expense of intracellular volume. There is more evidence of CNS depression and/or irritability than can be explained by the primary process; this is due to cellular dehydration in the CNS. The doughlike or brawny characteristic noted when examining tissue turgor is fairly characteristic of hypernatremia, but initially its presence is highly variable. This finding may become more apparent as rehydration occurs. The doughy turgor is believed to be related to a change in the characteristics of the elastin and collagen fibers resulting from the high ionic strength of the ambient fluid.

The laboratory data base must include an elevation of serum Na^+ in excess of 155 mEq/liter to be significant, but it may also include elevated CSF protein concentration, hypocalcemia, elevated $[Cl^-]_s$, and reduced $[HCO_3^-]_s$. The urine may be concentrated, or in the presence of hypernatremic dehydration, surprisingly the urine may show an osmolarity of only 75–400 mOsm/liter (specific gravity 1.001–1.015). The EKG usually shows no characteristic change, but the EEG may be diffusely abnormal, sometimes with seizure pattern, in the absence of other CNS disease.

Management. The goal in managing hypernatremia is to provide an excess of fluid over solute at a rate that will reduce the $[Na^+]$ to a normal range in approximately 48–72 hours. Although correction of elevated $[Na^+]$ theoretically could be accomplished with an electrolyte-free solution (using glucose to maintain osmolarity), such an approach generally results in too rapid a decrease in $[Na^+]$, with consequent cellular overhydration. The rapid shift of water into the brain may create new CNS manifestations, especially seizures. If rehydration without sodium is to proceed slowly to avoid CNS difficulties, repair of the volume deficit is inordinately slowed. Actually, an adequately hydrated individual with hypernatremia can be treated intravenously by judicious administration of 5% dextrose in water or orally with essentially electrolyte-free fluids. (See Chapter 4 for more details of treatment.)

DECREASE IN $[Na^+]$

Cause. As might be expected, many of the causes of hyponatremia are the opposite of those producing hypernatremia. In general, the causes of either condition can be divided into those producing differential losses or retentions of water and solute (Table 5-1). The conditions created when the change in body water exceeds a proportional change in body solute, either as loss or gain (the upper horizontal row in Table 5-1), are more common than those generated by either loss or retention of solute in excess of water. Thus when hyponatremia (or hypernatremia) occurs, it is more likely to be the result of change in body water in excess of change in body solute rather than change in solute in excess of change in water.

Relatively few cases of hyponatremic dehydration secondary to gastroenteritis occur in the United States, but in those areas of the world where serious malnutrition is more common, the frequency of hypona-

Table 5-1
Serum Sodium as a Function of Changes in
Losses and Retention*

	Excess Loss	Excess Retention
Water < solute	Hypernatremia	Hyponatremia
Solute < water	Hyponatremia	Hypernatremia

* Changes in body fluids resulting from body fluid losses in which water loss exceeds solute loss (producing hypernatremia) and in which solute loss exceeds water loss (producing hyponatremia). Equivalently, retention of fluids in which water retention exceeds solute retention produces hyponatremia, and retentions in which solute retention exceeds water retention produce hypernatremia.

tremia with gastroenteritis is much greater. The reason for this difference may be related to the differences in the responsible mechanisms. In the United States, hyponatremia from gastroenteritis arises primarily from net solute losses exceeding net water losses—the less common underlying mechanism. In the presence of severe malnutrition, there appears to be an underlying element of water retention in excess of solute retention prior to onset of dehydration. Then gastroenteritis may cause hyponatremia more frequently when associated with preexisting malnutrition.

Another infrequent but serious form of hyponatremia, with solute loss exceeding water loss, is that due to adrenal cortical insufficiency. The major solute lost is Na^+, and its loss exceeds that of water. It was previously stated that hyponatremia was more often associated with water retention in excess of solute retention than with solute loss in excess of water loss. Substantiating this statement is the fact that the hyponatremia of adrenal insufficiency is more often seen when the disease is not initially suspected and the associated dehydration is treated with a solution that is hypotonic in regard to electrolyte content. Such therapy produces water retention in excess of solute and thus fits into the more common mechanism generating hyponatremia.

The most common causes of hyponatremia (water retention > solute retention) are related to the ADH system, but in many individuals it is unclear at what point the system is being affected. A frequently used label under these circumstances is "inappropriate ADH activity," but the difficulty may be with sensor, messenger, or effector. The end result tends to be water retention in excess of solute retention, rather than solute loss in excess of water loss. Thus, of the various actions of ADH, the problem results more from excess water retained in the body than from Na^+ lost in the urine, although sodium losses must play some part in the picture.

The conditions in which the label inappropriate ADH activity has been applied include the following:

1. Chronic illnesses, including tuberculosis, cancer, and malnutrition. The hyponatremia in these conditions may well be related to a disorder at the sensing level of the ADH system. It may or may not be a related finding that the hyponatremia in these illnesses is asymptomatic in itself.

2. CNS lesions that have an irritative effect on the hypothalamic–posterior-pituitary axis and thereby act at the messenger level. Meningitis is a common example of a process that has at times been incriminated in the generation of inappropriate ADH activity. These episodes tend to be both acute and symptomatic.

3. Nonosmotic stimuli to the ADH message system. These include pain, stress, anxiety, burns, surgical procedures, and a variety of drugs and toxins. Surgical procedures, trauma, and serious acute infections all seem to provoke an ADH response and a resultant tendency to hyponatremia. Provision of electrolyte-poor or electrolyte-free fluids in such situations may enhance the degree of hyponatremia. Such cases are both acute and symptomatic.

Implications.   The results of hyponatremia depend on whether there is associated dehydration. If dehydration is present, there is relatively greater loss of ECF. This occurs because the lost Na^+ is primarily extracellular and the ICF then has a higher osmolarity, so that fluid shifts from the ECF into the cells. The predominance of ECF loss is also reflected in the vascular space; the reduced plasma volume leads to a higher prevalence of hypotension, poor renal function, and shock.

If dehydration is not present, and if the course is relatively acute, there is increasing difficulty in excreting fluid load, which leads to oliguria and eventually anuria. There is also clouding of the sensorium, and agitation may become prominent. The patient can appear acutely ill, but no well-defined physiologic mechanism has been elucidated to explain any of these findings. Contrary to expectations, serum ADH levels may be elevated. ADH elevation suggests that secretion of ADH may be the cause of the problem, because one would expect the result of hyponatremia to be low levels of ADH.

If the process is chronic and/or if it involves the sensing mechanism itself, there are few manifestations due to the hyponatremia per se, and it appears that there is a general reduction in the osmolarity of all body fluids. As the chronic process improves, there is a gradual increase in $[Na^+]$, probably reflecting an increase in cellular osmolarity.

Detection.   The historical data are of major importance in understanding the etiology of hyponatremia and planning rational management. If the patient has a chronic process and does not appear symptomatic, a watchful approach is justified. On the other hand, if the process is acute (which at times can be superimposed on a chronic process), and if the patient's symptoms may be related to the hyponatremia, then more active intervention is required.

The physical findings in symptomatic patients may include pallor, hypotension, tachycardia, confusion, anxiety, and hyporeflexia. The laboratory can provide both definitive and supportive information. The definitive value is a low serum $[Na^+]$. Although a value for $[Na^+]_s$ of less than 135 mEq/liter may be considered to define hyponatremia, there are rarely significant therapeutic problems unless the $[Na^+]_s$ is less than 125 mEq/liter. The supportive information may include mild azotemia, which suggests impaired renal perfusion and failure to establish diuresis of hypotonic urine in the presence of adequate hydration and hyponatremia.

Management. In the presence of dehydration and hyponatremia, fluid replacement should be calculated as usual, and then the quantity of additional Na^+ to be added should be estimated on the basis of repairing half the concentration deficit in the first 24 hours. Such calculations are related to the total body water, as the hypotonicity affects all body fluids equally.

EXAMPLES

EXAMPLE 1.   A 2-year-old male infant weighing 14 kg appears to be 10% dehydrated (from gastroenteritis) and has a $[Na^+]_s$ of 120 mEq/liter. He is afebrile, and there is no evidence of other causes of fluid losses.

The fluid calculation provides a maintenance figure of 37.5 ml/kg for IWL, 47 ml/kg for urinary needs, and 30 ml/kg for ongoing gastrointestinal losses—a total of 115 ml/kg. If he is 10% dehydrated, it may be decided to repair two-thirds of that in the first day (65 ml/kg). The total of maintenance and repair is 180 ml/kg. Normally this fluid would be provided initially with a $[Na^+]$ of 75 mEq/liter, and after about 6 hours as a solution containing $[Na^+]$ = 45 mEq/liter and $[K^+]$ = 30 mEq/liter. Total fluids would be 180 ml/kg × 14 kg = 2520 ml.

To improve hydration quickly, one-third of the total fluid may be given in the first 6 hours and the remainder in the next 18 hours. First 6 hours: (⅓) × 2520 = 840/6 = 140 ml/hour. Next 18 hours: 2520 − 840 = 1680; 1680/18 = 93 ml/hour.

To calculate the additional Na^+, two-thirds of body weight is body water; (⅔) × 14 = 9.333 liters. Na^+ deficit = 140 − 120 = 20 mEq/liter. The first day's repair is one-half of deficit = 10 mEq/liter. Na^+ needed = 10 × 9.333 = 93 mEq/liter.

To calculate the added $[Na^+]$ in intravenous fluids, 93 mEq/2.52 liters = 37 mEq/liter.

The $[Na^+]$ in the initial fluid (for the first 6 hours) equals the basic amount plus added $Na^+ = 75 + 37 = 112$ mEq/liter, and in the remaining 18 hours, $45 + 37 = 82$ mEq/liter.

At the end of 24 hours, the patient should be reassessed, reexamined, and weighed again; new electrolyte values should be obtained. New calculations will be based on this reevaluation.

If there is no evidence of dehydration, the problem is more difficult, and there are two classes of patients who must be considered: those with hyponatremia but no clinical manifestations of the hyponatremia and those who are symptomatic as a result of the hyponatremia itself.

Without evidence of hyponatremic symptomatology and with known chronic illness, watchful waiting, careful weighing, evaluation of food and fluid intake and output, and possibly mild fluid restriction may be appropriate.

In the presence of symptoms and signs of hyponatremia following acute onset, the response should vary with the acuteness and severity of the problem. At one extreme is a program such as that indicated above for the asymptomatic individual. The next most active step is to restrict fluid intake markedly and add oral salt as indicated; if parenteral fluids are required, either isotonic saline ($[Na^+] = 155$ mEq/liter) or a multielectrolyte solution with $[Na^+] = 120$ mEq/liter and $[K^+] = 30$ mEq/liter can be used to meet the patient's total fluid needs. In the most critical situation, where time and fluid volume are limiting, hypertonic saline ($3\% = 500$ mEq/liter) is provided. The calculation of the amount required is similar to that in the preceding example, except that no maintenance or repair fluids are given and all oral intake is stopped.

EXAMPLE 2.   A 5-year-old girl has been given only 5% dextrose in water during and after surgical repair of a compound fracture and debridement of wounds suffered in an automobile accident. She appears well hydrated, but she is pale and hypotensive and has a rapidly diminishing urine output. Her $[Na^+]_s = 110$ mEq/liter. Her weight is 21 kg. Body water = 60% of body weight = $0.6 \times 21 = 12.6$ liters. Na^+ deficit = $140 - 110 = 30$ mEq/liter. Na^+ required initially is one-half the deficit × body water = $15 \times 12.6 = 189$ mEq. Volume of 3% NaCl (500 mEq/liter = 0.5 mEq/ml) = $189/0.5 = 378$ ml.

This salt solution will be administered in a period of 4–6 hours, and the patient will be reevaluated after that time. If improvement is noted, and if the new $[Na^+]_s = 125$ mEq/liter (the calculated value), the same amount of 3% NaCl could be given, or a less concentrated (but at least isotonic) salt solution containing the same total amount of Na^+ could be administered.

The difficult situation is that in which dehydration is not a problem but in which the history, physical examination, and laboratory findings indicate hyponatremia in a very ill person, although it is not possible to be certain to what degree (if any) the findings are the result of the hyponatremia. The use of hypertonic saline can be lifesaving if the patient is acutely hyponatremic; however, if the patient's low Na^+ is secondary to a more chronic condition,* the acute overload of the vascular system induced by a hypertonic infusion could be fatal. Under these circumstances it is usually of little benefit and of equal or greater risk to use large volumes of isotonic solution. Therefore the approach recommended is that one calculate the amount of hypertonic saline needed to correct the Na^+ deficit by 50% and then divide that amount into three portions, giving one-third in 2 hours, waiting 2 hours, reassessing, and proceeding with the next third if the patient is improving or at least is no worse. The same procedure is followed for the subsequent third of the calculated amount of 3% NaCl. The major problems that can arise are pulmonary edema and/or congestive failure. It is mandatory when trying to correct hyponatremia with parenteral fluids, and especially when giving 3% NaCl, to prohibit all oral intake and to discontinue all other intravenous fluids.

Potassium

Although potassium is the principal monovalent cation of the ICF and sodium is the principal cation of the ECF, that is about the extent of similarity between these two ions. The total K^+ of the body consists of that K^+ within the active metabolic cells (which is the largest fraction), a lesser amount in bone, and a small amount in the ECF. The amounts present in a 10-kg child are illustrated by Table 5-2.

Although cellular K^+ is related to discrete subcellular structures, it behaves metabolically as though it consists of three fractions: a stable fraction that cannot be lost if life is to continue (about 60%–70% of the ICF $[K^+]_i$) and two labile fractions, one that is readily labile (10%–15%) and one that is less readily labile (20%–25%). The readily labile K^+ varies with changes in intake of K^+, calories, Na^+, etc. Alteration in the quantity of labile $[K^+]_i$ does not appear to have any measurable impact on bodily functions. The labile fraction that is more difficult to change is the fraction that takes part in those conditions leading to K^+ deficiency, and it is depletion of this fraction that creates hypokalemia and leads to associated symptomatology.

It is impossible to measure the total K^+ of the body by available clinical methods and impossible to measure the concentration of K^+ in the ICF ($[K^+]_i$). Thus our knowledge of the state of K^+ metabolism in a particular patient is limited, because the ion is essentially an intracellular one, and we have no simple methods for determining intracellular ionic concentrations. A further restriction involved in consideration of K^+

---

* Some of the more important conditions in which asymptomatic hyponatremia may occur are miliary tuberculosis, tuberculous meningitis, chronic cardiac failure with prolonged diuretic therapy, diarrhea in the presence of chronic malnutrition, and debilitating malignancies.

Table 5-2
Potassium Distribution in the Body*

Body Composition	Weight or Volume (kg or liter)	[K⁺] (mEq/kg or mEq/liter)	(K⁺) (mEq)
Total body	10.0 kg	56	560
Body fat	1.5 kg	0	0
Lean body mass	8.5 kg		
Body solids	2.5 kg	16	40
Body water	6.0 liters		
ICW	3.5 liters	145	508
ECW	2.5 liters	5	12

* Illustration of the concept that the bulk of potassium in the body exists in the intracellular water, with a small amount in body solids (primarily in bone) and the smallest amount in the ECF.

metabolism within the cells is that the intracellular K^+ is not uniformly distributed in the subcellular structure. There is, as well, no direct proportionality between intracellular and extracellular concentrations of K^+ (see paragraphs on detection). As a result of these limitations, the discussion of hyperkalemia and hypokalemia is focused on the extracellular changes and effects. The terms hyperkalemia and hypokalemia refer to increased and decreased blood levels and do not necessarily reflect intracellular concentration of K^+.

HYPERKALEMIA

Cause. The concentration of K^+ inside the cell is 20–30 times the concentration of K^+ in serum. Any significant destruction of cells, loss of permeability by cell membranes, or decrease in function of the Na^+–K^+ pump (an energy-requiring process that maintains the concentration gradients across the cell wall) will result in a rapid and measurable rise in serum $[K^+]$. Normally the kidney excretes this added K^+ through its processes of filtration, reabsorption, and tubular secretion. However, should the loss from cells exceed the rate at which the kidney can excrete K^+, the serum $[K^+]$ must rise. Causes of hyperkalemia can be divided into those related to cellular K^+ loss and those related to impaired renal excretion of K^+.

Cells may be destroyed, damaged, or metabolically altered, releasing K^+ and producing hyperkalemia. Infarction, trauma (both accidental and surgical), burns, radiotherapy, and chemotherapy have all been responsible for sufficient cell destruction and cell damage to cause hyperkalemia. Metabolic states that can result in K^+ release from cells are generally catabolic; they include uncontrolled diabetes mellitus, especially with ketoacidosis, untreated adrenocortical insufficiency, and hyperthyroidism.

It must be remembered that even in those disease states where total body K^+ is depleted, there may be transient elevation of $[K^+]_s$. Those processes that are characterized by total K^+ depletion occur because the cells are losing K^+ rapidly. This K^+ goes into the ECF and then out in the urine. If there is temporary renal functional impairment (i.g., from dehydration), the cellular loss of K^+ continues, and serum $[K^+]$ can rise rapidly and even reach toxic levels.

Inadequate renal handling of K^+ can occur either because the load presented is excessive or because the kidney's excretory capacity is diminished. All the causes for excessive release of K^+ from cells can contribute more K^+ to the ECF than the kidney may be able to handle effectively. Another important source of extra K^+ is potassium provided orally or parenterally. In healthy people the potassium consumed orally is rarely of sufficient amount to produce significant elevation of $[K^+]_s$. The tissue of small infants can acquire relatively large amounts of K^+ (about 3 mEq/kg body weight per day) as a function of growth, and in older children and adults the healthy mature kidneys can excrete any K^+ not needed by cells.

An interesting experiment on newborn animals illustrates the important role played by tissue growth. Two groups of newborn rats were studied: in one group the rats were given known amounts of water with the same amount of potassium as in rat's milk; rat's milk was the diet of the second group. The second group showed no evidence of an increase in $[K^+]_s$, but those in the group given water and equal K^+ had marked hyperkalemia, and some died as a result. Without the protein and other nutrients of milk, the infant animals were not anabolic and did not grow; thus their tissues were unable to utilize the oral K^+. Because of immature functioning, the infant rat kidneys were unable to excrete the oral intake of K^+, and hyperkalemia resulted. When the animals were growing, the kidneys were not required to excrete the K^+ because it was taken up by the newly forming cells.

For many years it was thought that the bowel could not absorb toxic amounts of K^+; so oral administration of K^+ was considered to be safe. When specific K^+ therapy was considered important in fluid therapy, there was great reluctance to attempt parenteral administration because the safeguard of bowel absorption would be lacking. Subcutaneous clysis was considered the next best alternative, as it was thought that there would be slower absorption from these tissues and some sort of safeguard would still be present. Once it was appreciated that ionic equilibrium between plasma and normal subcutaneous tissue fluid was rapidly established and that the ions behaved as they would in any two fluids separated by a semipermeable membrane, intravenous administration was undertaken. It remains essential, however, to recognize that any K^+ provided orally or parenterally that is not taken up by cells must be excreted by the kidney, or it will accumulate in the ECF and produce hyperkalemia.

Adequate kidney function is necessary for proper regulation of serum $[K^+]$. In the absence of excessive tissue loss of K^+ and in the absence of added K^+ intake, hyperkalemia will not ensue even though renal function may be as low as 20% of normal. Below this level of function, hyperkalemia may begin to be a problem on a usual level of potassium intake. With somewhat better function (but still less than normal), hyperkalemia may occur if K^+ supplement is given or if tissue damage or breakdown occurs. Thus it is crucial that some clinical assessment of renal function be undertaken before K^+ administration to any patient.

Transient hyperkalemia may occur in persons without tissue breakdown and with normal renal function if K^+ is administered in too large an amount or is given too rapidly. Limits (although somewhat arbitrary) have been established for parenteral K^+ therapy: (1) The total amount of K^+ should not exceed 3–4 mEq/kg body weight per day. (2) The concentration should not exceed 30–40 mEq/liter of infusing solution. Both of these rules can be modified under special circumstances, but one must be certain why it is being done and what risks are entailed in doing so.

EXAMPLE. A 33-kg 10-year-old child is being treated for diabetic ketoacidosis. After 4 hours of treatment with insulin and a solution of NaCl and $NaHCO_3$, the serum $[K^+]$ is 4.0 mEq/liter. The child is voiding adequately, and there is no history of renal disease. BUN is normal, and the urine contains no protein, red blood cells, white blood cells, or casts. The chief resident physician suggests that 100 mEq of K^+ be added to the remaining intravenous fluids for that 24 hours (approximately 3000 ml). This would provide a concentration of 30 mEq/liter and would not exceed 3 mEq of K^+ per kilogram of body weight. The first-year resident in charge of the patient is called away before he has an opportunity to write the order. Because it is an extremely busy service and a particularly frantic day, the resident is distracted from writing the order for the K^+ for about 18 hours. Eventually the resident recalls the incident and proceeds to write the order when there are only 300 ml of fluid left to run for that 24-hour period. What order should be written?

Feeling chagrined (and not thinking too well) the resident writes the order: "Add 100 mEq K^+ to remaining I. V. fluids." The nurse proceeds to do this. Shortly thereafter the patient is found dead in bed. The concentration of potassium in the infusion was found to be in excess of 250 mEq/liter.

The proper order would have been, "add 10 mEq of K^+ to the remaining 300 ml of fluid," and then the final concentration would have been about 33 mEq/liter. Although the patient would not have received the total

Table 5-3
EKG and Serum Potassium*

Serum [K⁺]	Sequence of EKG Manifestations (primarily seen in limb lead II)
7–9 mEq/liter	Elevation and peaking of T wave
	Widening of QRS complex
	Loss of P wave
8–10 mEq/liter	Broad QRS complex, proceeding to sine wave pattern
>10–11 mEq/liter	Cessation of electrical activity

* Effects of elevation in serum potassium on the EKG are shown for increasing levels of serum potassium. These effects and serum potassium ranges must be considered approximations, because the concentrations of other ions in the serum and the concentration of potassium intracellularly also affect the changes in the EKG.

amount of K^+ that had been planned, there would have been no practical way to accomplish that at that late time.

Implications.   Hyperkalemia may suggest several things: unusual cell catabolism, cell damage, cell destruction, excessive intake, or abnormal renal function—acute or chronic, functional (as in shock), or structural. The etiology must be ascertained for rational management. The direct effects of the hyperkalemia itself are primarily seen in cardiac function. Transmission of cardiac impulses is dependent on (among other things) the potential generated by the ratio of intracellular to extracellular potassium. If one assumes an intracellular $[K^+]$ of 150 mEq/liter and an extracellular $[K^+]$ of 5 mEq/liter, a ratio of 30:1 would exist normally. A rise or fall in intracellular $[K^+]$ of 25 mEq/liter would change the ratio to 35:1 or 25:1; but a 3-mEq/liter rise of extracellular $[K^+]$ would create a ratio of about 20:1. A change in the ICF:ECF ratio of $[K^+]$ from 30:1 to 20:1 is sufficient to create changes in cardiac impulse transmission that will be reflected in the EKG (see Fig. 4-3).

The changes noted on the EKG are not directly related to $[K^+]_s$ because of the variability of intracellular $[K^+]$ and the concentrations of other ions involved in neuromuscular excitability, such as Ca^{++}, Mg^{++}, Na^+, and H^+. However, the sequences of EKG changes and their relationships to approximate $[K^+]_s$ levels are relatively well understood (Table 5-3).

Detection.   Other than those historical, physical, and laboratory findings that are consonant with the basic etiologic process, there are few findings related to hyperkalemia except the serum [K⁺] and the EKG. One should examine the serum and EKG when the patient has a history of (or when there are findings of) the following: anuria, oliguria, severe dehydration, extensive trauma, burns, prolonged surgery, shock, any period of hypotension, severe sepsis, transfusion reaction, intense radiotherapy or chemotherapy for solid tumors or leukemia, massive internal bleeding including gastrointestinal bleeding, acute nephritis, or azotemia from any cause. It is remarkable how high the $[K^+]_s$ can become at times without any external evidence of hyperkalemia.

Management. Once hyperkalemia is recognized in a patient, it can constitute a true medical emergency. One of the first tasks of the physician is to examine the EKG for evidence of cardiac toxicity. If minimal changes have occurred, such as an elevated and peaked T wave without QRS-complex or P-wave abnormality, one can afford to temporize at least long enough to ascertain the background and determine whether the $[K^+]_s$ is still rising or has plateaued. Specific therapy may involve four separate mechanisms: diluting the ECF, creating chemical antagonism to the membrane effects of K⁺, increasing the cellular uptake of K⁺, and removing K⁺ from the body. The armamentarium for these endeavors includes NaCl and $NaHCO_3$ solutions, glucose solutions, calcium gluconate, cation-exchange resins (Kayexalate), peritoneal dialysis, and extracorporeal dialysis.

Although there are differences of opinion about which therapy is most appropriate in terms of sequence, timing, and efficacy, there is sufficient consensus to suggest at least one approach. The initial treatment, if severe cardiotoxicity is present, is to give a 10% solution of calcium gluconate* intravenously. The amount recommended is 0.05–0.15 g of the salt per kilogram of body weight; this is equivalent to 0.5–1.5 ml of the 10% solution per kilogram of body weight (5–15 mg of Ca⁺⁺). It would be appropriate to choose a 1.0-ml/kg initial dose. This should be given very slowly intravenously while continuously monitoring cardiac rate (and EKG, if possible), using bradycardia as evidence of a "toxic" effect of the calcium. The calcium acts as a direct antagonist to the cardiac effects of potassium, and immediate improvement in the EKG should be apparent. There will be no change in the $[K^+]_s$.

The next modality may be glucose, saline, or bicarbonate solutions. Glucose tends to reduce serum [K⁺] by increasing cellular uptake of K⁺ and by dilution of the ECF. Some authors recommend simultaneous administration of insulin with hypertonic glucose (20%–50% glucose intravenously using 0.5 g/kg with 0.1 unit of regular insulin per kilogram). If

---

* Ten milliliters of 10% calcium gluconate = 1 g of calcium gluconate = 93 mg of elemental calcium.

Table 5-4
Modalities for Immediate Treatment
of Hyperkalemia*

Calcium gluconate: 0.1 g/kg; 1 ml/kg (10% solution)
Glucose: 0.5 g/kg ± insulin 0.1 unit/kg
NaCl: isotonic, 10 ml/kg; 3%, 3 ml/kg
NaHCO$_3$: 2 mEq/kg
Kayexalate: 0.5 g/kg

---

* Summary of medications that can be used to treat
hyperkalemia. The most effective for immediate treatment are calcium gluconate and glucose. For long-term
management, the exchange resin Kayexalate is the only
useful agent short of dialysis.

either a large volume of 5% glucose or hypertonic glucose is to be used,
the cardiac status should be evaluated carefully, because the resulting
increased plasma volume will increase the venous return significantly.
The average child (nondiabetic) can metabolize glucose at about 1 g/
kg/hour. Thus it is reasonable to administer 0.5–1 g/kg as an initial intravenous "push" (2.5–5.0 ml of 20% glucose per kilogram or 10–20 ml of
5% glucose per kilogram), and a good starting point is to give 1 ml of 50%
glucose per kilogram. There is no strong evidence as to the value of adding
insulin in nondiabetic persons, but if one chooses to give insulin, 0.1
unit/kg can be given with the glucose.

Sodium chloride can be given as an isotonic solution (0.85%) or as a
hypertonic solution (3%). In either case the action is primarily to dilute the
ECF; there is also a slight cardiac anti-K$^+$ effect from the increase in [Na$^+$].
If isotonic NaCl is used, 10 ml/kg can be given relatively rapidly. More or
less the same effect can be obtained with 3% NaCl at 3 ml/kg. The total
amount of fluid given is less with 3% NaCl, but the impact on the plasma
volume is about the same, from the point of view of both cardiac work and
potassium dilution, since the fluid shift that is required to attain osmotic
equilibrium when giving 3% NaCl at 3 ml/kg amounts to an additional 7
ml/kg.

Alternatively, an equivalent amount of Na$^+$ can be given as NaHCO$_3$.
The recommended amount is 2 mEq/kg. The effects of the Na$^+$ are the
same, but there is potentially an additive effect in reducing [H$^+$]$_s$, which
may also antagonize the cardiac muscle effects of K$^+$ to some extent.
These treatments are summarized in Table 5-4.

All these measures have relatively brief effects, and none removes
K$^+$ from the body, although use of Na$^+$ and glucose solutions may produce some diuresis (if renal function is present) and thereby lead to some
additional K$^+$ excretion. The first measure available for significant elimination of K$^+$ from the body is use of a cation-exchange resin (Kayexalate).

This material can be given orally or rectally as a 20% suspension in a 5% glucose solution. The amount to be given is 0.5 g/kg, and this can be repeated two or three times in 24 hours. Administration of the resin either orally or rectally can be undertaken as soon as the hyperkalemia becomes known. From 4 to 12 hours may be required for the resin to produce a significant fall in $[K^+]_s$. In the interim, the short-term approaches involving Ca^{++}, glucose, or $NaCl$ should be started. If there is progressive deterioration in the EKG or continuing rise in $[K^+]_s$, peritoneal dialysis is appropriate. When hyperkalemia is accompanied by other fluid and electrolyte disorders and when it may be a severe and prolonged process, peritoneal dialysis should be instituted as soon as possible and continued as long as the problem persists. In those institutions in which extracorporeal dialysis is available and is used effectively for children, that method of K^+ removal may also be considered. Extracorporeal dialysis probably offers a slight advantage over peritoneal dialysis in K^+ removal, but it also carries a greater risk for the patient.

HYPOKALEMIA

Whether total body (K^+) is decreased, normal, or increased, reduced renal function may produce an elevated serum $[K^+]$. Similarly, because of possible alteration in renal function, a normal level of $[K^+]_s$ gives no indication of the adequacy of total body (K^+). By contrast, a low level of $[K^+]_s$ is always indicative of reduced body (K^+). When hypokalemia is present, it is certain that total K^+ deficiency exists. This occurs because the intracellular supply of K^+ is very large compared to the amount of K^+ in the ECF, and the equilibria are such that as long as any easily mobilizable K^+ is left in the cell, serum $[K^+]$ will be maintained at least at a normal level. Serum $[K^+]$ falls only when the $(K^+)_i$ is down to the point where the less labile K^+ is beginning to be depleted. The reverse, however, is not true, as total K^+ deficit may be present in association with low, normal, or elevated levels of $[K^+]_s$, depending on the amount and rate of K^+ intake and on renal function.

Cause. As is suggested by the preceding paragraph, the cause of hypokalemia is total body K^+ deficiency (with the added proviso that K^+ intake is small and renal function is adequate). Total body K^+ deficiency occurs because of excessive losses through the gastrointestinal tract or the kidneys without adequate replacement. Gastrointestinal fluids all contain significant amounts of K^+, so that any large loss of such fluids can, over a period of time, produce a serious K^+ deficit. Diarrhea, vomiting, early ileostomy drainage, continuous gastrointestinal suction, and gastrointestinal fistulas have all been implicated as etiologic factors. A rare form of chronic diarrhea that may have a congenital basis and that is associated with a propensity to develop metabolic alkalosis also can result in marked hypokalemia. Of particular interest is the vomiting associated with pyloric or duodenal obstruction. Gastric secretion loss leads to a direct loss of K^+ and H^+, resulting in metabolic alkalosis with hypokalemia. The acid–base imbalance increases the loss of K^+ from cells, and urinary K^+ losses are marked; thus there is further depletion of K^+ from the body.

Increased urinary K^+ excretion may occur because the kidney has increased amounts of K^+ presented to it via the plasma (amounts derived from other parts of the body) and/or because the renal tubular cells are unable to conserve K^+. In metabolic alkalosis all of these mechanisms apply. In general, cells will lose K^+ during metabolic alkalosis, and renal tubular cells exchange increased amounts of cellular K^+ for the Na^+ of the tubular fluid when there is a decrease in $[H^+]$, as occurs in this acid–base disorder.

The factors that directly affect the loss of K^+ from cells are disorders of acid–base equilibrium and adrenocortical hormones (especially aldosterone). Both metabolic alkalosis and metabolic acidosis result in loss of K^+ from cells. The mechanisms are probably different, but the kidneys play a significant role in each situation, although the details of these interactions remain unclear. The biochemical reactions that lead to K^+ loss as a result of increased aldosterone activity or aldosterone-like activity are also poorly understood. Nevertheless, it is well recognized that hyperaldosteronism, whether endogenous in origin or resulting from administration of mineralocorticoid hormones, results in K^+ deficiency and increased amounts of K^+ in the urine.

Although it is not certain whether the effect of aldosterone on K^+ excretion is primarily at the level of the cell or at the level of the renal tubule,* there are other problems that are known to affect the kidney directly; these include drugs with renal tubular actions (essentially the diuretics) and renal diseases. The diuretics generally interfere with reabsorption of Na^+, but to a greater or lesser extent they also increase K^+ excretion. Those agents that inhibit H^+ excretion by the tubule tend to enhance K^+ losses to the largest extent. Since individual responses to specific drugs will vary to some degree, it is difficult to predict the impact of a particular drug on K^+ handling in a specific patient.

The renal diseases that lead to K^+ depletion are tubular processes that depress the urinary acidification mechanisms. When H^+ cannot be

---

* The effects of aldosterone may be identical at both sites, since the renal tubular cell may behave as any other body cell in this regard, the difference being that when any other cell loses K^+ it goes into the ECF, and when the renal tubular cell loses K^+ it goes into the urine.

exchanged for filtered Na^+, the K^+–Na^+ exchange increases, and greater K^+ losses occur. Renal tubular acidosis is the most common condition in this category. When functional renal tubular damage has occurred in association with severe obstructive uropathy, prolonged severe dehydration with marked oliguria or anuria, marked hypotension or shock, transfusion reactions, or renal toxic agents, then recovery from such an episode may be accompanied by marked losses of K^+ in the urine, resulting in K^+ deficiency and hypokalemia.

The ketoacidosis of diabetes mellitus warrants additional mention, because this process leads to K^+ depletion through several mechanisms operating simultaneously. Insulin deficiency interferes with cell metabolism, and K^+ may be lost from the cell on that basis. Metabolic acidosis occurs, and it further increases cellular loss of K^+. An osmotic diuresis resulting from hyperglycemia leads to losses of water, Na^+, and K^+, and the resulting dehydration increases aldosterone activity, thus adding another kaliuretic effect to the process. When the dehydration becomes severe enough, renal function may decrease, reducing urinary losses of K^+; but the cellular loss of K^+ continues, and hyperkalemia may occur. However, once fluid therapy is instituted and renal function improves, the urinary K^+ loss again increases, and hypokalemia becomes evident, reflecting the whole body K^+ deficiency.

Implications. The significance of hypokalemia is primarily that it represents marked or severe depletion of the K^+ content of cells. The cellular deficiency of K^+ is manifested as impairment in cellular function. It is assumed that cell functions of many varieties and in all body organs are affected, but those dysfunctions that manifest themselves as clinical problems involve skeletal muscle, cardiac muscle, smooth muscle, renal tubules, and possibly the brain. The functional changes are reflected as follows: in skeletal muscle as weakness, which may be quite profound; in cardiac muscle as flattened or negative T waves, prolongation of the Q-T interval, and widening of the QRS complex; in smooth muscle primarily as paralytic ileus; in the kidney tubules as an inability to concentrate urine, with resulting polyuria, and as an increased tendency to excrete H^+ and reabsorb HCO_3^-, manifested by acid urine and metabolic alkalosis.

Detection. A history that is consistent with any of the causes of potassium deficiency should raise the possibility of hypokalemia. Among the most common are severe diarrhea, pyloric stenosis, and diabetes mellitus. The physical findings of muscle weakness, diminished or absent bowel sounds, and abdominal distension are all suggestive of a hypokalemic state. The laboratory results that are supportive include a urine specific gravity below 1.015 (osmolarity < 400 mOsm/liter), the presence of polyuria, evidence of metabolic alkalosis (especially when accompanied by acid or neutral urine pH), and, of most importance, $[K^+]_s$ of less than 3.5 mEq/liter. It should be remembered that in the presence of dehydration or reduced renal function, the initial $[K^+]_s$ may be normal or elevated, but it can become quite low once dehydration is corrected and renal function is restored.

Management. Potassium replacement is the principal therapy, assuming that other appropriate treatment is directed toward the underlying causative condition. Because the cells have a limited rate at which they can restore their K^+ content, and because transient hyperkalemia can be produced by too high a K^+ concentration in intravenous fluids, arbitrary limits on parenteral K^+ have been proposed as 3–4 mEq/kg/day and 30–40 mEq/liter of intravenous fluids. Similar precautions are indicated for oral administration of added K^+. However, these limits can be modified for K^+ given either orally or parenterally when there are large and continuing losses of K^+ that cannot be corrected immediately. One can begin K^+ treatment using the accepted guidelines. If there is little evidence of improvement in the patient's condition or in the level of $[K^+]_s$, a cautious increase in the amount of K^+ being administered is reasonable, provided there is careful monitoring of the $[K^+]_s$ and the EKG. As much as 10 mEq/kg has been given under such unusual circumstances.

Calcium

To some degree each of the ion species of plasma may be bound to the amphoteric serum proteins. For the divalent cations, especially Ca^{++}, the amount bound to serum protein accounts for about half of the total quantity of the ion present in the plasma. The extent of binding varies somewhat with $[H^+]$, but it varies strikingly with protein concentration.

Figure 5-1 is a modification of the McLean-Hastings nomogram relating ionized Ca^{++} to total Ca and serum protein concentrations. Recent studies indicate that actual measurement of the ionic Ca^{++} itself yields values somewhat divergent from those predicted from this nomogram. This may be especially true in newborns. Therefore, when it is possible to measure the Ca^{++} concentration directly, this is preferable to predicting its concentration on the basis of total [Ca] and total serum protein concentration.

Regulation of calcium metabolism involves level of intake, intestinal absorption, renal excretion, and the actions of parathormone, calcitonin, and vitamin D metabolites, particularly 1,25-dihydrotachysterol, or 1,25-$(OH)_2D$. Regulation of serum concentrations of Ca^{++} and regulation of

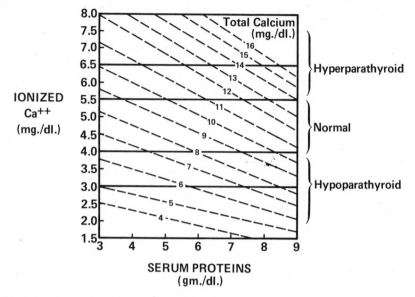

Fig. 5-1. Ionized calcium, total calcium, and serum proteins. Illustration of the relationships among ionized calcium, total calcium, and serum protein concentrations. This is drawn somewhat differently than the traditional representation of these relationships to emphasize the significance of ionized calcium in terms of parathyroid function. For example, using a total calcium concentration of 9 mg/dl, if the serum proteins were 8 g/dl the ionized calcium would be below 4 mg/dl and thereby in the hypoparathyroid range. If the serum proteins were 3 g/dl, with the same total calcium, the ionized calcium would be over 5.5 mg/dl, and this would be in the lower hyperparathyroid range.

serum concentrations of phosphorus (represented as [HPO_4^{--}], the principal form of inorganic phosphorus in serum*) are so closely linked that this discussion will include factors related to both Ca^{++} and HPO_4^{--}. Although complete understanding of the roles of parathormone, vitamin D, and calcitonin in regulating Ca^{++} and HPO_4^{--} metabolism is lacking, enough is known to provide a rational interpretation of many of the observed phenomena.

There are three substances, besides the ions themselves, that have a major controlling effect: parathormone, vitamin D derivatives, and calcitonin. There are four major organs involved, in addition to the thyroid-parathyroid, that are affected by, and in turn affect, the Ca^{++} and HPO_4^{--}

---

* Inorganic phosphorus exists in the serum as phosphate ions. At the normal [H^+] of serum, 40 nEq/liter (pH 7.4), there exist both HPO_4^{--} and $H_2PO_4^-$ in a ratio giving an effective negative change of about 1.8. Such a ratio indicates that the major form of phosphate ion in the serum is HPO_4^{--}; therefore HPO_4^{--} is used in the text but should be interpreted as a mixture of HPO_4^{--} and H_2PO_4.

equilibria: liver, kidney, bone, and gut. The interactions are listed in Table 5-5 and are diagrammed in Figures 5-2 and 5-3.

Parathormone, which is produced in the parathyroid in response to either reduced $[Ca^{++}]_s$ or elevated $[HPO_4^{--}]_s$, has the following effects: it raises $[Ca^{++}]$ by increasing resorption of bone mineral (Ca and P); it enhances distal tubular calcium reabsorption while blocking proximal reabsorption of Ca and P; it plays some part in increasing absorption of Ca and P from the gut and stimulating the kidney to produce the active metabolite of vitamin D: $1,25\text{-}(OH)_2D$. Parathormone generally tends to lower $[HPO_4^{--}]_s$, even though P absorption from the gut is enhanced and P is also increased by resorption of bone; however, the blocking of proximal tubular reabsorption of P tends to dominate the other effects, so that phosphaturia is increased and serum $[HPO_4^{--}]$ falls.

Vitamin D may derive from plant origin as ergosterol or from animal origin as 7-dehydrocholesterol. Each form requires ultraviolet radiation to convert it to an active substance: ergocalciferol, D_2, or cholecalciferol, D_3. In the liver, hydroxylation takes place to form 25-OH-D, which is many times more potent than either D_2 or D_3. However, a subsequent hydroxylation takes place in the kidney and produces either a much more potent product, $1,25\text{-}(OH)_2D$, or an essentially inactive form, $24,25\text{-}(OH)_2D$. Which of these two forms is produced by the kidney depends on the state of Ca and P equilibrium in the body fluids. Phosphorus appears to have the dominant role; when it is normal or increased, the inactive form $24,25\text{-}(OH)_2D$ is made. When the P is low, the active form $1,25\text{-}(OH)_2D$ is the hydroxylation product. As noted earlier, parathormone also stimulates the production of $1,25\text{-}(OH)_2D$. Vitamin D, or more properly its derivative $1,25\text{-}(OH)_2D$, acts to raise serum concentrations of Ca^{++} and HPO_4^{--}. This results from the action of the vitamin in increasing absorption of Ca and P from the gut, increasing reabsorption of Ca and P by the renal tubule, and (conjointly with parathormone) increasing resorption of bone.

Calcitonin, which is actually a peptide with 32 amino acids, is produced by cells found in the parathyroid, thyroid, and thymus glands. The main actions of calcitonin are to lower total serum Ca (both bound and ionized) by inhibiting the actions of $1,25\text{-}(OH)_2D$, lower resorption of bone, lower absorption from the gut, and lower reabsorption from the renal tubules.

HYPERCALCEMIA

Since total serum calcium is what is usually measured in the clinical laboratory, even though the ionized calcium is the physiologically significant moiety, this discussion will consider elevation in terms of total calcium.

Table 5-5

Factors Involved in Regulation of Calcium and Phosphorus*

Organ/Ion	Parathormone	Vitamin D	Calcitonin
Liver		→ conversion of vitamin D to 25-OH-D	
Bone	Resorption of bone	Resorption of bone	Suppressor resorption
Kidney	Blocks proximal reabsorption of Ca and P; increases distal reabsorption of Ca; stimulates production of 1,25-(OH)₂D	→ conversion of 25-OH-D to 24,25-(OH)₂D or 1,25-(OH)₂D, which increases reabsorption of Ca and P	Blocks reabsorption of Ca and P
Gut	Increases absorption of Ca and P directly or indirectly	Increases absorption of Ca and P	Blocks absorption of Ca and P
Normal Ca and P			
Ca↑ P↓ }		→ stimulation of production of 24,25-(OH)₂D	
Ca↓ P↑ }	Stimulates production	→ stimulation of production of 1,25-(OH)₂D	→ stimulation of release

* Illustration of the interrelationships of the effects of parathormone, vitamin D, and calcitonin on calcium and phosphorus metabolism in the various organs of the body. For example, conversion of vitamin D to 25-OH-D occurs in the liver, and both vitamin D and parathormone are necessary for resorption of bone. In the kidney, parathormone blocks proximal reabsorption of calcium and phosphorus, increases distal reabsorption of calcium, and stimulates production of 1,25-(OH)₂D.

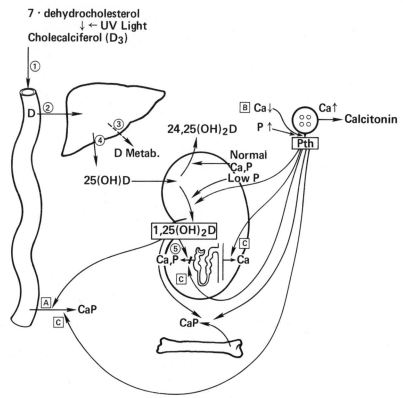

Fig. 5-2. Vitamin D metabolism. Diagrammatic representation of metabolism of vitamin D and its effects on calcium and phosphorus. The circled numbers represent points at which abnormalities can produce disease: (1) Decreased intake of vitamin D will produce D-deficient rickets. (2) Malabsorption of vitamin D will also produce D-deficient rickets. (3 and 4) Liver abnormalities in vitamin D metabolism that can produce a form of rickets that requires increased amounts of vitamin D or other compounds for correction; in this case 25-OH-D would be therapeutic. (5) Lack of responsiveness of the renal tubule to 1,25-(OH)₂D and what may be hypophosphatemic D-resistant rickets. The letters in the squares represent the events that occur in the absence of 1,25-(OH)₂D activity on calcium reabsorption in the bowel. When that occurs (as shown at A), serum calcium falls (as shown at B), with the result that parathormone is stimulated; this, in turn (as shown at C), increases calcium reabsorption in the kidney but blocks proximal tubular calcium and phosphorus reabsorption and stimulates calcium and phosphorus absorption from the bowel. The net result is return of serum calcium toward normal, but diminished serum phosphorus.

CELLULAR ACTIONS OF
PARATHORMONE AND CALCITONIN

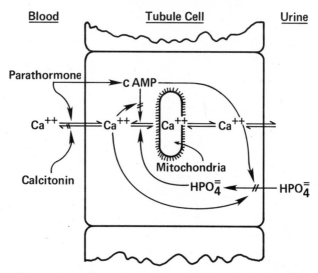

Fig. 5-3.   Cellular actions of parathormone and calcitonin. Some of the postulated interactions among parathormone, calcitonin, calcium, and phosphorus are shown in this schematic diagram of a renal tubular cell. Parathormone increases the transfer of calcium from the blood to the tubular cell and simultaneously increases cyclic AMP activity. The cyclic AMP blocks phosphorus reabsorption. The lowered cellular phosphate reduces the tendency of cytoplasmic calcium to move into the mitochondria; thereby cytoplasmic calcium is increased. It also tends to block phosphate reabsorption, and at the same time it may be transferred back to the blood when reabsorption from the urine increases its cytoplasmic concentration further.

Cause.   One of the common reasons for elevation of serum calcium is that serum proteins are elevated, either as part of dehydration or as part of some disease process (e.g., multiple myeloma). In such circumstances the ionized calcium is normal. Another common reason for elevation of [Ca] is hyperparathyroidism; in this case ionizable $[Ca^{++}]$ is also increased above the normal range, as serum concentrations are usually in the normal range. Vitamin D intoxication (or overdosage) is the third common cause of hypercalcemia. The situation in which excessive amounts of vitamin D are frequently given is in the treatment of vitamin-D-resistant rickets. The amount of vitamin D required to heal vitamin-D-resistant rickets is about the same amount required to produce intoxication. Sudden immobilization, particularly as it is often associated with trauma to bone or fractures of bones, leads to marked mobilization of bone Ca^{++}. This will be accentuated if the person has been receiving moderate amounts of vitamin D—

as most children in the United States do in their vitamin-D-fortified milk. Under such circumstances, more Ca^{++} may be mobilized than the kidney can excrete, so that an elevated $[Ca^{++}]$ results.

Maternal hypoparathyroidism during pregnancy can result in fetal compensation, with hyperparathyroidism and resultant hypercalcemia occurring in the infant shortly after birth. Another form of hypercalcemia in infancy has been termed idiopathic, but it may be a hypersensitivity to amounts of vitamin D that do not produce toxicity in other infants. Characteristic facies and subvalvular aortic stenosis may be present. In the past, some of these patients were English babies who were actually getting quite large amounts of vitamin D because of a higher level of fortification in food than was necessary. In older individuals, hypersensitivity to vitamin D may occur with sarcoidosis or tuberculosis.

Other rare causes of hypercalcemia include tumors (especially with metastases to bone), thyroid disorders, and use of thiazide diuretics.

Implications.   The most serious effect of elevated $[Ca^{++}]_s$ is on the kidney. Initially, the insult is manifested as loss of concentrating ability, with resultant polyuria. If uncorrected, the hypercalcemia can result in progressive renal damage, with loss of glomerular function that can become permanent. Such long-term change is often accompanied by intrarenal calcification of the renal tubule, particularly in the proximal tubule where the initial reabsorption of glomerular filtrate takes place. Whether the calcification is the cause of the progressive renal damage or simply a concomitant is unclear. Calcification can occur in other locations in the body, but in general this process is not itself destructive.

Changes also include neuromuscular irritability characterized by decreased tendon reflexes and bradycardia. Other changes are apparent in the EKG, including shortening of the Q-T interval.

Detection.   A history of high intake of vitamin D or a sudden immobilization, such as in a body cast (especially after trauma), should suggest the possibility of hypercalcemia. Serum $[Ca^{++}]$ should also be measured regularly during management of vitamin-D-resistant rickets. A history of renal calculi should always alert one to the possibility of hyperparathyroidism with hypercalcemia. The symptomatology consists of nausea, anorexia, vomiting, headache, mental confusion, irritability, lethargy, fatigue, constipation, pruritus, polyuria, and polydipsia. There is little on physical examination other than bradycardia and decreased reflexes that is specific for hypercalcemia; so the laboratory becomes the only means of establishing an elevation of $[Ca^{++}]_s$. Low urinary specific gravity that is not appropriate to the patient's condition and the presence of unexplained polyuria should raise the suspicion of hypercalcemia. Serum $[Ca^{++}]$ is the definitive test, and when sending blood for that determination one should also request determination of serum proteins, alkaline phosphatase, and serum inorganic phosphorus. These latter values will assist in evaluating the possibility that the elevated $[Ca^{++}]_s$ may be related either to increased protein concentration or to hyperparathyroidism. The EKG changes are not specific enough to be diagnostic.

Management. There are two elements to the treatment of this electrolyte abnormality, in addition to management of the underlying illness: reducing the intake of vitamin D and calcium and lowering the serum Ca^{++} concentration. Regardless of severity, reductions in intake of vitamin D and calcium are appropriate. Reduction in serum calcium can be accomplished in several ways, depending on the severity of the problem. If the elevated $[Ca^{++}]_s$ is less than 13 Mg/dl,* forcing fluids orally or intravenously, reducing Ca^{++} intake, and stopping all sources of vitamin D will usually suffice. With moderate elevation of $[Ca^{++}]_s$ to 13–15 mg/dl, oral phosphates, prednisone or dexamethasone, intravenous saline, and the diuretic furosemide can be used. Calcitonin (1–5 units/kg/day) has also been used successfully. Elevation of $[Ca^{++}]_s$ higher than 15 mg/dl require prompt treatment. In addition to the use of relatively large amounts of intravenous saline and furosemide (1 mg/kg as a single injection), mithramycin (25 μg/kg intravenously) has been used in adults, but its use has not yet been reported in children. Peritoneal dialysis should also be considered. EDTA can be used intravenously if great caution is exercised (being certain to use the sodium salt without Ca^{++}), as it may lower the $[Ca^{++}]_s$ rapidly and produce cardiac and respiratory arrest; it also has other toxic manifestations. EDTA is administered intravenously in glucose or saline at a concentration of less than 7 mg/ml and in a dose of 50 mg/kg (1.5 g/m²) over a period of 3–4 hours. Serum $[Ca^{++}]$ should be checked frequently, the EKG should be monitored carefully, and calcium gluconate should be immediately available for use as an antagonist if the need arises.

HYPOCALCEMIA

Decreased serum calcium concentrations are significant primarily in terms of the concentration of the unbound ion, Ca^{++}. As mentioned in the general discussion of calcium, ionic concentration can be estimated from total calcium, and serum protein values can be estimated by use of a nomogram. However, actual measurements of ionized calcium do not correlate well with the nomogram estimates, especially in the newborn.

---

* Serum calcium may be expressed as milligrams/deciliter or as milliequivalents/liter. In expressing any value, the number used with the former units will be twice the number used to express the value in the latter units: e.g., 10 mg/dl = 5 mEq/liter.

As a result, it is particularly valuable to obtain measured values for $[Ca^{++}]$, the ion, in hypocalcemic infants.

Cause and Implications.   The causes of hypocalcemia can be classified in terms of organs involved or substances involved. The organs that can be responsible for low $[Ca^{++}]_s$ include the following: (1) the parathyroid gland, because of lack of production of parathormone (hypoparathyroidism); (2) the intestinal tract, since malabsorptive conditions may result in blocked absorption or complexing of calcium, with subsequent loss in stool; (3) the kidney, either because it does not respond to parathormone (pseudohypoparathyroidism) or because it has other tubular disease interfering with calcium reabsorption and subsequent hypercalciuria; (4) the bone, which has the major body stores of calcium, so that increased avidity for Ca^{++} or decreased release of Ca^{++} can produce a lowered $[Ca^{++}]_s$.

The major substances that play a role in maintaining serum calcium are parathormone, calcium, phosphorus, calcitonin, and vitamin D. The interactions of these substances are described in the introductory discussion on calcium. Calcitonin is ordinarily not involved in hypocalcemia. The other substances may be involved simultaneously, as in neonatal tetany, which appears to result from a relative lack of parathormone, from a relative reduction in the kidneys' ability to excrete phosphorus (resulting in elevated serum phosphorus levels), and from poor absorption of calcium when the infant is fed milk with a high ratio of phosphorus to calcium. Maternal hyperparathyroidism may play a role in this condition in some infants.

In an infant or child, rickets can result from lack of vitamin D intake, although this is rare in the United States because almost all milk is now adequately fortified with vitamin D. When vitamin-D-deficiency rickets does occur, the reduced absorption of calcium from the intestinal tract leads to stimulation of the parathyroids. The increased activity of parathormone increases the serum calcium to normal or near normal levels and depresses the serum phosphorus. If there is concomitant low intake of calcium, the serum calcium may still be depressed after these compensations take place. Another circumstance that can produce hypocalcemia in association with simple rickets arises when the amounts of vitamin D activity imparted to the rachitic child are too small, either as exposure to increased sunlight or as prescription of an amount of vitamin D that is too small for full therapeutic response. When either of these events occurs, the rate of deposition of calcium in bone exceeds the increased absorption from the intestine, and hypocalcemia becomes evident.

Other forms of rickets (D-dependent, D-resistant, renal insufficiency with secondary hyperparathyroidism) will manifest hypocalcemia of varying degrees, depending on the intake of calcium, vitamin D, and phosphorus and on the duration of the disease and the degree of renal impairment. The elevation of serum phosphorus may be more impressive than the reduction in serum calcium; so it is important to examine the concentrations of calcium and phosphorus simultaneously when one is concerned about a problem with either ion.

Hypoparathyroidism may occasionally result from thyroid surgery, but more often it is idiopathic in origin. As a cause of hypocalcemia, it becomes increasingly important with increasing age. In children there is a high degree of correlation between hypoparathyroidism and moniliasis. Hypoparathyroidism also occurs as part of a complex disorder involving abnormal function of the adrenal cortex and other endocrine glands. Thymic hypoplasia with hypoparathyroidism (the DiGeorge syndrome) is an important clinical entity to consider, because the finding of low serum calcium may lead to discovery of the immunologic deficiency.

Detection. Hypocalcemia should be suspected whenever there is a sudden alteration in the functioning of the neuromuscular system: tremor, tetany, convulsions, coma, hyperirritability, carpopedal spasm, or laryngospasm. Other physical findings include skeletal abnormalities of rickets and positive Trousseau, Chvostek, and/or peroneal signs.

A history of inadequate vitamin D intake, symptoms of renal insufficiency or malabsorption, frequent infections, convulsions, or monilial infection should alert one to the possibility of hypocalcemia. Among the laboratory findings that may suggest low $[Ca^{++}]_s$ are elevated phosphorus, hypoglycemia (the pathophysiology of this relationship is unclear), elevated $[K^+]$ with low $[Na^+]$ (seen in adrenal insufficiency), and hypomagnesemia. Actual determination of serum calcium, especially the calcium ion, is the sine qua non for establishing the presence of hypocalcemia.

Management. Acute treatment for symptomatic hypocalcemia is with calcium gluconate (10%) given intravenously. An initial injection of 2 ml/kg can be given slowly while monitoring cardiac rate for evidence of bradycardia. Other calcium salts can be given orally; their effects will be slower, although more prolonged. Calcium lactate is commonly used. Calcium chloride has a higher proportion of calcium, but it can produce serious metabolic acidosis, and so it is usually not recommended.

Reduction of phosphorus intake and increases in intake of calcium, vitamin D, the metabolites of vitamin D, derivatives of these compounds, and parathormone all have a role in the long-term management of one or

another of the conditions creating hypocalcemia. However, other resources should be consulted regarding such treatment programs.

Magnesium

The divalent cation Mg^{++} is primarily an intracellular ion that appears
to have important functions in cellular homeostasis, although these functions are not yet well defined. The mean plasma concentration varies in
different series from about 0.8 to 1.0 mM/liter (1.6–2.0 mEq/liter). Mg^{++},
like Ca^{++}, is bound to serum proteins, and about 70% of the serum Mg^{++}
is present in the ultrafiltrate (not bound). Both Ca^{++} and Mg^{++} are probably bound to the same sites on these proteins, although Ca^{++} is more
highly bound than Mg^{++}. Of the ultrafiltrable Mg^{++}, about 20% is com-
plexed to nonprotein anions, and thus only 50% exists as free ions in the
serum.

In tissue such as skeletal muscle, the values are about 36 mM/kg
fat-free dry tissue, which would be equivalent to an intracellular water
concentration of approximately 12 mM/liter. Bone represents the other
major site of Mg^{++} concentration in the body, with one study reporting 233
mM/kg fat-free dry bone.

There does not appear to be a clear-cut relationship between acute
changes in serum Mg^{++} and either intracellular concentration or bone
concentration. Serum $[Mg^{++}]$ gives no indication of whether total body
Mg^{++} deficiency exists. Furthermore, changes in serum Mg^{++} seem to
have poorly defined physiologic effects in man. In general, Ca^{++} and Mg^{++}
are absorbed from the gut and excreted by the kidney in similar fashions
and modified by similar hormonal factors.

HYPERMAGNESEMIA

Cause. The most prominent situation associated with increased
serum $[Mg^{++}]$ is acute renal failure. The other significant cause of hypermagnesemia is iatrogenic, when Mg^{++} is used as a therapeutic agent.
Problems commonly arise when magnesium is being given repeatedly for
hypertension, as in eclampsia or nephritis, and when renal function is
impaired because of the underlying process. Accumulation of magnesium
in the serum occurs under these circumstances and produces
hypermagnesemia.

Implications. The symptomatology arising from elevated levels of
serum $[Mg^{++}]$ is primarily related to the nervous system. Some of the
effects occur as the desired sequelae of treatment, such as sedation and
hypotension. The others are not therapy-related, except as they may
occur as the result of overtreatment. These findings are nausea, vomiting,

stupor, coma, respiratory depression, areflexia, voiding difficulty, and conduction defects in the heart characterized by arrhythmias and prolongation of the Q-T interval in the EKG.

Detection. Serum levels are the only reasonable way to be certain of an elevation in serum Mg^{++}.

Management. The use of Ca^{++} salts intravenously seems to be the most appropriate mode of management for hypermagnesemia.

HYPOMAGNESEMIA

Since serum $[Mg^{++}]$ does not necessarily reflect body $[Mg^{++}]$, the causes and implications of low serum $[Mg^{++}]$ are somewhat variable.

Cause. The causes of hypomagnesemia are several: (1) the primary etiology in adults is alcoholism, and hypomagnesemia has been reported primarily in relation to delirium tremens; (2) malabsorption syndromes have also been associated with reduced serum $[Mg^{++}]$; (3) cirrhosis of the liver; (4) hyperaldosteronism; (5) hyperparathyroidism; (6) diuretics (especially furosemide, ethacrynic acid, thiazides, and mercurials) have been associated with hypomagnesemia; (7) in diabetes mellitus, serum $[Mg^{++}]$ may behave in a manner similar to serum $[K^+]$, the low values not appearing until after fluid and insulin therapy are under way; (8) other factors found in association with low $[Mg^{++}]$ include drugs such as gentamicin, viomycin, and capreomycin, hyperthyroidism, vitamin-D-resistant rickets, and excessive lactation.

Implications. Tetany that responds to Mg^{++} therapy is the most commonly reported symptom. However, tetany due to hypocalcemia with normal $[Mg^{++}]$ also responds to Mg^{++} therapy. Therefore it is not entirely clear how significant low $[Mg^{++}]$ is in tetany, particularly since some patients have shown no neuromuscular findings with quite low serum $[Mg^{++}]$. Other CNS findings such as delirium, confusion, and athetosis have been reported to be associated with hypomagnesemia, but these relationships are not well established. There appear to be no significant cardiovascular effects in man from hypomagnesemia unless it is associated with total body Mg^{++} deficiency. In the latter situation, tachycardia and a variety of arrhythmias have been reported. It is interesting that digitalis effects, including toxicity, are enhanced by Mg^{++} deficiency.

Detection. In tetany that is not associated with low levels of Ca^{++}, hypomagnesemia should be suspected and serum determinations made. Because of the variability in symptomatology associated with low $[Mg^{++}]$, the only approach to evaluating the plasma levels is direct analysis.

Management. It has been known for some time that Mg^{++} administration has a vasodilatory effect and that this may improve renal hemodynamics during the hypertensive period of acute glomerulonephritis. Mg^{++} has also been used to treat eclampsia seizures and as a sedative. However, in none of these situations has there necessarily been hypomagnesemia. In fact, serum levels of 2–3 mM/liter are necessary for optimal effect. $MgSO_4$ is the compound generally used, and careful monitoring of the deep tendon reflexes (with notation of any decrease) serves to guard against overdosage; but serum levels need to be obtained at regular intervals.

For hypomagnesemia, a recommended amount of Mg^{++} is 0.1 ml/kg (0.2 mEq/kg) of a 25% solution given every 6 hours. For hypertension, $MgSO_4 \cdot 7H_2O$ may be given intramuscularly using a 0.2-ml/kg dose of 50% solution every 4–6 hours. Intravenously, up to 10 ml/kg using a 1% solution may be given slowly.

Chloride

During the past 30 years the role of the chloride ion in body fluid physiology has been interpreted primarily as passive. With the requirement of electroneutrality to be satisfied, and with Na^+ being the major cation and Cl^- the major anion of the ECF, it has been generally accepted that Na^+ is the ion that is usually actively transported and that Cl^- follows more or less passively. This is not a universal situation in all tissues, and recent information has been interpreted to suggest that Cl^- is actively transported in the renal tubule. For clinical patient care, one can assume a passive role for Cl^- without creating significant problems or discrepancies. In addition to varying proportionately with $[Na^+]$, $[Cl^-]$ tends to vary inversely with $[HCO_3^-]$. Because the two anions Cl^- and HCO_3^- make up more than 80% of the ECF anions, as one increases, the other must decrease, and vice versa, unless the total cation concentration changes. The concentrations of the other anions (proteins, phosphate, organic acid anions, and sulfate) may also change in response to alterations in $[Cl^-]$ or $[HCO_3^-]$, but generally the range of concentrations for these other anions is small on an absolute basis and thus does not have a major impact on Cl^- and HCO_3^- concentrations. Often the anions other than Cl^- and HCO_3^- are considered as a group, since they are seldom measured individually when evaluating electrolyte disorders. Those situations in which variations in these anions become important will be discussed in subsequent sections.

At the present time the major reason for determining $[Cl^-]$ is to estimate the concentration of unmeasured anions and to validate the values for the measured ion concentrations.

EXAMPLE. The following values are determined for a patient:

$$Na^+ = 165 \text{ mEq/liter} \qquad Cl^- = 141 \text{ mEq/liter}$$
$$K^+ = 5.0 \text{ mEq/liter} \qquad HCO_3^- = 12 \text{ mEq/liter}$$
$$(C_x^{++})^* = 8.0 \text{ mEq/liter} \qquad (A_x^-)\dagger = ? \text{ mEq/liter}$$

First one must evaluate the information to be certain that it is internally consistent. The usual method of checking the results is to determine the value of the total milliequivalents/liter for cations, assume the total anion value is the same, subtract the $[Cl^-]$ and $[HCO_3^-]$ from the total anion concentration, and evaluate the reasonableness of the remaining value in terms of the unmeasured $[A_x^-]$, which is normally between 20 and 30 mEq/liter.

In this example, assuming a value of 5 mEq/liter for $[Ca^{++}]$ and 3 mEq/liter for $[Mg^{++}]$, the total cation concentration is 178 mEq/liter (165 + 5 + 5 + 3). This must also be the figure for anions; so $[A_x^-]$ must equal 25 mEq/liter (178 − 141 − 12). That value for $[A_x^-]$ is appropriate; therefore one can assume that the laboratory values are probably correct and that the person has hypernatremia with metabolic acidosis (and a $[Cl^-]$ that is elevated because of both the increased $[Na^+]$ and the decreased $[HCO_3^-]$).

EXAMPLE. The following values are determined for a patient whose BUN = 15 mg/dl:

$$[Na^+] = 130 \text{ mEq/liter} \qquad [Cl^-] = 80 \text{ mEq/liter}$$
$$[K^+] = 4.0 \text{ mEq/liter} \qquad [HCO_3^-] = 22 \text{ mEq/liter}$$
$$[Ca^{++}] = 5 \text{ mEq/liter} \qquad [A_x^-] = ? \text{ mEq/liter}$$
$$[Mg^{++}] = 3 \text{ mEq/liter}$$

What is the patient's problem? The total cation concentration is 142 mEq/liter. The $[A_x^-]$ value must be 40 mEq/liter if the other ion concentration values are correct (142 − 80 − 22 = 40). A value of 40 mEq/liter for $[A_x^-]$ is abnormally high. Therefore one must first assess the probability that this is a correct value. $[A_x^-]$ is increased to this extent only if there is some elevation of SO_4^{--}, HPO_4^{--}, serum proteins, or organic acid anions. The anion equivalence of serum proteins is about 16 mEq/liter. Unless serum proteins have doubled in concentration, which is a remote possibility, proteins will not account for this elevation of about 15 mEq/liter in $[A_x^-]$. It is unlikely that $[HPO_4^{--}]$ would be elevated with a normal $[Ca^{++}]$. Organic acids are generally not elevated when the $[HCO_3^-]$ is normal, as they function as stronger acids than carbonic acid in body fluids; so if they were increased, they would be expected to displace

* C_x^+ refers to those cations not shown: Ca^{++} and Mg^{++}.
† A_x^- refers to those anions not shown: protein, phosphate, sulfate, and the anions of organic acids, lactate, pyruvate, acetate, etc.

HCO_3^-, converting it to H_2CO_3, which in turn would become H_2O plus CO_2, with the CO_2 being expired. $[SO_4^{--}]$ is usually increased only in the presence of renal failure; with a normal BUN, $[SO_4^{--}]$ is unlikely to be abnormal. Therefore one must suspect that there is an aberrant laboratory value, and it is most probably either $[Na^+]$ or $[Cl^-]$, unless one has reason to suspect a marked elevation in $[HCO_3^-]$, which could occur with either marked metabolic alkalosis or severe respiratory acidosis, each of which should be suspected on the basis of clinical findings. Repeat determinations of the serum electrolyte values yields the following results: $[Na^+] = 135$ mEq/liter and $[Cl^-] = 100$ mEq/liter. The interpretation, then, is a normal electrolyte pattern. Total cations equal 147 mEq/liter (135 + 4 + 5 + 3), and $[A_x^-] = 147 - 22 - 100 = 25$, which is a normal value for $[A_x^-]$.

HYPERCHLOREMIA

Cause. The most common reason for $[Cl^-]$ to be increased is in compensation for an increase in $[Na^+]$ or a decrease in $[HCO_3^-]$ or both. Since these are discussed in the sections on $[Na^+]$ and in Chapter 6, Acid–Base Phenomena, no further discussion is given here. One situation in which increased $[Cl^-]$ can be considered primary occurs when there is an unusually large load of Cl^- presented to the body. This can result from either external or internal factors. Externally, an infusion of large amounts of Cl^- without associated buffer anions such as HCO_3^- is common when saline (NaCl) solutions are given intravenously. Large amounts of NH_4Cl given as a diuretic agent may also result in hyperchloremia. The kidney can usually handle a Cl^- load, but if renal function is reduced, either in terms of tubular acidification of urine or in terms of the total kidney, a Cl^- excess can occur. Under such circumstances, use of NaCl solutions without HCO_3^- (or lactate) or use of NH_4Cl can result in primary hyperchloremia. Saltwater drowning (nonfatal) can also produce hyperchloremia because of the very high $[Cl^-]$ in seawater.

Internal loads of Cl^- have been created when ureters have been diverted into the bowel, with urinary Cl^- being recirculated.

Implications. Metabolic acidosis, prolonged severe respiratory alkalosis (most unusual), or hypernatremia can be the accompaniments of hyperchloremia; these are all discussed in other sections. Hyperchloremia in the absence of any of these other findings should suggest the possibility of laboratory error. With very low serum protein levels, the $[Cl^-]_s$ may be increased 10–15 mEq/liter, although a decrease in $[Na^+]_s$ is more likely under these circumstances.

Detection. A history of NH_4Cl ingestion, nonfatal seawater drowning, infusions of $NaCl$ in the presence of reduced renal function, or ureteral transplantation to the bowel may suggest the presence of hyperchloremia. Physical findings of hyperchloremia per se are not known to exist.

Essentially, laboratory estimation of $[Cl^-]_s$ is the method for establishing changes in the concentration of this ion. Elevations in $[Cl^-]_s$ can be expected in the presence of hypernatremia or metabolic acidosis.

Management. It is rare that specific therapy must be directed toward elevations in $[Cl^-]_s$. Hypernatremia or metabolic acidosis should be the focus of attention when they are present. If excessive Cl^- has been administered to a patient, use of buffered solutions and/or discontinuation of the Cl^- load will usually correct the problem.

HYPOCHLOREMIA

Cause. Decreases in $[Cl^-]_s$, as with elevations, can usually be considered secondary to some other phenomenon. The most frequent disorders associated with hypochloremia are metabolic alkalosis, hyponatremia, azotemia, and chronic respiratory acidosis.

Essentially, anything that lowers $[Na^+]_s$ or increases the concentration of any anion other than Cl^- can result in hypochloremia. Two diseases that also exhibit low $[Cl^-]_s$ are cystic fibrosis (particularly when sweating is pronounced) and congenital diarrhea with alkalosis (a rare but recognized clinical entity).

Implications. In the majority of instances the presence of hypochloremia is explicable by decreased $[Na^+]_s$, elevated $[HCO_3^-]_s$, or laboratory error. When none of these three is the basis of low $[Cl^-]_s$, one must consider the possibility of elevation of other anions. Inorganic phosphate may increase, as in azotemia or hypoparathyroidism, but a doubling of its concentration would produce an increase of only 2–3 mEq/liter and thus a reduction in serum chloride of only 2–3 mEq/liter. If $[SO_4^{--}]_s$ is increased, as in azotemia, or if the organic acids are increased, as in diabetic ketosis, there will be a significant decrease in $[HCO_3^-]_s$ because the SO_4^{--} and organic acids are stronger acids than HCO_3^-. The result is that HCO_3^- falls when these ions increase in concentration, and the decrease in $[Cl^-]_s$ is not as marked as it might be otherwise. Elevation of serum proteins (see subsequent section) may be associated with reduced $[Cl^-]$, but this rarely exceeds 10 mEq/liter.

Detection. The presence of vomiting or chronic diarrhea, salt restriction, diuretic therapy (particularly with thiazides), prolonged use of corticosteroids, other conditions leading to K^+ deficiency (with resulting metabolic alkalosis), or cystic fibrosis may indicate a likelihood of hypochloremia. No specific physical findings are helpful other than those associated with the preceding conditions.

At the level of laboratory findings, low $[Na^+]_s$ or elevated $[HCO_3^-]_s$ is likely to be associated with low $[Cl^-]_s$, but determination of $[Cl^-]$ specifically is necessary to establish a finding of hypochloremia.

Management. In the most common situation in which hypochloremia is noted (metabolic alkalosis with or without associated K^+ deficiency), there is a temptation to consider the use of Cl^- itself to correct the disorder. However, in the majority of instances, correction of any existing dehydration and of any potassium deficiency with solutions containing no buffer anion (e.g., NaCl, KCl) is most efficacious.

Serum Proteins

Serum proteins are not usually considered ionic substances, since their physiologic roles are much more closely related to other properties and characteristics of these large molecules. These molecules are amphoteric (i.e., they act as both cations and anions simultaneously), but their net charge is negative; so, effectively, they behave as anions. The serum proteins are a group of compounds, each with somewhat different ionic characteristics, and all are less dissociated from their accompanying ions than are the elemental ions; this is especially true for the interaction between proteins and the divalent cations. The extent of binding of ions to serum proteins is sufficient to reduce the measured osmolarity of plasma or serum about 10% below the value that would be obtained if all the ionic substances of the plasma were completely dissociated. Because of these characteristics, it is impossible to convert serum protein concentrations directly to milliequivalents/liter. For the clinical setting, a value of 2.43 mEq/liter for each gram of protein per deciliter is assumed. Thus 6.5 g/dl = 16 mEq/liter, and one can reasonably assume a direct proportionality between these two values, i.e., 3.25 g of protein per deciliter = 8 mEq/liter.

Another major difference between serum proteins and the other ionic substances of plasma is in their distributions in body fluids. The other anions and the cations are found throughout the ECF at about the same concentrations as in plasma. The small differences that exist are the direct result of the relative impermeability of the vascular walls to the serum proteins that limits their concentration in the extravascular ECF. The other ionic substances diffuse readily across the vascular wall and are distributed in such a manner as to compensate for restriction of the proteins' anionic properties to the vascular system. The proteins found in serum are present at very low concentrations in the interstitial fluid and are also found in the lymph and in the liver. The total amounts of these proteins in the body are distributed so that about half are present in the plasma and the other half in other locations. Because of this distribution and because of the difference in the volumes of blood plasma and interstitial fluid, the resulting concentration is much higher in plasma than in interstitial fluid.

In health there is equilibrium between the osmotic pressure of the plasma drawing water into the vascular system and the hydrostatic pressure forcing water out of the system. The result is that there is little net shift of water between the vascular and interstitial parts of the ECF. However, if venous pressure rises or serum protein concentration falls, or if both occur, there will be a net shift of fluid into the interstitial phase of tissues (edema, ascites, etc.) and a diminution in plasma volume. If the concentration of proteins is markedly increased in the blood, the result is a greater difference in osmotic pressures (the difference is termed the oncotic pressure when referring to the osmotic pressure of the serum proteins)* between the vascular and interstitial compartments, with a tendency to draw water into the vascular space. This osmotic effect is eventually countered by an increase in hydrostatic pressure within the vascular system as its volume expands.

Other Anions

Disorders of $[HPO_4^{--}]$ are discussed in the section on calcium and in the section on azotemia, as the concentration of this ion is dependent on those factors affecting the divalent cations Ca^{++} and Mg^{++}, as well as on renal function. $[HCO_3^-]$ is discussed in Chapter 6 on acid–base disorders, as this anion cannot change in concentration without altering the acid–base situation in some manner. Other anions such as SO_4^{--} and the organic ions such as lactate and pyruvate are considered in the section on azotemia, as their concentrations become significant in this condition more frequently than in any other.

RENAL FAILURE

The complex compositional changes in body fluids that occur in renal failure involve many of the individual ionic alterations discussed in the previous section, but the interactional aspects of these changes and the

---

* The osmotic pressure of plasma is the result of the total solute of plasma. The osmotic pressure of interstitial fluid is lower than that of plasma by an amount equal to that resulting from the plasma proteins. The term oncotic pressure is used when referring to the value of the specific osmotic pressure of plasma that is due to proteins. Example: osmotic pressure of plasma = 280 mOsm/liter; osmotic pressure of interstitial fluid = 278 mOsm/liter. Therefore the oncotic pressure is 2 mOsm/liter (280 − 278).

necessity of considering total management warrant separate discussion. The major emphasis in this section is on acute renal failure, with some additional comment on the added problems of chronic failure.

In a careful study of acute renal failure in Israel, the overall incidence was about 5 cases per 100,000 population per year. The highest age-specific rate was found in children in the first year of life (20/1000,000); the mortality in the same age group was about 55%.

Uremia (an increase of urea in the blood) and azotemia (an increase of all nitrogenous metabolic products in the blood) are both terms that have been used to characterize the syndrome of renal failure, but they have different definitions; and although it is less commonly used, azotemia is the preferred term. Renal failure has also been defined by the terms anuria (no urine output) and oliguria (less than 180 ml/m²/24 hours). However, although markedly reduced urine output is the usual concomitant of renal failure, it is not an invariable occurrence, as polyuria can and does occur in the presence of a severely reduced GFR.

Acute renal failure (ARF) has also been termed acute tubular necrosis. This latter term refers to the destruction of tubular epithelium that is usually seen as part of the pathologic picture. The term acute tubular necrosis also reflected the presumed pathophysiology for the oliguria. One theory was that urine flow was decreased because of blockage of the tubule by cellular debris; another concept was that the extensive cellular damage resulted in total or near total back-diffusion of the glomerular filtrate from the lumen of the tubule back into the interstitial tissue and then into the blood. There are still proponents of each of these views, but there is a growing tendency to consider a third possibility: that the basic process is a marked reduction or absence of glomerular filtration. The cause for the reduction in the filtering process is presumed to be a loss of filtration pressure, and some authors have used the term vasomotor nephropathy for ARF. This is related to the marked decrease in blood flow to the cortical nephrons seen in ARF. The factors involved in changing cortical blood flow in ARF remain unknown, and although it has been hypothesized that the renin-angiotensin system is involved, the experimental evidence to date does not support this hypothesis.

Etiology

The underlying problems that may lead to ARF can be divided into prerenal, renal, and postrenal. Hypovolemia is the major prerenal problem. Reduced blood volume in children occurs most frequently as the result of dehydration. Blood loss is the next most common event producing hypovolemia. Postoperatively, ARF may occur for several reasons: hypotension during the surgical procedure, hemorrhage, and marked fluid restriction may individually or collectively contribute to postoperative ARF. Sepsis and congestive heart failure are the other major causes of prerenal ARF; sepsis is especially important when gram-negative organisms are involved. Although they are rare in children, the metabolic problems of hypercalcemia, hypokalemia, and hyponatremia may precipitate ARF.

The most frequently encountered renal type of ARF is that termed toxic, which is the classic acute oliguric failure; the term is essentially synonymous with the older term acute tubular necrosis. In the Israeli study this type of ARF accounted for better than one-third of all cases, and for all ages it involved a 65% mortality. This form of ARF includes failure due to intravascular hemolysis, drug intoxication, myoglobinuria, and chemical poisons. Whether the ARF that is secondary to extensive trauma, hypotension, or crush injuries fits into the category of toxic ARF is debatable. Other renal forms of ARF have been termed parenchymatous; they include those cases resulting from acute glomerulonephritis, lupus erythematosus, interstitial nephritis, pyelonephritis, and a variety of systemic diseases with renal involvement. Unusual situations such as the ARF following intravenous pyelograms in diabetes or multiple myeloma fit into this latter category. The hepatorenal syndrome may also be considered in the parenchymatous group, but this remains problematic. Renal artery and vein occlusions also probably belong with the renal forms of ARF.

The postrenal causes of ARF are seen with high obstruction (above the bladder) occurring in the person with a single kidney, but the processes producing high obstruction can also occur bilaterally in persons with two kidneys. Bladder or outlet obstructions have also been implicated in ARF.

Chronic renal failure may be either the end result of ARF or, more commonly, an insidious and slowly developing process, usually secondary to renal parenchymatous disease processes or long-standing obstructive problems. In children the congenital disorders including renal cystic diseases, other dysplasias, hypoplasia, and obstruction are prominent underlying processes. Chronic glomerulonephritis is the most common acquired illness producing chronic renal failure.

Manifestations

In ARF the problems encountered relate to the azotemia, disturbances in fluid balance, and ionic disorders. ARF is also accompanied by disorders of nitrogen, lipid, and carbohydrate metabolism. These disorders include elevation in concentration of many nitrogenous products, urea, creatinine, and many guanidino compounds; the lipid changes result

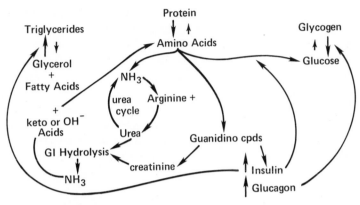

Fig. 5-4. Uremia and nutrient metabolism. Schematic metabolic interrelationships among lipid, protein, and carbohydrate are drawn to illustrate some of the effects of elevated urea concentrations as seen in renal failure. The arginine derived from the urea cycle may combine with amino acids to produce the guanadino compounds. These, in turn, may be responsible for the increase in insulin, which in turn stimulates the production of triglycerides and the conversion of amino acids to glucose, as well as the utilization of glucose for energy. The resulting hypoglycemia may increase glucagon activity, depleting liver glycogen. The value of synthetic diets containing specific keto acids or hydroxy acids is indicated on the left-hand side of the diagram; it results from combination with ammonia to produce new amino acids.

in increases in pre-β-lipoproteins and hypertriglyceridemia; the carbohydrate abnormalities include reduced glucose tolerance, hyperglycemia, lower glycogen stores, increased gluconeogenesis, hyperinsulinemia, and hyperglucagonemia. Associated findings include enteric circulation of urea and creatinine, with hydrolysis providing free amino groups that can combine with appropriate keto or OH^- acids to produce amino acid synthesis. Some of the possible interrelationships of these reactions are shown in Figure 5-4.

The central focus of these reactions appears to be protein catabolism. Most investigators believe that the poorly defined toxic effects of axotemia are related to some series of metabolic products resulting from these catabolic processes. In addition, many of the abnormal metabolic concomitants of azotemia can be corrected or ameliorated by restriction of protein intake or by other ways of improving protein metabolism, e.g., special amino acid diets.

A fluid balance problem is often a precipitating factor; as discussed in the section on management, it must be corrected as soon as it is identified. Thereafter, body fluid status will depend on whether the renal failure is polyuric or oliguric in type. In the rarer polyuric renal failure, the tendency to dehydration is constant, and careful monitoring of output and daily weight is necessary to assure adequate replacement. In the oliguric or anuric ARF, it is equally important to measure urinary output and weight. Fluid replacement is given to provide for the continuous IWL and whatever urine output occurs. The volume of maintenance fluids is the sum of the fluid for IWL plus that for measured urine output minus the metabolic water; the amount of water created by metabolism of nutrients (metabolic water) is about 0.1 ml per kilocalorie utilized. Weight is allowed to decrease about 0.5%–1.0% per day, as these persons are usually in a catabolic state. Failure to allow for a gradual weight loss will ultimately produce a state of overhydration frequently accompanied by hyponatremia.

The initial ionic disturbance that is most serious is elevation of serum $[K^+]$. If tissue damage from burns, trauma, or surgery has preceded the ARF, or if hemolysis is the underlying mechanism, the loss of large amounts of K^+ from cells may cause the serum $[K^+]$ to rise rapidly and create a medical emergency. In the absence of sudden cellular K^+ losses, serum $[K^+]$ will rise more gradually as a result of tissue catabolism and because of any K^+ that is in the fluid or nutrient intake. The results of hyperkalemia are discussed in the section of Chapter 5 on ionic disorders.

Since one can be relatively certain that in the oliguric types of ARF the serum $[K^+]$ will rise to toxic levels, it is more effective to work at managing this problem expectantly rather than after the fact. There are two basic approaches to preventing hyperkalemia in ARF: reducing intake and complexing the ion in the gastrointestinal tract.

The rise in serum $[K^+]$ can be related to the breakdown of cells with their high concentration of K^+ and the body's inability to dispose of that substance through the renal excretory process. In the presence of protein catabolism (cell breakdown) and markedly compromised renal function, it would seem likely that elevated plasma concentrations of most other cellular constituents or their metabolic products would also appear. Urea, creatinine, and potassium all meet those criteria, but phosphate is the anionic substance of most importance that manifests this rise in the serum. Elevation of serum inorganic $[HPO_4^{--}]$ leads to increased secretion of parathormone and in turn to demineralization of bone. If renal failure becomes chronic, renal hyperparathyroidism is a serious complication. Reduction of phosphorus intake and complexing of phosphorus in the gastrointestinal tract are two methods for controlling this disorder. Tetany with lowered serum calcium may also be secondary to the hyperphosphatemia.

The other serious ionic disorder is elevation of extracellular $[H^+]$. Metabolic acidosis is thus another of the manifestations of ARF and is also related to protein catabolism. Breakdown of many of the amino acids yields an excess of H^+, and in the absence of renal removal, they accumulate and create acidemia. Both reduced protein intake and provision of buffer salts are measures used to counter this problem.

Management

Therapy of ARF may be divided into three areas: management of the underlying or etiologic problem, medical maintenance treatment during the period of ARF, and dialysis, either peritoneal or extracorporeal.

When the underlying process is diagnosed and is treatable, the therapy program should be specifically directed toward correction of that disease state. Since dehydration, which often is not recognized, is frequently a primary or secondary factor in the development of ARF, it is imperative to hydrate the patient up to at least a normovolemic state; and it is often wise to create a slight degree of hypervolemia, not exceeding 5% of body weight, except in the presence of congestive heart failure, when hypervolemia is to be avoided.

Obtaining the weight of the patient is mandatory prior to beginning fluid therapy, and weighing should be repeated every 12–24 hours thereafter. Even if the patient is connected to various medical paraphernalia, weight can be obtained, with the various attachments being recorded so that subsequent weighings can be done under similar circumstances. Once appropriate hydration has been obtained, weight should be allowed to decrease 0.5%–1.0% per day.

The amount of fluid to be given in the first 12–24 hours is based on the estimated degree of dehydration, plus maintenance fluid to replace the IWL, plus fluid equivalent to the measured urine or drainage losses, minus the water created by oxidation of nutrients (0.1 ml/kcal). The patient is then weighed, and if there is no evidence of overhydration or other untoward symptoms from the fluid therapy, an additional 50 ml/kg can be given over the following 12-hour period. This 50 ml/kg (approximately 5% of body weight) is in addition to what would ordinarily be given in that half day. It is frequently useful to monitor central venous pressure when planning to provide maximal fluids. The rationale for this additional fluid load is to be certain that normovolemia has been attained, since it is very difficult to accurately assess levels of dehydration of 5% or less. By giving this added fluid, one can be relatively certain that even unrecognized dehydration will be corrected.

The composition of these initial fluids should be calculated as for other problems:

1. Fluid for repair of dehydration should be an isotonic salt mixture. In this case, all of the cation is Na^+, as there is no mechanism for excretion of the K^+ that will be released from cells as protein catabolism oc-

curs. The anions should be Cl^- and HCO_3^-; a reasonable ratio comparable to that in body fluids would be 3–4 parts of Cl^- for 1 part of HCO_3^-.

2. Fluid for IWL replacement should be 5%–10% dextrose in water.

3. Fluid that is given to replace urine and other losses in ARF can be given as equal parts of the salt solution described in paragraph 1 and the dextrose solution mentioned in paragraph 2. The reason for this compromise is that without an analysis of the ionic contents of these excreted or secreted fluids, their compositions are difficult to assess. However, experience indicates that a half-strength salt solution is likely to be reasonably close to the actual values. For long-term treatment, laboratory analyses of urine and other fluids being lost in ARF for their Na^+, K^+, and Cl^- concentrations are useful procedures. When these laboratory values are known, appropriate alteration of the fluids being administered can be carried out. (An example is provided in Part III.)

Another measure that has been used in the past during the initial period of ARF is administration of mannitol or furosemide to induce a diuresis. Although it was originally believed that these might "open up" the kidney, most investigators now believe that there is little therapeutic benefit from such measures. Even though a diuresis may be obtained, GFR does not seem to be affected, and the course of the ARF presumably is not altered. There is still some dispute about these approaches at the clinical level, even though there may be at least hypothetical reasons contraindicating such therapy.

Long-term or maintenance management consists of providing minimal protein intake (approximately 1 g/kg/day), encouraging caloric intake up to the maintenance level for the child, restricting K^+ and PO_4^{--} intakes, and using gastrointestinal sorbents such as Kayexalate for K^+ removal (0.5 g/kg/day) and aluminum hydroxide for PO_4^{--} removal (1 or 2 tablets per meal). Maintenance fluid is equivalent to IWL plus urine output (measured) minus water of oxidation. Weight is allowed to fall 0.5%–1.0% per day.

Dialysis, especially peritoneal dialysis in children, has proved to be very effective and should be started early. Successful peritoneal dialysis makes dietary management somewhat easier, as the restrictions on protein, K^+, PO_4^{--}, and water can be relaxed somewhat. Peritoneal dialysis, short- and long-term extracorporeal dialysis, and renal transplantation are all important aspects of long-term therapy. However, they are beyond the scope of this book. (For further details, see Lieberman E: Clinical Pediatric Nephrology. Philadelphia, PA, Lippincott, 1976.)

EXAMPLE. A 5-year-old child weighing 20 kg appears to be in ARF; after being severely dehydrated he appears to be about 5% dehydrated. Urine output is about 25 ml every 8 hours.

1. Initial 24 hours:

Volume

  For dehydration = 50 ml/kg = 1000 ml

  For IWL   = 34 ml/kg =   680 ml

  For urine   =   75 ml

  Total   = 1755 ml

  Calories = 75 kcal/kg =

  1500 kcal   − 150 ml

                      1605 ml

Composition

  $[Na^+]$ = 150 mEq/liter × 1000 ml = 150 mEq

  $[Cl^-]$ = 100   = 100 mEq

  $[HCO_3^-]$ = 50   = 50 mEq

  10% dextrose × 680 ml   = 68 g

  $[Na^+]$ 75 × 75 ml   =   6 mEq

  $[Cl^-]$ 50   =   4 mEq

  $[HCO_3^-]$ 25   =   2 mEq

Final composition

$$[Na^+] = \frac{150 + 6\ \text{mEq}}{1605\ \text{ml}} = 97\ \text{mEq/liter}$$

$$[Cl^-] = \frac{100 + 4}{1605\ \text{ml}} = 65\ \text{mEq/liter}; [HCO_3^-] = 32\ \text{mEq/liter (by difference)}$$

$$\text{Glucose} = \frac{60\ \text{g}}{1605\ \text{ml}} = 3.7\%$$

  2. The next 12 hours, assuming urine volume remains the same and the patient is otherwise unchanged:

Volume

  The "extra" = 50 ml/kg × 20 kg = 1000 ml*

  IWL for 12 hours = $^1/_2$(34 ml/kg) =   340

  Urine for 12 hours = $^1/_2$(75)   =   37.5

  Total   = 1377.5

  H_2O of oxidation = $^1/_2$(50)   = −75

                     1302.5 or ~ 1300 ml

Composition

  Same as initial 24 hours: Na^+ = 150 mEq

                         Cl^- = 100 mEq

  * This is given to be certain that hydration is adequate; it is expected to produce a 5% overhydration.

$$HCO_3^- = 50 \text{ mEq}$$

Dextrose = $10\% \times 300$ ml	= 30 g
$[Na^+] = 75$ mEq/liter $\times 37.5$ ml	= 3 mEq
$[Cl^-] = 50$ mEq/liter $\times 37.5$ ml	= 2 mEq
$[HCO_3^-] = 25$ mEq/liter $\times 37.5$ ml	= 1 mEq

Final composition

$$[Na^+] = \frac{150 \text{ mEq}}{1300 \text{ ml}} = 115 \text{ mEq/liter}$$

$$[Cl^-] = \frac{102 \text{ mEq}}{1300 \text{ ml}} = 78 \text{ mEq/liter}$$

$$[HCO_3^-] = \frac{30 \text{ g}}{1300 \text{ ml}} = 2.3\%$$

   3. Fluids for hours 36–48:

Volume

  None

  IWL for 12 hours = +340

  Urine for 12 hours = +37.5

  H_2O of oxidation = $\underline{-75}$

  Total   302.5 ml or $\sim$ 300 ml (22 ml/hour)

Composition: There is essentially no electrolyte content; so the total fluid can be given as 10% glucose (dextrose).

   4. Fluid for day 3 is essentially double that of the previous 12 hours (providing the same rate/hour), i.e., 520 ml for 24 hours = 22 ml/hr.

6

Acid–Base Phenomena*

Achieving a unified approach to acid–base disturbances is in some ways simpler and in some ways more complex than dealing with the other problems of water and salt balance. It is simpler because it involves primarily one ion—the hydrogen ion. It is more complex because this ubiquitous ion is present in body fluids at such small concentrations that

---

* This chapter is modified from the article "Acid Base Phenomenon and the Hydrogen Ion," by W. B. Weil, which appeared in *The Journal of Pediatrics*, Vol. 83, September 1973, pp. 350–371.

less familiar terminology is used and because the concepts of buffering, weak acids and bases, and dissociation are included.

DEFINITIONS

Traditionally in clinical medicine the pH has been used to signify the state of acid–base equilibrium. This measurement has value from the viewpoint of physical chemistry, and it has the advantage of familiarity. However, it has obscured for the clinician the real significance of the hydrogen ion, since pH is the negative logarithm of $[H^+]$. Therefore it seems appropriate to examine acid–base disorders directly in terms of H^+ rather than in terms of the negative logarithm of $[H^+]$.

In aqueous solutions, such as body fluids, hydrogen ions are found hydrated with one molecule of water, and they should be represented as the hydronium ion, designated H^+H_2O, H_3O^+, OH_3^+, or H_2OH^+. However, after recognizing this, it will be simpler to discuss hydrogen ions as if they were not hydrated and represent them as H^+. Similarly, the concentration of the ion will be shown as $[H^+]$.

Nanoequivalents

As an ion, hydrogen has such potent effects on all enzymes that only minute concentrations of the ion are tolerable in living systems. In the ECF of man the concentration of hydrogen ion, $[H^+]$, is 0.000040 mEq/liter, in contrast to $[Na^+]$, which is 140 mEq/liter, and $[K^+]$, which is 5 mEq/liter.

To avoid the use of so many zeros in expressing $[H^+]$, the term nanoequivalent is employed. One nanoequivalent/liter (nEq/liter) is 0.000000001 Eq/liter or 0.000001 mEq/liter. Thus the usual $[H^+]$ in plasma or ECF can be expressed as 40 nEq/liter.

Relation between $[H^+]$ and pH

As previously mentioned, pH is the negative logarithm of the $[H^+]$ when the latter is given as equivalents/liter. In plasma the average $[H^+]$ is 40 nEq/liter or 0.000000040 Eq/liter, which can also be written 40×10^{-9} Eq/liter. Then the pH equals the negative logarithm of 40×10^{-9}

$= - \log 40 \times 10^{-9}$; separating this
$= - (\log 40 + \log 10^{-9})$; removing parentheses
$= - \log 40 - \log 10^{-9}$; obtaining log values
$= - (1.6) - (-9)$; removing parentheses
$= - 1.6 + 9$; completing the arithmetic
$= 7.4$

Table 6-1
[H$^+$] and pH Values*

[H$^+$]						pH					
20						7.70					
	25						7.60				
	40	30	35				7.40	7.52	7.46		
		50	60	70				7.30	7.22	7.16	
		80	100	120				7.10	7.00	6.92	
			160		140				6.80		6.86

* Values of hydrogen ion concentration and pH are given in staggered rows and columns in order to facilitate reading corresponding values.

Doubling [H$^+$] to 80 nEq/liter would be equivalent to a pH of 7.1:

$$pH = -\log 80 \times 10^{-9}$$
$$pH = -\log 80 + \log 10^{-9})$$
$$pH = -(1.9) - (-9)$$
$$pH = 7.1$$

Thus doubling the [H$^+$] drops the pH 0.3 units.

As a general rule, in the range of body [H$^+$], doubling or halving the [H$^+$] decreases or increases the pH value by 0.3 units. These relationships are summarized in Table 6-1. The corresponding pH for each [H$^+$] is shown on the right in the appropriate position. The values 160 nEq/liter for [H$^+$] and pH = 6.80 represent about the highest [H$^+$] the body can tolerate. The lowest level of [H$^+$] in the ECF that is compatible with life is approximately 20 nEq/liter. This is equivalent to a pH of 7.7. Man can survive an eightfold variation in extracellular [H$^+$] (20–160 nEq/liter), which is four times the degree of variation tolerable for [Na$^+$] (100–200 mEq/liter) and about the same as the tolerable eightfold variation in [K$^+$] (1.5–12 mEq/liter).

The [H$^+$] in the ICF has not been mentioned, even though its concentration in the cells is even more critical for survival than is its concentration in the ECF. Hydrogen ions are not evenly distributed inside cells or between cells, and thus no single value is possible. However, for considering total body physiology, an overall value of intracellular [H$^+$] of 80 nEq/liter (pH = 7.1) can be assumed as a reasonable approximation without altering the physiologic considerations.

Acids and Bases

Even though the concentration of free or ionized hydrogen ions in body water is minute, the total amount of potentially ionizable hydrogen in the body is vast. The distinction is based on the fact that high per-

Table 6-2
Buffers Found in Blood or Urine

$$H_2CO_3 \rightleftharpoons H^+ + HCO_3^-$$
$$H_2PO_4^- \rightleftharpoons H^+ + HPO_4^{--}$$
$$NH_4^+ \rightleftharpoons H^+ + NH_3$$
$$H\ Protein^* \rightleftharpoons H^+ + Protein^-$$
$$H\ Hgb \rightleftharpoons H^+ + Hgb^-$$

The general equation can be written $HA \rightleftharpoons H^+ + A^-$

* H Protein should be represented as H Protein^{n-}, and Protein$^-$ should be Protein$^{(n-)-}$ because the anion (protein) has a net negative charge, but the exact quantification of this charge is difficult to describe because of the heterogeneity of the various proteins involved. The symbols shown in the table are used for simplicity.

centages of hydrogen ions (which are cations) are associated with anions or uncharged compounds, and under appropriate circumstances some of the H^+ can dissociate from these anions or uncharged compounds. Examples of these relationships are shown in Table 6-2. The preponderant form is the associated form shown on the left. The dissociated H^+ and the anions or uncharged compounds are on the right. The double arrow indicates that the reaction can go in both directions.

Any compound, charged or not, that can give up a hydrogen ion is termed an acid. A weak acid gives up, donates, or dissociates its hydrogen ion to a very slight extent, and a strong acid gives up or dissociates its hydrogen ion readily. The extent to which a compound dissociates a hydrogen ion is a constant for each compound, i.e., each compound has its own dissociation constant K.* A weak acid will have a small dissociation constant, and a strong acid will have a large one.† For weak acids the degree of dissociation is extremely small, and the hydrogen present in the form shown on the left of each equation is present in amounts 1 million to 1 billion times the amount of hydrogen present as the dissociation ion, H^+. Thus, in the Bronsted terminology for acids (the one to be used here), the compounds on the left side of Table 6-2 are termed weak acids, i.e., they

* Technically, correct terminology for use in body fluids requires the use of the designation K', because without the prime marker the designation for the dissociation constant K refers only to infinitely dilute solutions. In the same fashion that it is possible to consider $[H^+]$ in terms of pH, it is also possible to consider K' by using pK', which is the negative logarithm of K'. For example, if the dissociation constant of acetic acid is 0.00002, the pK' is 4.7 (0.00002 is 2×10^{-5}) the log is log $2 + \log^{-5}$, or $0.3 + (-5) = -4.7$; the negative log is 4.7).

† The pK' for a weak acid will be a larger number than the pK' for a strong acid. Acetic acid, with a pK' of 4.7, is a stronger acid than $H_2PO_4^-$, with a pK' near 7. Thus HPO_4^{--} will have greater affinity for H^+ than will the acetate anion CH_3COO^-.

give up their hydrogen very reluctantly.* By contrast, HCl is a strong acid, and in an aqueous solution it will essentially completely dissociate to $H^+ + Cl^-$.

An ion or compound shown on the far right in Table 6-2 is one that can accept a hydrogen ion when the reaction goes from right to left. Such a substance is therefore termed a base, or a hydrogen ion acceptor. Thus the three components of the fundamental acid–base equation are an acid (a hydrogen ion donor), hydrogen ion, and a base (a hydrogen ion acceptor). Since every acid must have a related base, the pair is considered as an acid and its conjugate base.

Buffers

The importance of acids and their conjugate bases in medicine is that several weak acids and their conjugate bases constitute a series of buffer systems that tend to stabilize the acid–base balance or hydrogen ion concentration of body fluids.

Appreciation of a buffer system requires an understanding of the mass action law. In the description of the dissociation constant K', it is inherent that in the reaction

$$HA \rightleftarrows H^+ + A^-$$

there is a stable state for the reaction under a given set of circumstances. The result is that the product of $[H^+]$ and $[A^-]$ is a constant fraction of the $[HA]$. Another way to write this is

$$K' = \frac{[H^+][A^-]}{[HA]}$$

Therefore, if one adds a large amount of A^- (the conjugate base) to a solution of HA, the $[H^+]$ must decrease and the $[HA]$ increase to keep the ratio of the product of $[H^+]$ and $[A^-]$ divided by $[HA]$ a constant. That these changes in concentration occur in this manner can be derived from the mass action law.

Another way to consider this, using the major extracellular buffer pair H_2CO_3/HCO_3^-, is to examine this reaction:

$$H_2CO_3 \rightleftarrows H^+ + HCO_3^-$$

Bicarbonate, carbonic acid, and carbon dioxide are important as a buffering system in man for two reasons: The chemical reaction functions in what may be termed an open system, i.e., gaseous carbon dioxide can

---

* Actually, H_2CO_3 is a relatively strong acid, but in the presence of dissolved CO_2, as in body fluids, the effective activity of $H_2CO_3 + CO_2$ (dissolved) places this in the weak acid category.

leave the system through the lungs. Additionally, most of the carbon dioxide is present as dissolved CO_2 rather than as carbonic acid, so that the total mixture of CO_2 and H_2CO_3 behaves as if it had a pK' of 6.1 rather than as it would if all the CO_2 were H_2CO_3. Were all of the CO_2 present as H_2CO_3, the system would function at the true pK' of H_2CO_3, which is 3.5.

The equation for the bicarbonate system in man should be written:

$$Pco_2 \uparrow \times S \rightleftarrows CO_2(d) + H_2O \rightleftarrows H_2CO_3 \rightleftarrows H^+ + HCO_3^-$$

The significance of the additional terms on the left is as follows: (1) the term Pco_2 represents the partial pressure of carbon dioxide in the blood and in equilibrium with the partial pressure of CO_2 in the alveolus. The term relating these two is the solubility constant S. (2) The $\uparrow$ indicates that the CO_2 as a gas can escape from the system because this is an "open" system. The bicarbonate buffer has increased capacity to buffer body fluids and play a very significant role in maintaining acid–base homeostasis. (3) The term $CO_2(d)$ represents the carbon dioxide dissolved in body fluids but not hydrated to become H_2CO_3. The amount of CO_2 present as $CO_2(d)$ is about 80 times more than the amount present as H_2CO_3 (1.185 versus 0.015 mM/liter).

It is the combination of these three factors that must be understood to appreciate the usefulness of the bicarbonate buffer for the body. Carbonic acid at its actual pK' cannot exist in body fluids to any great extent. Because the carbonic acid formed can rapidly become carbon dioxide, and because the carbon dioxide can be eliminated quickly in the lungs, this reaction can have potent effects on acid–base equilibrium. It should be obvious that if there is a respiratory problem limiting the body's ability to vary or to maintain an appropriate Pco_2, the buffering capacity of the ECF will be seriously impaired.

For convenience, when used in this book, $[H_2CO_3]$ will be equivalent to the sum of the $CO_2(d)$ and the H_2CO_3 present in the fluid. Furthermore, the $[H_2CO_3]$ will often be used interchangeably with Pco_2, since

$$S \times \quad Pco_2 \quad = CO_2(d) + H_2CO_3 = [H_2CO_3]$$
$$0.03 \times 40 \, mm \, Hg = 1.185 + 0.015 = 1.2 \, mM/liter$$

as used in this book.

Returning to the reaction

$$H_2CO_3 \rightleftarrows H^+ + HCO_3^-$$

if one adds bicarbonate ion (HCO_3^-) to a solution containing these substances, the reaction is shifted to the left, the $[H^+]$ decreases (the pH rises), and some of the added HCO_3^- becomes H_2CO_3, as predicted by the mass action law. However, the H_2CO_3 then goes on to dissociate to H_2O and CO_2, and the CO_2 is removed from the system by respiration. The loss of CO_2 (and respiratory control of CO_2 concentration) modifies the quantities of reactants and products that are involved in the H_2CO_3/HCO_3^- system, but the basic principle of the law of mass action is as applicable to this equation as to any other. An addition of H^+ will shift the equation to the left, the $[HCO_3^-]$ will decrease, and the increase in $[H^+]$ will not be as great as the amount of H^+ added, since some of it will have been converted to H_2CO_3. Finally, addition of H_2CO_3 will cause the reaction to shift to the right, and the amounts of H^+ and HCO_3^- will increase, so that the new total for H_2CO_3 will be less than the sum of the initial amount plus that added. Thus weak acids and their conjugate bases act to modify the effects of additions of H^+, A^-, and HA on the final $[H^+]$ of the solutions. A weak acid and its conjugate base that can do this are termed a buffer pair, or more simply a buffer. The efficiency of a buffer depends on the proximity of its dissociation constant to the hydrogen ion concentration of the solution in which it exists and on the concentration of the buffer (the more buffer that is present, the more hydrogen ion it can accommodate).

A typical titration curve for a hypothetical buffer with a pK' of 7.4 ($K' = 1.6 \times 10^{-9}$) is shown in Figure 6-1. $[H^+]$ and pH are shown on the abscissa, and the quantity of acid or base added is shown on the ordinate. Addition of acid is in an upward direction, and addition of base is shown in a downward direction.

When the buffer pair exists at the point of its maximum buffering capacity, the amount present as the acid will be equivalent to the amount present as the base, and the $[H^+]$ will correspond to the value of K' (the pH will be equal to the pK'). In this situation, relatively large additions of H^+ or A^- produce minimal changes in $[H^+]$. This point is shown by the X in Figure 6-1. If 20 units of acid or base are added at this point, the $[H^+]$ will increase about 15 mEq/liter and decrease 12 mEq/liter (shown as points A_1 and B_1) for addition of acid and base, respectively. If further acid or base is added, 20 units of acid or base will produce an increase in $[H^+]$ of 105 mEq/liter for acid or a decrease of 18 mEq/liter for base. Thus the further the initial $[H^+]$ is from the K' of the buffer, the more profound will be the change in $[H^+]$ produced by addition of a specific amount of acid or base.

Two factors in body fluids modify the simple buffer relationships described thus far. Body fluids contain a mixture of buffer pairs with different K' values, and the H_2CO_3/HCO_3^- pair exists in a relatively open system; i.e., as additional H_2CO_3 is formed, it will be converted to CO_2 and H_2O, and the CO_2 will in turn be removed from the body by the lungs as expired CO_2. Thus a rise in $[H^+]$ or $[HCO_3^-]$ does not produce the

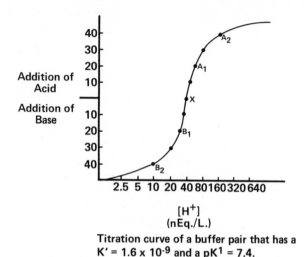

Titration curve of a buffer pair that has a K' = 1.6 x 10⁻⁹ and a pK¹ = 7.4.

Fig. 6-1. Titration curve of a buffer pair illustrating the phenomenon common to all buffers: at a hydrogen ion concentration that corresponds to their equilibrium constant, additions of significant amounts of acid or base will have minimal effect on the hydrogen ion concentration.

expected degree of rise in the opposite component of this buffer pair, but it produces changes in all the nonbicarbonate buffers. For example, addition of HCO_3^- to body fluids will produce a transient increase in H_2CO_3 (Pco_2); but more important, the nonbicarbonate buffers (Table 6-2) will shift to the right because of the overall reduction in $[H^+]$, and any rise in H_2CO_3 that is produced will be quite quickly eliminated by its conversion to CO_2 and pulmonary removal. Similarly, a rise in H_2CO_3 (or Pco_2) will increase $[H^+]$, with a slight rise in $[HCO_3^-]$; but more important, the other buffer pairs will be shifted to the left by the increased $[H^+]$.

The buffers of body fluids can be divided into those in the ECF and those in the ICF. The buffers in cells include cellular proteins, amino acids, phosphoric ester compounds, and bicarbonate. In the ECF, hemoglobin within the red cells, serum proteins in the plasma, phosphate, and bicarbonate are the major buffers. The relative values of the buffers present in whole blood are given in relation to the measured concentration of HCO_3^- in Table 6-3. The total buffering capacity of whole blood with a normal hemoglobin level will be equivalent to that of a solution with $[HCO_3^-]$ of 48 mEq/liter.

No such quantification of buffer values is known for the ICF, but after addition of an H^+ load to the ECF, allowing for equilibrium to be established, about half of the buffering that takes place in the whole body will occur in the ECF and about half in the ICF. It should be recognized that

Table 6-3
Relative Values of Buffers of Blood*

Bicarbonate	26 mEq/liter
Phosphate	2 mEq/liter
Plasma proteins	3 mEq/liter
Hemoglobin†	17 mEq/liter
	48 = buffer base (mEq/liter)

* The sum of the buffer anions in whole blood is termed the total buffer base. Deviation from the normal value of buffer base is termed base excess, and this may be positive (a true excess) or negative (actually a base deficit).

† The buffer base value for whole blood varies with the hemoglobin concentration.

when anions in cells accept H^+ from the ECF, they release a cation to the ECF to maintain electroneutrality; initially the cation exchanged will be primarily Na^+ and then K^+. The exchange of extracellular H^+ for intracellular cations is not equal, because some intracellular compounds may change their composition and in the process change their buffering capacity.

PHYSIOLOGIC CONTROLS

Although the buffer systems of the body can accommodate a day's net production of H^+ by the body,* prolonged survival is impossible without mechanisms for excretion of H^+ and regeneration of buffer. The two major control control systems of the body for regulating buffer concentrations are the respiratory and the renal excretory systems.

Respiratory Regulation

Respiratory control affects only the bicarbonate system directly. However, in a solution containing several buffer pairs, the common ion effect, from the mass action law, keeps them all in equilibrium; so there is an indirect effect on all buffers by the respiratory mechanism.

The fundamental reaction involved in respiratory control is

$$CO_2 + H_2O \rightleftarrows H_2CO_3 \rightleftarrows H^+ + HCO_3^-$$

* This assumes that metabolically produced CO_2 is removed by the lungs.

The concentration of carbon dioxide in body fluids is directly related to the partial pressure of gaseous carbon dioxide in the alveoli of the lungs.

Therefore the following events will produce the changes listed:

1. Increased respiratory effectiveness (increased alveolar ventilation) will produce the following:

Decreased partial pressure of CO_2 in alveoli
Decreased concentration of plasma CO_2
Shift of the reaction to the left (by the mass action law)
Decreased $[H^+]$ (elevation of pH)

This reaction can produce rapid alteration of $[H^+]$, but it does not serve as a primary mechanism for removal of H^+, as some of the bicarbonate ion is consumed in the process while the other buffer pairs are shifted to the right, and thus total buffer base will not change. Furthermore, the decrease in $[H^+]$ will not be equivalent to the decrease in P_{CO_2}, since the shift of the nonbicarbonate buffer pairs to the right will add some H^+ to the common pool.

2. Decreased respiratory effectiveness (decreased alveolar ventilation, as in emphysema and pulmonry edema) will produce the following:

Increased partial pressure of alveolar CO_2
Increased concentration of plasma CO_2
Shift of the reaction to the right (by the mass action law)
Increased $[H^+]$ (decreased pH)

This reaction, although potentially doubling or tripling the P_{CO_2} ($40 \rightarrow 80$–120 mm Hg), will also produce a small increase in bicarbonate concentration and a decrease in nonbicarbonate buffer bases (again by the common ion $[H^+]$ effect), so that total buffer base will not change.

These two respiratory changes can occur as primary events; the first reaction will produce respiratory alkalosis, and the second will produce respiratory acidosis. The same reactions can occur as secondary or compensatory reactions. Thus, if a patient is acidemic (excess $[H^+]$, low pH) for any reason, increased respiratory effectiveness will tend to decrease $[H^+]$ and restore pH toward normal. Similarly, decreased respiratory effectiveness will be useful in compensating for existing alkalemia (decreased $[H^+]$, high pH).*

Thus the respiratory system can rapidly change $[H^+]$, either as a primary disturbance or as a modifying compensatory function; but in this

* The terms acidemia and alkalemia refer to increased and decreased $[H^+]$ in the blood. Acidosis refers to a physiologic process in which H^+ is increased or HCO_3^- is decreased. Alkalosis refers to other physiologic processes in which H^+ is decreased or HCO_3^- is increased.

latter role, respiratory changes can correct [H^+] but cannot restore the concentration of H^+ acceptors, the buffers of the body (total buffer base).

EXAMPLES

EXAMPLE 1. A child becomes very excited because he fears having blood drawn. He is presumably healthy, except for phimosis, but his serum values are $P_{CO_2} = 30$ mm Hg (normal = 40) and [H^+] = 32 nEq/liter (normal = 40). How can these be explained? Referring to the reactions

$$CO_2 + H_2O \rightleftarrows H_2CO_3 \rightleftarrows H^+ + HCO_3^- \tag{1}$$
$$HA \rightleftarrows H^+ + A^- \tag{2}$$

the excitation may well have produced hyperventilation, with increased removal of CO_2. Then equation (1) will shift to the left, dropping both [H^+] and [HCO_3^-]. However, at the same time, reaction (2), representing all the nonbicarbonate buffers, will be affected by the reduced [H^+] and will shift to the right, releasing some H^+, but not as much as was removed by equation (1), and increasing the other buffer bases, so that the total buffer base will not change. The net result will still be a decrease in [H^+] and a decrease in P_{CO_2}.

EXAMPLE 2. A child undergoes surgery requiring controlled respiration. The anesthetist determines the rate and depth of respiration as well as the gas mixture being used. After a period of time, the anesthetist draws blood to determine how the patient is progressing. He finds a normal oxygen tension but a pH of 7.1. What might he expect the CO_2 tension to be?*

A pH of 7.1 corresponds to [H^+] of 80 nEq/liter (from Table 6-1). This represents acidemia. If there are no metabolic problems such as hypoxia and there has been no time for any renal response, it may be presumed that the acidemia is due to respiratory acidosis. The P_{CO_2} can be calculated from the [H^+] and an assumed [HCO_3^-]. In the equation $K' = [H^-][HCO_3^-]/[H_2CO_3]$, [$H_2CO_3$] can also be considered as P_{CO_2}. Then rearrangement yields [H_2CO_3] ~ $P_{CO_2} = [H^-][HCO_3^-]/K'$. If [$HCO_3^-$] has not changed, then $P_{CO_2} = [H^+] \times C$, where C is an arbitrary constant equal to [HCO_3^-]/K'. From this equation it should be apparent that doubling the [H^+], from 40 to 80 nEq/liter, will be the result of doubling P_{CO_2} from 40 to 80 mm Hg. Therefore the anesthetist can assume a value for P_{CO_2} of approximately 80 mm Hg.

Renal Regulation

In contrast to respiratory control, the kidneys change [H^+] more slowly, but they can also restore the concentration of A^-, the buffer anion, or conjugate base.

---

* Normally, either P_{CO_2} or [HCO^-_3] would also be determined to obtain the P_{CO_2} directly or indirectly knowing [H^+] and [HCO^-_3].

Table 6-4

Tubular Mechanism for H^+ Secretion*

Blood	Tubular Cells	Urine

$$CO_2 + H_2O$$
$$\downarrow$$

H_2CO_3† $\longrightarrow$ H_2CO_3

$$\downarrow$$

$$HCO_3^- + H^+$$

$HCO_3^- \longleftarrow \rule{2cm}{0.4pt}\rceil \qquad \lceil \rule{2cm}{0.4pt} \longrightarrow H^+$

$(Na^+ \longleftarrow \rule{4cm}{0.4pt} \qquad \longleftarrow \rule{3cm}{0.4pt} Na^+)$‡

    * The reactions that take place in the tubular cells represent dissociation of carbonic acid, with movement of hydrogen ion into the urine in exchange for sodium and then reabsorption of sodium and bicarbonate ions into the blood.

    † H_2CO_3 represents H_2CO_3 and dissolved CO_2 of the blood as well as that produced in the body cells and then diffused into the blood.

    ‡ An active exchange process that satisfies electroneutrality and returns Na^+ to the body from glomerular filtrate.

    The kidneys excrete H^+ in several ways. First, they have the capacity to excrete free H^+. Actually, the renal tubules can increase $[H^+]$ 1000-fold over its concentration in the ECF: from 40 nEq/liter (as in plasma and glomerular filtrate) to 40,000 nEq/liter (as in a final urine with a pH of 4.4). However, this removes a very small part of the body's daily production of H^+, as 40,000 nEq/liter is only 0.04 mEq/liter, and daily H^+ production averages 2–3 mEq/kg body weight per day in infants and 1–1.5 mEq/kg/day in adults.

    Even though the amount of H^+ excreted directly is quantitatively of little significance, the reaction leading to the increased $[H^+]$ in the tubular fluid is of prime importance. The reaction in the healthy tubular cells begins with CO_2, both CO_2 produced metabolically in the tubular cells and CO_2 derived metabolically from other tissues, since such CO_2 readily diffuses into the blood and then into the tubular cells from the blood. CO_2 produced metabolically anywhere in the body can thus be used by the tubular cells for the reaction shown in Table 6-4. This reaction makes H^+ available for other reactions in the urine (vide infra) and also restores the hydrogen acceptor (buffer anion or conjugate base) HCO_3^- to the blood and thereby to the ECF.

    Excretion of H^+ as part of an undissociated weak acid is the other mechanism for elimination of H^+ from the body; this is quantitatively the most important reaction for excretion of H^+. Excretion of H^+ as an undissociated weak acid is dependent on the availability of free H^+ in the tubular urine. The conjugate bases for these weak acids are derived either by tubular metabolism or by glomerular filtration.

Healthy kidney tubular cells are capable of producing NH_3 from glutamic acid. The NH_3 thus formed then diffuses into the urine and reacts as a hydrogen ion acceptor (base). The dissociation constant for the reaction $NH_4^+ \leftrightarrows NH_3 + H^+$ is sufficiently high that in acid urine the reaction is shifted markedly to the left and the H^+ is present almost entirely in the form NH_4^+. Thus as H^+ excretion needs to be increased, the urine will contain larger amounts of the weak acid NH_4^+. The concentration of the base NH_3 determines the rate of NH_3 formation by the tubular cells—to the extent the cells have that capacity. The more H^+ there is in the urine, the greater will be the rate of combination of H^+ and NH_3. The faster the NH_3 is removed by conversion to NH_4^+, the greater will be the production rate of NH_3 by the tubules. However, it requires several days for NH_3 production to reach a maximum rate for any individual.

The second source of conjugate bases in the urine is from the glomerular filtrate. At the $[H^+]$ of blood, phosphate is present primarily as the conjugate base HPO_4^{--}, and it is present in glomerular filtrate in that form. As the glomerular fluid passes through the length of the tubule, $[H^+]$ may increase. In urine with high $[H^+]$, HPO_4^{--} combines with H^+ because the following reaction is shifted to the left:

$$H_2PO_4^- \rightleftarrows H^+ + HPO_4^{--}$$

This allows excretion of additional H^+ in the undissociated form as the weak acid $H_2PO_4^-$. Other substances that function in a manner similar to phosphate are the ketone anions (acetoacetate$^-$ and β-hydroxybutyrate$^-$), and creatinine, all of which will accept H^+ at the $[H^+]$ of acid urine.

In the healthy state, renal excretion of H^+ and regeneration of HCO_3^- are balanced against the ingestion and production of H^+ pursuant to metabolic processes and the consumption of HCO_3^- as a buffer anion. If necessary, the renal mechanism can be speeded up or slowed down to compensate for unusual increases or decreases in H^+ production.

The kidney itself can be a primary cause of depletion or elevation of buffer base (metabolic acidosis or alkalosis), or nonrenal problems may create alterations in the body content of H^+ or A^-; in both situations these are termed metabolic acidosis or alkalosis.

Thus in the equation $K' = [H^+] [HCO_3^-]/[H_2CO_3]$, when change in the numerator is the primary disorder, the disturbance is called metabolic; when change in the denominator is the primary alteration, the disturbance is termed respiratory.

Table 6-5
Regulation of Extracellular [H$^+$]*

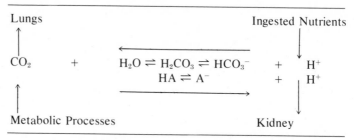

* This illustrates the general acid–base reactions of the body as they relate to the bicarbonate buffer as well as other body buffers. Carbon dioxide tends to be generated by metabolic processes and removed by respiratory effort through the lungs. Hydrogen ions are generated by the metabolism of ingested nutrients and lost to the body through the kidneys; these two processes tend to shift reactions to the left, whereas metabolic processes and renal loss of hydrogen ion tend to shift the general reaction to the right.

Summary of Physiologic Controls

In summary, the regulation of [H$^+$] in the ECF of the body can be represented as a balance of forces working on common chemical equations (Table 6-5). In general, the forces shown above the equations tend to drive them to the left by mass action effects, and the forces shown below the equations tend to drive them to the right. When everything is balanced, there is [H$^+$] of 40 nEq/liter, [HCO$_3^-$] of 24 mEq/liter, [H$_2$CO$_3$] of 1.2 mM/liter, Pco$_2$ of 40 mm Hg, and buffer base of $\sim$ 48 mEq/liter.* For infants the normal values tend to approach [H$^+$] = 40 nEq/liter, [HCO$_3^-$] = 20 mEq/liter, [H$_2$CO$_3$] = 1.0 mM/liter, and Pco$_2$ = 33 mm Hg.

CLINICAL STATES

In clinical settings four basic disturbances of acid–base physiology are recognized: metabolic acidosis, metabolic alkalosis, respiratory acidosis, and respiratory alkalosis. These disorders do not occur in pure form, as they usually become partially compensated by respiratory alteration in Pco$_2$ in the primary metabolic disorders and somewhat more slowly

* The actual normal value of buffer base varies with hemoglobin concentration, as hemoglobin is the principal nonbicarbonate buffer base.

compensated by renal alteration in $[H^+]$, $[HCO_3^-]$, and other buffer base concentrations in primary respiratory problems. In addition, there can exist mixed metabolic and respiratory disturbances in which both metabolic and respiratory changes may be primary factors.

The term metabolic acidosis or metabolic alkalosis is used when there is a net addition to body fluids or a net loss from body fluids of H^+ or a reciprocal change of any buffer base (HCO_3^-, HPO_4^{--}, etc.). Respiratory acidosis or alkalosis is used when there is a primary change in PCO_2 (or H_2CO_3), as in emphysema, pulmonary edema, or hyperventilation of CNS origin.

From changes in blood $[H^+]$ alone, one can diagnose acidemia or alkalemia but cannot determine whether the initiating physiologic disorder is metabolic or respiratory. However, if $[H^+]$ and PCO_2 or $[HCO_3^-]$ are known, the type of physiologic disturbance can be defined for most patients. However, there are clinical situations in which two acid–base disorders may exist simultaneously. When metabolic acidosis exists concomitantly with respiratory alkalosis, it is difficult to distinguish this from the compensation that may occur in either situation. It is necessary to consider the physiologic limits that exist for the compensatory responses when attempting to identify those mixed disorders in which one type of acidosis (metabolic or respiratory) is combined with the other type of alkalosis.

In the simple metabolic disorders, $[H^+]$ is primarily affected, and PCO_2 changes in the opposite direction for compensation. The increase in $[H^+]$ can occur as a result of an actual increase in H^+ or as a result of a loss of buffer base, reflected by a decrease in $[HCO_3^-]$. In a closed system, an increase in $[H^+]$ would increase $[H_2CO_3]$ and PCO_2; but the body is an open system, and an increase in $[H_2CO_3]$ is quickly dissipated as expired CO_2. The only time this would not occur in man would be if increased alveolar perfusion and/or ventilation were not possible (e.g., machine ventilation, severe pulmonary disease). In such a situation the disturbance would be termed a mixed metabolic and respiratory acidosis.

In respiratory acidosis or alkalosis, the primary change is in PCO_2, and the change in $[H^+]$ is in the same direction as the change in PCO_2. The compensation for respiratory disorders is accomplished by change in the buffer base concentration and is recognized by a change in $[HCO_3^-]$ in a direction similar to the change in PCO_2 and $[H^+]$. These relationships are shown diagrammatically in Table 6-6.

Examples

In regard to the following examples, these are the normal values: $PCO_2 = 40$ mm Hg, $[H^+] = 40$ nEq/liter, $[HCO_3^-] = 24$ mEq/liter.

Table 6-6
P_{CO_2}, $[H^+]$, and $[HCO_3^-]$ in Physiologic Disorders*

Physiologic Disorder	P_{CO_2}	$[H^+]$	$[HCO_3^-]$
Metabolic acidosis†	↓	↑	↓
Metabolic alkalosis†	↑	↓	↑
Respiratory acidosis‡	↑	↑	↑̖
Respiratory alkalosis‡	↓	↓	↓̖
Mixed metabolic and respiratory acidosis§	↑	↑	↓
Mixed metabolic and respiratory alkalosis§	↓	↓	↑

Note: ↑ = primary increase, ↓ = primary decrease, ↑̖ = compensatory increase, ↓̖ = compensatory decrease.

* As can be seen, when the changes in acid–base disorder are metabolic in origin, the change in hydrogen ion is opposite in direction to the change in bicarbonate ion. When the changes are respiratory, the changes in hydrogen ion and bicarbonate are in the same direction. Mixed disorders are also distinguishable, because they change hydrogen ion and P_{CO_2} in the same direction but bicarbonate in the opposite direction.

† The changes in $[H^+]$ and P_{CO_2} are in opposite directions in the metabolic disorders. The changes in $[H^+]$ and $[HCO_3^-]$ are also in opposite directions.

‡ The changes in $[H^+]$ and P_{CO_2} are in the same direction, and the change in $[HCO_3^-]$ is also in the same direction.

§ The changes in $[H^+]$ and P_{CO_2} are in the same direction, but the change in $[HCO_3^-]$ is in the opposite direction.

EXAMPLE 1. Infant with diarrhea:

P_{CO_2} = 30 mm Hg
$[H^+]$ = 50 nEq/liter
$[HCO_3^-]$ = 14.4 mEq/liter
Pattern: P_{CO_2} ↓, $[H^+]$ ↑, $[HCO_3^-]$ ↓
Clinical state: metabolic acidosis

EXAMPLE 2. Infant with pyloric stenosis:

P_{CO_2} = 45 mm Hg
$[H^+]$ = 30 nEq/liter
$[CO_3^-]$ = 36 mEq/liter
Pattern: P_{CO_2} ↑, $[H^+]$ ↓, $[HCO_3^-]$ ↑
Clinical state: metabolic alkalosis

EXAMPLE 3. Child with status asthmaticus:

P_{CO_2} = 70 mm Hg
$[H^+]$ = 60 nEq/liter
$[HCO_3^-]$ = 28 mEq/liter
Pattern: P_{CO_2} ↑, $[H^+]$ ↑, $[HCO_3^-]$ ↑
Clinical state: respiratory acidosis

EXAMPLE 4. Child early in salicylate intoxication:

P_{CO_2} = 20 mm Hg
$[H^+]$ = 24 nEq/liter
$[HCO_3^-]$ = 20 mEq/liter
Pattern P_{CO_2} ↓, $[H^+]$ ↓, $[HCO_3^-]$ ↓
Clinical state: respiratory alkalosis

EXAMPLE 5. Infant with Respiratory Distress Syndrome:

P_{CO_2} = 60 mm Hg
$[H^+]$ = 100 nEq/liter
$[HCO_3^-]$ = 14.4 mEq/liter
Pattern P_{CO_2} ↑, $[H^+]$ ↑, $[HCO_3^-]$ ↓
Clinical state: mixed respiratory and metabolic acidosis

Calculation of Values

In some laboratories only two of the three primary variables P_{CO_2}, $[H^+]$, and $[HCO_3^-]$ are provided by direct analysis, and the third value is obtained by calculation. In addition, at times total buffer base may be given instead of $[HCO_3^-]$, and a hemoglobin concentration should be available with this, as the major buffer of the nonbicarbonate group of buffers is hemoglobin. A nomogram is included in the Appendix for calculations when buffer base is to be considered. The remainder of this discussion is limited to P_{CO_2}, $[H^+]$, and $[HCO_3^-]$.

When the value for pH is provided, but $[H^+]$ is desired, conversion may be made using Table 6-1; or if the pH is close to 6.8, 7.1, 7.7, or 8.0, $[H^+]$ can be calculated quickly, because a change of 0.3 pH units is equivalent to doubling or halving the $[H^+]$, using pH 7.4 = $[H^+]$ of 40 nEq/liter. Thus pH = 7.1 (a drop of 0.3 pH units from pH = 7.4) would mean a doubling of $[H^+]$ = 40 nEq/liter, or a value of $[H^+]$ = 80 nEq/liter. Similarly, a pH = 7.7 (a rise of 0.3 pH units) would be equivalent to halving $[H^+]$ = 40 nEq/liter, or $[H^+]$ = 20 nEq/liter. A pH of 6.8 (two drops of 0.3 pH units) would equal two doublings of $[H^+]$, or $40 \times 2 \times 2 = 160$ nEq/liter.

P_{CO_2} and $[H_2CO_3]$ are also easily interchangeable. Remembering that $[H_2CO_3]$, as used herein, is actually $[H_2CO_3 + CO_2(d)]$, $[H_2CO_3]$ can be obtained from P_{CO_2} by multiplying the P_{CO_2} value by 0.03, its solubility coefficient. In a reverse manner, P_{CO_2} can be calculated from $[H_2CO_3]$ by dividing $[H_2CO_3]$ by 0.3. For example:

P_{CO_2} = 60 mm Hg; $[H_2CO_3]$ = 0.03 × 60 = 1.8 mEq/liter
P_{CO_2} = 20 mm Hg; $[H_2CO_3]$ = 0.03 × 20 = 0.6 mEq/liter
$[H_2CO_3]$ = 1.5 mEq/liter; P_{CO_2} = 1.5/0.03 = 50 mm Hg
$[H_2CO_3]$ = 0.9 mEq/liter; P_{CO_2} = 0.9/0.03 = 30 mm Hg

INTRACELLULAR CHANGES

The preceding discussion is applicable to chemical reactions in all the body water—intracellular and extracellular. However, the primary regulation and compensating functions affect the ECF directly and the ICF in an indirect manner. The primary reasons for this distinction are that (1) cell membranes are relatively impermeable to anions, (2) they exchange cations by an active process, and (3) they are relatively permeable to small uncharged molecules. Thus HCO_3^- crosses cell membranes very slowly and H_2CO_3 (CO_2) quite rapidly. Therefore, respiratory changes in Pco_2 affect the interiors of cells quickly, but the renal changes in $[H^+]$ and $[HCO_3^-]$ do not affect cellular fluids as quickly as they change the ECF. The impact of this will be shown in the examples that follow.

ILLUSTRATIVE CASES

EXAMPLE 1. A 10-kg infant with a history of diarrhea for 3 days is admitted to the hospital with moderately severe dehydration and noticeable hyperventilation. The initial serum values reported by the laboratory are the following: Na^+ = 136 mEq/liter, Cl^- = 110 mEq/liter, K^+ = 4.4 mEq/liter, pH = 7.10, "total CO_2" = 6.6 mEq/liter,* Pco_2 = 20 mm Hg.† The following values can be derived: $[H^+]$ can be found either by recalling that doubling the normal value of 40 nEq/liter produces a drop of 0.3 pH units or by consulting Table 6-1. The value is 80 nEq/liter. $[H_2CO_3]$‡ may be found by multiplying Pco_2 by its solubility coefficient, 0.03. The resultant value is 0.6 mM/liter.

In addition, since K' is a constant, any variable in the following equation can be calculated if the other two are given:

$$\frac{[H^+][HCO_3^-]}{[H_2CO_3]} = K'; \qquad K' = 800 \times 10^{-9}$$

In an adult or older child the normal values (in equivalents or moles/ liter are

* The "total CO_2" content, a common laboratory term, represents the sum of $[HCO_3^-] + [H_2CO_3 + CO_2(d)]$ in the plasma or serum. Therefore, one should subtract the value of $[H_2CO_3 + CO_2(d)]$ from this to obtain the correct figure for $[HCO_3^-]$. However, for clinical purposes this is a small correction, and ignoring it will not affect clinical management.

† More recently, laboratories are beginning to report Pco_2 values instead "total CO_2." If any two of the three values or their alternates ($[H^+]$) or pH, [total CO_2] or $[HCO_3^-]$, and Pco_2 or $[H_2CO_3]$) are provided, the other term or its alternate can be calculated.

‡ Remember that this is really $[H_2CO_3 + CO_2(d)]$.

$$\frac{(40 \times 10^{-9})(24 \times 10^{-3})}{(1.2 \times 10^{-3})} = 800 \times 10^{-9}$$

For purposes of calculation, one can ignore the exponents and use

$$\frac{(40)(24)}{(1.2)} = 800$$

The denominator on the left is frequently expressed in terms of P_{CO_2} rather than H_2CO_3; because the units of measurement are changed, the value of the constant is altered. The normal values for the variables and the constant for an older child or adult become

$$\frac{(40)(24)}{(40)} = 24$$

and for an infant, they are

$$\frac{(40)(20)}{(33.3)} = 24$$

Although the variables on the left have different normal values for infants, the constant is the same at all ages because the units of measurement are the same.

In the example of the 10-kg infant, if $[H^+] = 80$ nEq/liter and $P_{CO_2} = 20$ mm Hg are known, $[HCO_3^-]$ can be calculated:

$$\frac{(80)[HCO_3^-]}{(20)} = 24; \qquad [HCO_3^-] = 6 \text{ m Eq/liter*}$$

If $[H^+]$ and "total CO_2" are known, P_{CO_2} can be calculated:

$$\frac{(80)(``6.6")}{(P_{CO_2})} = 24; \qquad P_{CO_2} = 22 \text{ mm Hg*}$$

Finally, should $[HCO_3^-]$ and P_{CO_2} be known, $[H^+]$ can be calculated:

$$\frac{[H^+](6.0)}{(20)} = 24; \qquad [H^+] = 80 \text{ nEq/liter}$$

* Note that the difference between $[HCO_3^-]$ calculated and the "total CO_2" is the difference between 6.0 and 6.6 mEq/liter, and the error in calculating P_{CO_2} from "total CO_2" rather than from $[HCO_3^-]$ is 2 mm Hg.

Thus this child is acidemic, as defined by $[H^+]$ greater than 40 nEq/liter (pH < 7.4). This acidemia is the result of either increased amounts of H^+ or decreased amounts of HCO_3^- or both. If one examines the basic equation and its normal values for the infant,

$$CO_2 + H_2O \rightleftarrows H_2CO_3 \rightleftarrows H^+ + HCO_3^-$$

$$(33) \qquad\qquad (1.2) \qquad (40) \qquad (24)$$

one notes that the $[H^+]$ is elevated and the $[HCO_3^-]$ is decreased. The pattern of changes is that of metabolic acidosis, and the decrease in Pco_2 represents an attempt by hyperventilation to compensate for the increased $[H^+]$ by moving the reaction further toward the left. Had compensatory hyperventilation not occurred, but the $[HCO_3^-]$ remained the same, $[H^+]$ would be

$$\frac{[H^+](6)}{(1.2)} + 800 \qquad \text{or} \qquad \frac{[H^+](6)}{(40)} = 24$$

$[H^+] = 160$ nEq/liter, and pH = 6.80. Thus this patient's acid–base balance can be said to represent partially compensated metabolic acidosis. It is only partially compensated because the patient remains acidemic.

    Therapeutically, the fluid management for example 1 would be calculated as follows:

Maintenance:
Insensible water loss = 40 ml/kg/day   (slight increase due to hyperventilation)

Urinary water loss   = 50 ml/kg/day

Gastrointestinal loss = 30 ml/kg/day   (moderately severe diarrhea)

Total   = 120 ml/kg/day

Repair:
10% dehydration = 100 ml/kg
Provide 60 ml/kg on first day and 40 ml/kg on second day
Day 1 repair = 60 ml/kg
Total fluid, first 24 hours = 120 + 60 = 180 ml/kg
For the 10-kg child, 10 × 180 = 1800 ml

    The fluid given to replace the IWL and the urinary loss will be given as 5% dextrose in water. The fluid used for the gastrointestinal losses and for repair will be an isotonic salt solution.* The total fluid will consist of equal parts dextrose in water (IWL + renal) (50 + 40) and isotonic salt solution (gastrointestinal + repair) (30 + 60).

---

* The term *salt* in this chapter, as in the others, does not necessarily refer to sodium chloride but to a balanced salt solution that may contain a mixture of anions and cations.

The initial composition of the salt solution will contain primarily Na^+, Cl^-, and HCO_3^-. Potassium will not be used for the first few hours or until it is clear that serum K^+ is not elevated and renal function is reasonable. Since the total solution is to be one-half salt, the $[Na^+]$ will be approximately 75 mEq/liter. The sum of Cl^- and HCO_3^- must equal 75, but the proportion of each remains to be determined.

HCO_3^- is given because it is a H^+ acceptor and can thus both reduce the elevated $[H^+]$ and restore the buffer anion concentration. Attempts have been made to calculate the amount of HCO_3^- necessary to return both these entities to their normal concentrations and then to provide this quantity; several empirical and theoretical formulas are available for such calculations. There are four reasons for not employing them. First, the continued effects of diarrhea and the rate of metabolic production of H^+ are unpredictable. Second, healthy kidneys can excrete H^+ and restore buffer base, when provided with an adequate amount of fluid for maintenance and renal function. The third reason relates to the rate of respiratory response to changes in $[H^+]$. If HCO_3^- is infused rapidly, the decrease in hyperventilation may not keep pace, and alkalemia may result. The fourth reason relates to the problem of anions entering cells. Entry of HCO_3^- into cells, because it is an anion, will be a slow process. The following situation can occur as a result of this difficulty. Given a person with metabolic acidosis, the pretreatment acid–base status of the ECF and ICF may be:

	Extracellular	Intracellular
$[H^+]$	80 (40)	120 (80) nEq/liter
$[HCO_3^-]$	9 (24)	6 (12) mEq/liter
Pco_2	30 (40)	30 (40) mm Hg
(pH)	7.1 (7.4)	6.92 (7.1)

Normally the interior of the cell is more acid than ECF, and this is usually true in metabolic acidosis as well. If this person were given HCO_3^- in an amount calculated to correct $[HCO_3^-]$, the values could become:

	Extracellular	Intracellular
$[H^+]$	40	160 nEq/liter
$[HCO_3^-]$	24	6 mEq/liter
Pco_2	40	40 mm Hg
(pH)	(7.4)	(6.8)

With rapid infusion of bicarbonate into the ECF, increasing the ECF buffer, the $[H^+]$ will fall and the stimulus to hyperventilation will decrease, with a subsequent rise of H_2CO_3 (or Pco_2) toward normal. In the cells, only the last reaction will occur rapidly, i.e., the P_{CO_2} will rise toward 40 mm Hg (H_2CO_3 to 1.2 mEq/liter). The HCO_3^- will not increase in this period of time; so the reaction $CO_2 + H_2O \rightleftarrows H_2CO_3 \rightleftarrows H^+ + HCO_3^-$ will be shifted to the right. This means that more H_2CO_3 will be present to contribute H^+, but there will be no additional buffer base to accept the H^+; therefore $[H^+]$ will rise (pH will fall), and the cellular contents will become more acidic.

If an elevated $[H^+]$ is harmful, it is likely to be more harmful in cells, where most critical chemical reactions take place. Thus rapid infusion of HCO_3^- in metabolic acidosis may produce an increase in the acidosis of the cells. If renal function is adequate, the kidneys will ordinarily correct metabolic acidosis at a rate such that an increase in intracellular acidosis will not occur. In the absence of reasonable renal function, HCO_3^- or another H^+ acceptor would have to be infused to correct the acidosis.

In the present case, as in most cases of metabolic acidosis, administration of some H^+ acceptor is useful. The quantity of HCO_3^- that may be given safely is comparable to the proportion of buffer anion to total anion in blood. In the blood the concentration of the buffer base is about one-third the total anion concentration. In the serum, the concentration of buffer anions (HCO_3^- and protein) is about one-fourth the anion concentration. Thus about one-third to one-fourth of the anion can be HCO_3^- or another H^+ acceptor. The total anion concentration in this case is 75 mEq/liter; so the $[HCO_3^-]$ can be approximately 15–25 mEq/liter, and the remaining 50–60 mEq/liter of anion will be Cl^-.

The final solution should be $Na^+ = 75$, $Cl^- = 55$, and $HCO_3^- = 20$ mEq/liter, with glucose 2.5%; and this fluid should be given more rapidly in the first few hours. If the infant is in shock or appears to be close to being in a shocklike state, 10–20 ml/kg of the initial solution should be given very rapidly using a syringe and "pushing" the fluid in over a period of 10–30 minutes. If shock is not a problem, one-third of the 24-hour fluid may be given in 6 hours or half of it in 8 hours. The remainder should then be given more slowly over the remainder of the 24-hour period.

The initial order should specify an intravenous infusion of 100 ml/hour for 6 hours of a solution containing $Na^+ = 75$ mEq/liter, $Cl^- = 55$ mEq/liter, $HCO_3^- = 20$ mEq/liter, and glucose = 2.5%. Then, provided the serum K^+ is not elevated and urine output is apparent, 65–70 ml/hour for 18 hours of a solution containing $Na^+ = 50$ mEq/liter, $K^+ = 25$ mEq/liter, $Cl^- = 55$ mEq/liter, $HCO_3^- = 20$ mEq/liter, and glucose = 2.5%.

These two orders will provide 1800 ml in a 24-hour period of a solution that is half-isotonic for sodium and potassium and that contains K^+ at 3 mEq/kg, which does not exceed a $[K^+]$ of 30 mEq/liter and which contains glucose in excess of 3 g/kg.

For the second 24-hour period, the fluids required will be based on maintenance needs of IWL = 40 ml/kg, renal loss = 50 ml/kg, and gastrointestinal loss = 10 ml/kg (diarrhea slowed), as well as remaining repair fluid of 40 ml/kg, for total fluid of 140 ml/kg, of which 90 ml/kg will be a glucose solution and 50 ml/kg will be a salt solution. For this 10-kg infant, the total is 1400 ml.

The cation concentration of the total solution is calculated on the basis of the ratio of salt-containing solution to the total amount of fluid to be given. In this example, it is the ratio of 50 ml/kg of salt solution to 140 ml/kg of total fluid. This is multiplied by the cation concentration of an isotonic salt solution (150 mEq/liter). The calculation is (50/140) × 150 = 53 mEq/liter. The cations will again be divided between Na^+ and K^+, and the anions between Cl^- and HCO_3^-.

Avoiding fractional values, the total solution will contain Na^+ = 30 mEq/liter, K^+ = 25 mEq/liter, Cl^- = 40 mEq/liter, HCO_3^- = 15 mEq/liter, and glucose = 2.5%–5.0% and will be given at a rate of 1400 ml/24 hours = approximately 58 ml/hour.

Formulations of Na^+, K^+, Cl^-, HCO_3^-, and glucose such as these are rarely available exactly as calculated, and ordinarily one can select a solution from those available in most hospitals to approximate as closely as possible the calculated concentrations. If there is no commercial solution that approximates what is needed, the pharmacy can prepare such a mixture.

In addition, frequent reexamination of the patient and repeat weight and serum chemical values at the end of 24 hours should indicate reasonable progress toward normality. If this is not the case, reassessment of the entire situation should be made before ordering additional fluids.

At the end of 48 hours, most such infants can be started on oral feedings.

EXAMPLE 2. A 4-week-old infant weighing 3.0 kg (birth weight = 3.5 kg) presents with a history of increasing vomiting since 1 week of age. A small firm mass is palpable in the epigastrium. The vomitus does not contain bile. The child appears quite dehydrated and thin. The laboratory values obtained are Na^+ = 137 mEq/liter, K^+ = 3.0 mEq/liter, Cl^- = 82 mEq/liter, pH = 7.52, Pco_2 = 50 mm Hg, and BUN = 35 mg/dl. Derived values are $[H^+]$ = 30 nEq/liter (from Table 6-1, pH = 7.52), $[HCO_3^-]$ = 40 mEq/liter (from 30 $[HCO_3^-]$/50 = 24; $[HCO_3^-]$ = 50 × 24/30 = 40 mEq/liter).

Since $[H^+]$ is below the normal value of 40 nEq/liter, the infant is alkalemic. $[HCO_3^-]$ is markedly elevated. Pco_2 has risen slightly to compensate for the reduced $[H^+]$, and so the situation can be described as partially compensated metabolic alkalosis (Table 6-5).

The potassium is low and may become much lower when hydration is improved. The mild azotemia probably represents reduced renal function secondary to the dehydration. The fluid calculation is as follows:

Maintenance:
IWL = 40 ml/kg
Renal loss = 50 ml/kg
Gastrointestinal loss = 10 ml/kg (slight increase due to nasogastric suction)
Repair = 100 ml/kg; 75% to be given in first 24 hours
Total glucose solution = 40 + 50 = 90 ml/kg
Total salt solution = 10 + 75 = 85 ml/kg
Total solution per kilogram = 175 ml/kg
Total fluids = 175 ml/kg × 3 kg = 525 ml/24 hours
Composition of total solution: Na^+ = 50 meq/liter, K^+ = 25 meq/liter, Cl^- = 75 meq/liter.

Note that no buffer anion such as HCO_3^- is given, since the $[H^+]$ is already low and the buffer anion concentration is already elevated.

Again, the fluid would be given more rapidly initially: 33 ml/hour × 8 hours; then 16 ml/hour × 16 hours.

EXAMPLE 3. A 5-year-old boy presents with fever, increased respiratory effort, and mild dehydration; he became ill in the previous 48 hours. Among other studies, his serum values are determined: Na^+ = 144 meq/liter, K^+ = 4 meq/liter, Cl^- = 96 meq/liter, "total CO_2" = 32 meq/liter, pH = 7.22 (H^+ = 60 neq/liter).

In this laboratory, pH was reported, but it can quickly be converted to $[H^+]$ from Table 6-1. Pco_2 can be calculated:

$$\frac{60 \times 32}{Pco_2} = 24$$

$$Pco_2 = 80 \text{ mm Hg}$$

This patient has acidemia ($[H^+]$ increased), but in this case the Pco_2 is also elevated, and the increased $[H_2CO_3]$ increased the $[H^+]$. The $[HCO_3^-]$ originally rose because of dissociation of $H_2CO_3 \rightarrow H^+ + HCO_3^-$ and has been increased further by the kidney to reduce the $[H^+]$.* Had the renal compensation not begun, the $[HCO_3^-]$ would have been 28 meq/liter, and the elevation of Pco_2 to 80 mm Hg would have created $[H^+]$ of 70 neq/liter (pH = 7.16). Thus this patient can be considered to have partially compensated respiratory acidosis.

Under usual conditions, one treats primary respiratory acidosis by methods designed to correct the respiratory problem itself. No special

---

* In respiratory acidosis the rise in Pco_2 increases $[H_2CO_3^-]$ and in turn increases $[H^+] + [HCO_3^-]$. Concomitantly, the increased $[H^+]$ reacts with other buffer bases, converting them to the weak acids; so the total buffer base does not change.

acid–base correction is attempted by the use of fluid therapy, since the amount of buffer anion, or H^+ acceptor, is already present in normal or increased concentration. There may be situations, as in infantile respiratory distress syndrome, where increasing the buffer anion further could be beneficial. This remains an equivocal situation, however.

EXAMPLE 4.   A 2-year-old girl is admitted to the hospital hyperpneic and with a history of ingestion of an unknown amount of aspirin a short time previously. Her initial serum values are $Na^+ = 135$ mEq/liter, $K^+ = 4$ mEq/liter, $Cl^- = 95$ mEq/liter, $HCO_3^- = 18$ mEq/liter, $Pco_2 = 25$ mm Hg, salicylate level = 70 mg/dl; $([H^+] \times 18)/25 = 24$; $[H^+] = 33$ nEq/liter (pH = 7.48).

The patient has alkalemia (reduced $[H^+]$) with reduced Pco_2, indicating respiratory alkalosis. At this point the reduction in $[HCO_3^-]$ would appear to represent a partial compensation to maintain $[H^+]$. Therefore, at this time, administration of additional HCO_3^- or another H^+ acceptor would be contraindicated. However, if the child had been seen later after the ingestion of the aspirin, the salicylate intoxication would have produced increasing $[H^+]$ and further reduction of the buffer anion concentration as a result of increased production of stronger acids as part of the metabolic response to salicylate intoxication. The values in the serum might then have become $Na^+ = 136$ mEq/liter, $K^+ = 4$ mEq/liter, $Cl^- = 110$ mEq/liter, $HCO_3^- = 8$ mEq/liter, $Pco_2 = 18$ mm Hg, $H^+ = 54$ nEq/liter (pH = 7.27).

This situation would then appear as metabolic acidosis and would be treated as in example 1. In actual fact, this represents a mixed disturbance (metabolic acidosis and respiratory alkalosis), but the metabolic acidosis dominates the situation at this time. However, caution must be observed as the $[HCO_3^-]$ rises, since the primary hyperventilation from the salicylate may persist and a respiratory alkalosis may reappear as the buffer base increases.

SUMMARY

A unitary concept for considering acid–base disorders has been presented in terms of hydrogen ion concentration. The concepts of metabolic and respiratory acidosis and alkalosis have been interpreted in terms of hydrogen ion concentrations and the basic respiratory and renal regulating system governing hydrogen ion metabolism and excretion. Four illustrative cases have been described, representing each of the classic situations of metabolic acidosis and alkalosis and respiratory acidosis and alkalosis.

Although consideration of these problems in terms of the hydrogen ion is relatively new and requires some reorientation of our classic thinking about these problems, such an orientation should ultimately prove simpler and more in keeping with our understanding of the other cations and anions of the body fluids.

PART III

Specific Clinical Disorders

7
Primary Medical Problems

ASSESSMENT SCHEMA FOR FLUID PROBLEMS

Assessment of a patient with a disturbance in fluid and electrolyte homeostasis must involve three elements: (1) volume abnormality, (2) composition abnormality, and (3) acid–base abnormality. These elements will be evaluated in the order given, and therapy is generally given priority in the same order.

As an example of this process, consider a dehydrated child with hypernatremia and metabolic acidosis. The first concern is to assess the degree of dehydration and the child's maintenance fluid requirements. These will determine the total volume of fluid to be given in a 24-hr period. Then one must consider the other aspects of the child's status to determine whether this total volume should be modified and/or given at variable rates. If the child has experienced peripheral vascular collapse or might easily develop it, the fluids should be given more rapidly initially. If the child has heart disease, cardiac failure, or cerebral edema, the total volume should be decreased or the replacement given over a longer period of time.

223

Once the fluid volume and rate of administration have been established, the electrolyte composition should be considered. If there is no remarkable electrolyte disturbance, the replacement (repair) fluid should consist of an essentially isotonic salt solution (a combination of anions and cations totaling 150 mEq/liter or 300 mOsm/liter). The maintenance fluids should be mostly water, with glucose (5%) to establish an isotonic solution. If the volumes of both solutions are approximately equal, the final mixture will be about half isosmotic for salt (total cations or anions = 75 mEq/liter) and for glucose (2.5%). Initially the 75 mEq of cation are generally all Na^+. If there are no urinary problems, the solution should be changed after 3–6 hr to a solution containing 45 mEq/liter Na^+ and 30 mEq/liter K^+. The anions may be 50 mEq/liter Cl^- and 25 mEq/liter "buffer anion," such as HCO_3^-, lactate$^-$, or HPO_4^{--}. After making these initial assessments, all other relevant factors should be evaluated to determine if any of these concentrations need to be modified.

In the presence of an electrolyte compositional problem, the first concern is the total solute concentration. This can be checked quickly by considering the concentrations of urea, glucose, and sodium. If the sum of the millimolar concentrations of urea plus glucose plus twice the sodium* is in the range of 250–320 mOsm/liter, no immediate action needs to be taken to alter the total solute concentration. If urea or glucose concentration is abnormal (whether or not the total solute is normal), specific therapy should be directed toward the cause of these abnormalities. If the total solute concentration is abnormally low, the salt content of the fluids may need to be adjusted upward. If the solute concentration is high because of an increase in the electrolyte component, a cautious reduction of the salt content of the fluids to be administered should be considered (see the section on Na^+; similarly, for abnormal concentrations of other ions, the appropriate section on that ion should be consulted).

Disorders of acid–base equilibrium are the last group of conditions that should be evaluated, for two reasons: these disturbances are less likely to impair function critically, and specific therapeutic measures are less often necessary, since self-correction usually occurs if sufficient fluid and salt are available and if renal and pulmonary functions are normal. In those conditions in which the extent of the disorder is extreme or where renal function is impaired, direct intervention may be required. If the disorder is respiratory in origin, treatment should be directed toward correcting the ventilatory response. If the problem is metabolic, some adjustment of the concentration of the buffer anion is indicated.

The case examples presented in Chapters 7 and 8 illustrate these assessments and the subsequent treatment priorities and processes under a variety of circumstances.

---

* [Na] × 2 is used to account in an approximate way for the anions as well as cations.

CASE 1: GASTROENTERITIS

A 2-month-old black female infant was admitted to the hospital with a 48-hr history of diarrhea. She had had 10–20 stools during each of the preceding 24 hr, and most of these had been green and watery, with small amounts of mucus and seedy material; in 2 stools frank red blood had been present. She had had no fever or respiratory symptoms. She had been anorectic, but had taken small amounts of a sugar solution containing 1 teaspoon of sugar in 3 ounces of water (about 5 g/100 ml). She did not void during the 6 hr prior to admission. She had had no medication and had not been ill previously. No other family members were ill or had been ill in recent weeks. The remainder of her history was unremarkable.

On physical examination she appeared to be alert and irritable, but she did not exhibit much spontaneous movement. She appeared adequately nourished and appeared to be about her stated age. Rectal temperature was 39.6°C; pulse was 140/min; respirations were 30/min; blood pressure was 80/40 mm Hg (right arm). Her length was 57 cm, and she weighed 4300 g. Her anterior fontanelle was depressed, her mucous membranes were dry, and she cried without tears. When the skin over her abdomen was pinched, it returned to its original position quite slowly. The remainder of the physical examination revealed no significant findings. Her laboratory values were as follows: hemoglobin = 12.5 g/dl; hematocrit = 35 vol%; WBC count = 12,100/mm^3 (35% neutrophils, 65% lymphocytes); Na$^+$ = 137 mEq/liter; K$^+$ = 4.0 mEq/liter; Cl$^-$ = 110 mEq/liter; total CO_2 = 12 mEq/liter; pH = 7.18; Pco$_2$ = 33 mm Hg; BUN = 30 mg/dl. A short time later a urine specimen was obtained and was reported as follows: color = yellow, clear; specific gravity = 1.027; pH = 5.5; sugar = 0; protein = 0; ketones = 0; formed elements = none present.

Problem List

1. Gastroenteritis
2. Dehydration with metabolic acidosis

Problem 1: Gastroenteritis

Assessment.   The 48-hr history of diarrhea without vomiting suggests an acute enteric infection; the presence of many watery green stools indicates a moderately severe process. Most such episodes are nonbacterial in etiology, and the presence of blood in two stools is compatible with a viral origin. However, a specific bacterial pathogen cannot be excluded without a stool culture. Other causes of diarrhea (e.g., malabsorption, food allergy, nonenteric infection) may need to be considered if the diarrhea does not subside promptly when oral intake ceases, but there is no evidence for them at this time. In any case, an acquired transient lactase deficiency may arise secondary to the enteric infection.

Plan

1. Stool cultures should be obtained to evaluate potential bacterial pathogens.
2. Blood for culture should be drawn for assessment of possible sepsis as an etiologic factor.
3. Urine for culture should be taken, as urinary tract infections can cause diarrhea in infants and because a normal urinalysis cannot exclude such infection in an infant.
4. Nothing should be taken by mouth; this should reduce stimulation and possible irritation of the gastrointestinal tract.
5. Parenteral fluids should be given (see problem 2).

Problem 2: Dehydration with Metabolic Acidosis

Assessment. The physical findings are indicative of moderate dehydration, and the weight is about 10% below that expected for the infant's length. With the lack of urine output for 6 hr and the above findings, one can estimate at least a 10% dehydration. The normal blood pressure, the lack of severe tachycardia, and the absence of any indication of peripheral vascular collapse suggest that the extent of the dehydration is not much above 10%.

The concentration of solute in body fluids is approximately $2 \times [Na^+] = 2 \times 137 = 274$ mOsm/liter, since the BUN is normal and there is no evidence for hyperglycemia. Thus there should be no need to modify the usual solute concentration of the infused solution. The composition of the ECF reveals a normal $[K^+]$ and no other evidence for an abnormality in composition; thus no special restraints are known to be necessary in regard to planning the composition of the intravenous fluids.

The $[H^+]$ is 66 mEq/liter (see Table 6-1); this indicates acidemia, but not severe acidemia. The relative reduction in CO_2 content ($20 \rightarrow 12$ mEq/liter) suggests that the acidemia is the result of a metabolic acidosis, partially compensated by some hyperventilation.

Parenteral Fluid Volume. Based on an assumed 10% dehydration, repair will require 100 ml/kg. Since the child is in good physical condition, 75 ml/kg will be given in the first 24 hr and the remaining 25 ml/kg during the second day.

Insensible water loss (IWL) for this age is about 40 ml/kg/day. The child's temperature is elevated about 2°C, which increases the metabolic rate 20% (10%/1°C). Thus the fluid required for IWL is $40 + (0.20)(40) = 40 + 8 = 48$ ml/kg.

Renal water requirement is about 50 ml/kg/day, given no unusual renal problems or abnormal solute loads. That value is appropriate for this child.

Gastrointestinal losses from the diarrhea may be expected to decrease when oral intake is stopped. However, until the stools do decrease, some estimate of their volume is required. Experiences with weighing diarrheal stools (in the United States) suggests that a usable average figure is about 35 ml/kg/day.

Thus on day 1 (initially) the total fluid requirements are as follows: repair = 75 ml/kg; IWL = 48 ml/kg; renal = 50 ml/kg; gastrointestinal = 35 ml/kg; total = 208 = 8.7 ml/kg/hr. If the diarrhea subsides, this volume may be reduced to 175 ml/kg = 7.3 ml/kg/hr. Multiplying each figure by the infant's weight gives 8.7 ml/kg/hr × 4.3 kg = 37.4 ml/hr (which can be rounded up or down), and 7.3 × 4.3 = 31.4 ml/hr.

Parenteral Fluid Composition. Until it appears certain that renal function will continue, potassium should not be included in the intravenous fluids. Thus about half the fluids (75 ml/kg for repair + 35 ml/kg for gastrointestinal losses) should contain isotonic [Na^+]. The final solution would then be $[(75 + 35)/(75 + 35 + 48 + 50)] \times 150$ mEq/liter $= \sim 0.5 \times 150 = 75$ mEq/liter Na^+.

The anions will also total 75 mEq/liter. If buffering is to be physiologic, about one-third of the anions should have a buffering capability. A [Cl^-] of 50 mEq/liter and a [HCO_3^-] of 25 mEq/liter will meet these requirements.

The next solution to be used, once it is known that the patient has a normal [K^+] and adequate renal function, is a solution containing K^+. The commonly used concentration is 30 mEq/liter.

Plan

1. Initial parenteral solution: 8.7 ml/kg/hr × 4.3 kg × 6 hr = 225 ml, with composition of Na^+ = 75 mEq/liter, Cl^- = 50 mEq/liter, HCO_3^- = 25 mEq/liter, and glucose = 2.5 g/dl. Infuse at 38 ml/hr until voided well or for 6 hr, whichever is later.

2. After the initial solution has been administered, determine the hemoglobin, hematocrit, Na^+, K^+, Cl^-, total CO_2, Pco_2, glucose, and BUN.

3. In the remaining 18 hr, if the patient is voiding and [K^+] is normal, volume = 8.7 ml/kg/hr × 4.3 kg × 18 hr = 675 ml. The composition will be Na^+ = 45 mEq/liter, K^+ = 30 mEq/liter, Cl^- = 50 mEq/liter, HCO_3^- = 25 mEq/liter, and glucose = 2.5 g/dl. The infusion will be continued at 38 ml/hr.

Progress Notes (24 hr)

PROBLEM 2: DEHYDRATION WITH
METABOLIC ACIDOSIS

Assessment. The child appears markedly improved; weight is 4.6 kg, and diarrhea has ceased. Dehydration as seen on physical examination is minimal, and temperature is 37°C. Repeat laboratory values are as follows: Na^+ = 140 mEq/liter; K^+ = 4.2 mEq/liter; Cl^- = 108 mEq/liter; total CO_2 = 17 mEq/liter; H^+ = 50 nEq/liter; Pco_2 = 35 mm Hg; glucose = 110 mEq/liter; BUN = 19 mg/dl.

Fluids: Since the child gained about 300 g and the planned repair was 75 ml/kg or 75 × 4.3 kg = 322 ml, the other maintenance estimates appear to have been reasonable.

For this 24-hr period the volume is as follows: repair = 25 ml/kg; IWL = 40 ml/kg; renal = 50 ml/kg; gastrointestinal = 0 ml/kg; total 115 ml/kg, or 115 × 4.6 kg = 530 ml, or

$$\frac{530 \text{ ml}}{24 \text{ hr}} = 22 \text{ ml/hr}$$

The composition of these fluids should be based on an isotonic "salt" mixture for the repair solution of 25 ml/kg and glucose in water for the IWL and renal water maintenance requirements (40 + 50 = 90 ml/kg). $[Na^+] + [K^+]$ = [25/(25 + 50 + 40)] × 150 mEq/liter ~ 33 mEq/liter.

Plan. Parenteral therapy for the second 24-hr period is as follows: Rate: 22 ml/hr × 24 hr. Composition: Na^+ = 20 mEq/liter, K^+ = 15 mEq/liter, Cl^- = 25 mEq/liter, HCO_3^- = 10 mEq/liter, glucose = 5 g/dl.

Progress Notes (48 hr)

PROBLEM 1: GASTROENTERITIS

Assessment. The child had no further stools and appeared alert and healthy. The stool, blood, and urine cultures were negative for any pathogens. The child's weight rose to 4.7 kg, which suggests adequate hydration; this was confirmed by the physical examination.

Plan. Begin giving the child oral clear fluids. If these are tolerated well for 12–18 hr, continue with the child's formula diluted with an equal volume of water for an additional 12–18 hr. If the child remains well, resume the child's original formula at that time. After 1 day of observation, discharge the child with appropriate instruction of the mother.

CASE 2: CARDIAC FAILURE

A 7-month-old male infant was admitted to the hospital because of lethargy, anorexia, and tachypnea that had lasted 48 hr. He had been seen in a cardiac clinic in another city when he was 2 months of age because of similar symptoms. At that time it was stated that he had congestive heart failure secondary to a moderately large ventricular septal defect; since then he has thrived poorly. He developed a respiratory infection 2 days prior to hospital admission. In the previous 48 hr he took milk and water but refused solid foods. His urine output was scanty.

The infant was being given digitalis; he was fed low-sodium milk and was maintained with an oral dose of furosemide, 1 mg/kg twice daily. However, he had vomited occasionally in the previous few days, and the parents were not certain how much of the medication he had retained or what his total fluid intake had been. His feet and lower legs had appeared to be slightly swollen, according to the parents.

On physical examination the infant weighed 6.3 kg and was 65 cm long. There was no cyanosis, but he looked anxious and fatigued, he was perspiring profusely, and he was markedly tachypneic (respiratory rate 60/min). There was flaring of the alae nasi and supraclavicular retraction. The lungs were noisy, with rales present bilaterally. The cardiac outline extended to the anterior axillary line on the left. There was a systolic thrill with a loud, harsh, pansystolic murmur over the entire precordium but loudest along the left sternal border. There was also a mid-diastolic rumble over the apical area. The liver edge was palpable 6 cm below the costal margin in the right midclavicular line. There was questionable edema of the eyelids and dorsa of the feet. The laboratory values were as follows: hemoglobin = 10.0 g/dl; hematocrit = 32 vol%; WBC count = 12,500/mm^3 (polymorphonuclear leukocytes 71%, lymphocytes 25%, monocytes 3%, eosinophils 1%); serum Na^+ = 124 mEq/liter; serum Cl^- = 80 mEq/liter; total CO_2 = 30 mEq/liter; total K^+ = 2.5 mEq/liter; BUN = 8 mg/dl. Urine values were as follows: specific gravity = 1.010; pH = 6.0; WBC count = 0–1/hpf; RBC count = 0–3/hpf; casts = 0–2/lpf; sugar = 0; acetone = 0; protein = 2.

Problem List

1. Cardiac failure
2. Hypokalemia and metabolic alkalosis
3. Hyponatremia
4. Growth retardation
5. Ventricular septal defect

Problem 1: Cardiac Failure

Assessment. The presenting symptoms and the physical findings are highly suggestive of cardiac failure, particularly since this diagnosis has been made before and the child is known to have a congenital cardiac lesion. A lower respiratory infection may also be present and may have precipitated the failure or may be the major element responsible for the infant's symptoms.

Plan

1. A chest x-ray should be obtained to evaluate cardiac and pulmonary status.
2. An electrocardiogram should be obtained to examine for digitalis effect, since this may be more marked with hypokalemia.
3. If indicated by steps 1 and 2, digitalis should be administered; the dosage will be dependent on the findings in step 2.
4. Furosemide should be administered: 1.5 mg/kg; 10 mg intravenously stat; this should provide some temporary reduction in circulating fluid volume.
5. Vital signs should be monitored every 30 min for a period of 6 hr.

Problem 2: Hypokalemia and Metabolic Alkalosis

Assessment. Hypokalemia and metabolic alkalosis are often seen together, and each may play a role in the development of the other. The presence of hypokalemia suggests a fairly extensive whole-body potassium deficiency and is probably related to the prolonged use of a diuretic that can produce renal K^+ loss. No supplemental K^+ was being given, and although the infant's formula was high in K^+, intake had been erratic.

The acid–base disturbance appears to be minimal alkalemia that is metabolic in origin, because the total CO_2 is elevated. The Pco_2 is also increased; this may be a secondary compensatory response, but on the basis of the pulmonary situation, it may also indicate some difficulty with gas exchange.

Plan

1. Intravenous fluids (see problem 3) should contain maximal tolerable amounts of K^+ (30–40 mEq/liter).
2. When oral fluids can be given and retained, these should also be high in potassium, such as milk and orange juice (intravenous fluids should be discontinued by then).

Problem 3: Hyponatremia

Assessment. The reduced $[Na^+]$ is most likely secondary to a markedly reduced Na^+ intake (Lonalac = 1.1 mEq/liter) and the prolonged use of a diuretic that increases Na^+ excretion. At times the degree of hyponatremia that can be produced by this combination may be much more marked. Sufficient fluid should be administered to meet the IWL needs. There is more than enough fluid present in the body already to provide for urine volume. Since the child needs Na^+ and K^+, the fluid will be given with these ions present; when the water is lost through the skin and lungs, the Na^+ and K^+ should remain to increase the concentrations of these ions in body water. IWL = 40 ml/kg/day for an infant of this size, although for his age slightly less would be appropriate.

Plan

1. Total fluids for 24 hr = 40 × 6 kg = 240 ml or 10 ml/hr. Rate: 10 ml/ hr × 24 hr. Composition: Na^+ = 110 mEq/liter, K^+ = 40 mEq/liter, and Cl^- = 150 mEq/liter.
2. Nothing should be given by mouth.
3. Weight determination and electrolyte administration should be repeated in 24 hr.

Problem 4: Growth Retardation

Assessment. Growth retardation is caused by inadequate calorie intake. Children with severe cardiac lesions may require more than the usual calorie intake for adequate growth.

Plan. When the child can begin to tolerate oral feedings, a milk with higher Na^+ content should be used, and the calorie concentration should be increased gradually from 20 kcal/ounce to 24–27 or even 30 kcal/ounce if this can be tolerated. These concentrations are available with commercial formulas, or they can be created from whole milk by addition of medium-chain triglycerides (MCT).

Problem 5: Ventricular Septal Defect

Because of repeated cardiac failure, this child's lesion should be repaired as soon as he can tolerate the procedure.

CASE 3: DIABETIC KETOACIDOSIS

An 11-year-old boy fell from his bicycle in the evening, but he was able to ride home. No external evidence of head injury was noted by his mother. He went to bed early, complaining of fatigue. He could not be aroused the following morning, and his parents thought his breathing was rapid and deep. He was then brought to the hospital; he was admitted to the neurosurgical service about 12 hr after he had fallen from his bicycle. No localizing neurologic signs were found. A lumbar puncture revealed a fluid under normal pressure, with no RBC, 4 WBC/mm³, a negative Pandy test, and a sugar level of 300 mg/dl. Physical examination showed a thin but not emaciated boy breathing deeply at a rate of 38/min. He appeared mildly dehydrated and could not be aroused even with painful stimuli. His blood pressure was 80/40 mm Hg; he weighed 32 kg and was 136 cm tall. The laboratory values were as follows: blood sugar = 442 mg/dl; acetone = 40 mg/dl; Na^+ = 134 mEq/liter; K^+ = 6.2 mEq/liter; Cl^- = 115 mEq/liter; total CO_2 = 9 mEq/liter; pH = 7.12 (H^+ = 80 nEq/liter); Pco_2 = 30 mm Hg. Urinalysis revealed a specific gravity of 1.040, with sugar strongly positive and acetone strongly positive.

Problem List

1. Hyperglycemia and glucosuria
2. Diabetic ketoacidosis

Problem 1: Hyperglycemia and Glucosuria

Assessment.   The increased glucose levels, the Kussmaul breathing, the elevated [H^+] in the blood, the serum acetone, and the spilling of sugar and acetone into the urine indicate diabetic ketoacidosis. The fatigue is probably the result of inability to utilize the circulating glucose because of lack of insulin. The body attempts to compensate for the decreased energy supply by increasing the breakdown of liver glycogen and by increasing gluconeogenesis from protein and increased utilization of fat. Ketone bodies obtained from triglycerides are also used as an energy source, but they accumulate more quickly than they can be metabolized, and this contributes to metabolic acidosis, as their pK is lower than that of H_2CO_3. Ketone acids have a low renal threshold and are detectable in the urine even when the plasma level is low. The ketone bodies are accompanied in the urine by depletion of electrolytes.

Insulin will be given by intravenous infusion of an initial dose of regular insulin, 0.1 U/kg or 3.2 U, followed by insulin administration at 0.1 U/kg/hr. Hourly blood sugar and other laboratory determinations will be done until the blood glucose is below 180 mg/dl. The rate of insulin infusion will be decreased at that time, and glucose will be added to the infusion.

Parenteral fluid volume.   An intravenous fluid solution containing Na^+, K^+, Cl^-, HCO_3^- should be given. The estimate of dehydration is 5%; therefore, repair fluids = 50 ml/kg. Maintenance fluids (basic): IWL = 40 − [(11/16)(20)] = 26 ml/kg; renal = 50 − [(11/16)(20)] = 33 ml/kg; gastrointestinal = 3 ml/kg. Because of solute diuresis due to hyperglycemia, the renal water requirement may be increased by 20%. Therefore, fluids for maintenance will equal 26 + (33 + 7) + 3 = 69 ml/kg. Total fluids = repair + maintenance = 50 + 69 = 119 ml/kg. For the first 24 hr, 119 ml/kg × 32 kg = 3808 ml or 3800 ml/day. This will be given so that one-third of the fluid is given in the first 6 hr: (1/3)(3800)/6 = 211 ml/hr for 6 hr. The remaining fluid will be given over an 18-hr period: (2/3)(3800)/18 = 140 ml/hr for 18 hr.

Parenteral fluid composition.   Repair + gastrointestinal = salt mixture; IWL + renal = glucose solution, 26 + 40 = 53 ml/kg; 53/119 × 150 mEq/liter = 67 mEq/liter for $[Na^+]$ or $[Na^+] + [K^+]$. The anions will also equal 67 mEq/liter: $[Cl^-]$ = 44 mEq/liter; $[HCO_3^-]$ = 23 mEq/liter.

For the first 6 hr, no K^+ will be given. Therefore, initially the composition will be Na^+ = 67 mEq/liter, Cl^- = 44 mEq/liter, HCO_3^- = 23 mEq/liter, and glucose = 2.5 g/dl to maintain isotonicity.

For the last 18 hr, a KH_2PO_4/K_2HPO_4 mixture will be used to provide both K^+ and PO_4^{--}, which are depleted in diabetic ketoacidosis. Thus the composition will be Na^+ = 37 mEq/liter, K^+ = 30 mEq/liter, Cl^- = 14 mEq/liter, PO_4^{--} = 30 mEq/liter, and HCO_3^- = 23 mEq/liter.

Plan

1. Fluid therapy for the first 6 hr will be as follows: Rate: 211 ml/hr × 6 hr. Composition: Na^+ = 67 mEq/liter, Cl^- = 44 mEq/liter, HCO_3^- = 23 mEq/liter, and glucose = 2.5 g/dl. For the next 18 hr fluid therapy will be as follows: Rate: 140 ml/hr × 18 hr. Composition: Na^+ = 37 mEq/liter, K^+ = 30 mEq/liter, Cl^- = 14 mEq/liter, PO_4^{--} = 30 mEq/liter, and HCO_3^- = 23 mEq/liter. The glucose concentration will be increased to 5% when blood sugar falls to 180 mg/dl.

2. Insulin infusion (regular insulin) will be as follows: initial bolus of 3.2 U followed by 3.2 U/hr until serum acetone has cleared, total CO_2 has reached 18 mEq/liter, or $[H^+]$ is down to 50 nEq/liter. Then the patient will be started on intermittent (9.6-hr) doses of subcutaneous regular insulin.

3. Blood values should be monitored hourly until blood glucose is controlled: glucose, Na^+, K^+, HCO_3^-, Pco_2. Additional lab tests: BUN, triglycerides.

Problem 2: Diabetic Ketoacidosis

Assessment. Acidosis is compensated by the actions of the buffer systems, by increased alveolar ventilation, and by increased renal excretion of ammonium and titratable acid. Respiratory compensation is near its maximum when the Pco_2 reaches 20 mm Hg. Bicarbonate is included in the intravenous fluids and will help to correct the acidosis.

Plan

1. Vital signs should be monitored every 30 min until stabilized.
2. Intravenous fluids should be administered as detailed for problem 1.

CASE 4: SALICYLATE POISONING

A 3½-year-old girl swallowed an unknown number of 5-grain (300-mg) aspirin tablets at 10:30 A.M. and was brought immediately to the emergency room by her parents. Her stomach was lavaged three times with 100 ml of physiologic saline, and 250 ml of fluid were recovered. She was then sent home. An hour later she vomited copiously and vomited several times during the afternoon. She refused food and fluids. When her father arrived home from work at 6 P.M. he noticed that she was breathing rapidly. The child was brought to the emergency room at midnight because her rapid breathing had continued and because she had begun to look "different."

Physical examination revealed a severely ill, moderately dehydrated child who weighed 13.5 kg. She was sluggish in her actions and had shallow, panting respirations at a rate of 42/min. Her rectal temperature was 38.8°C. The laboratory values were as follows: salicylates = 60 mg/dl; $Na^+ = 145$ mEq/liter; $K^+ = 3.8$ mEq/liter; $Cl^- = 116$ mEq/liter; total $CO_2 = 8$ mEq/liter; $Pco_2 = 18$ mm Hg; $H^+ = 54$ nEq/liter (pH = 7.24). Urinalysis yielded these findings: specific gravity = 1.015; pH = 5.0; trace of albumin; green reduction with Clinitest; negative Tes-Tape; nitroprusside (for urinary ketones) strongly positive; ferric chloride test on boiled urine was purple.

Problem List

1. Salicylate ingestion
2. Dehydration (10%) secondary to problem 1
3. Acid–base disorder

Problem 1: Salicylate Ingestion

Assessment. Salicylates have an antipyretic effect, apparently by inhibiting the synthesis of prostaglandins. However, when toxic doses of aspirin are ingested, fever may occur because oxidative phosphorylation is uncoupled, and the metabolic rate may be increased up to 40%. As a result of the increased metabolic rate, CO_2 production is increased. In addition, the respiratory center is directly stimulated by aspirin, which results in an increase in the depth and rate of respiration. This stimulation may overcompensate for the increased production of CO_2 and result in a respiratory alkalosis. In infants and young children salicylate intoxication may stimulate the production of organic acids (ketone bodies) and lead to metabolic acidosis. Depending on the ketonemia and the degree of respiratory alkalosis, the $[H^+]$ may be depressed, normal, or elevated. The progression of changes is usually in the order just listed.

The first acid–base change in salicylate intoxication is respiratory alkalosis. This results from direct CNS stimulation of respiration caused by the salicylate. The ensuing hyperventilation reduces the P_{CO_2}, shifting the buffer reaction to the left:

$$\uparrow CO_2 + H_2O \leftrightarrow H_2CO_3 \leftrightarrow H^+ + HCO_3^-$$
$$\xleftarrow{\hspace{3cm}}$$

and the $[H^+]$ falls. As compensation, the kidney will initially excrete HCO_3^- and produce alkaline urine. Metabolic acidosis develops very quickly as a result of the body's production of keto acids, which have lower pK than that of H_2CO_3 (in body fluids). This further reduces the $[HCO_3^-]$ by the release of H^+ from the keto acids. Thus the $[H^+]$ increases to a normal value, but then it continues to increase and creates acidemia. The urine then becomes acid in an attempt to conserve HCO_3^- and remove H^+ from the body fluids.

There is a complex of other effects, as shown in Figure 7-1. These reactions may result in alterations in blood sugar that may create either hypoglycemia or hyperglycemia.

Isotonic dehydration is common in such patients, but hypertonic dehydration may be present. Rehydration is especially important, since salicylates are excreted in the urine; maintenance fluids may be increased by 50%–100% to compensate for the higher metabolic rate.

This child appears about 10% dehydrated; she is compensating for metabolic acidosis by hyperventilation. The salicylate level measured about 14 hr after ingestion suggests a mild to moderate degree of intoxication (see Done AK: *Pediatrics* 26:800, 1960). The diagram given in the article by Done is useful for evaluating the significance of acute ingestion of salicylate, particularly when the amount is unknown. It applies to a single large ingestion when the time of that event can be reasonably ascer-

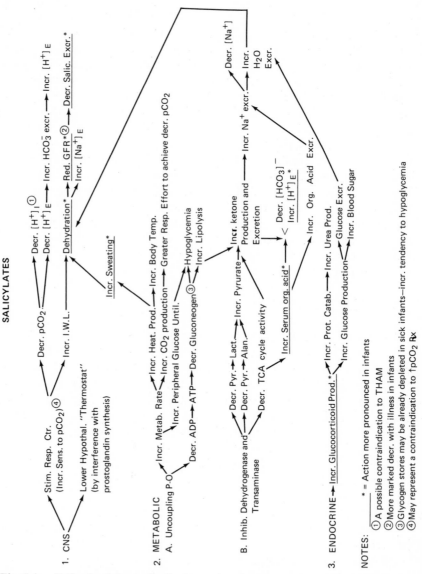

Fig. 7-1. Pathophysiology of salicylates, showing the four hypothetical pathways for development of the signs and symptoms of salicylate intoxication. These pathways are interconnected and may either reinforce each other, as with dehydration, or lead to opposite effects, as with [H⁺] initially or with blood glucose concentration. The certainty of many of the metabolic processes is not firmly established, and the time sequence of effects, as well as the dominant effect when there are opposing forces, cannot be determined from this diagram.

tained. The limitations of the diagram are that it cannot be used (1) when the salicylates have been given or taken over a period of time, (2) when the child is otherwise ill, because the impact of the illness must also be considered, and (3) when the child is under 12–18 months of age, because a given salicylate level appears to be more toxic in the infant than in the older child.

The degree of salicylism present in this child does not warrant dialysis or exchange transfusion as a mode of therapy. Development of CNS signs (such as coma and/or respiratory failure or fatigue) would be the indication for more intensive treatment than parenteral fluids.

Plan

1. Fluid therapy should be carried out as outlined for problem 2.
2. Vital signs should be monitored every 30 min for 16 hr.
3. Determination of salicylate level should be repeated every 6 hr.
4. Blood and urine sugar levels should be monitored, with blood sugar every 6 hr and urine sugar on each specimen.
5. Childhood poisoning and accidents should be discussed with the family.

Problem 2: Dehydration Secondary to Problem 1

Assessment. Physical examination showed a moderately dehydrated child, and this condition needs to be corrected. Maintenance fluids should be increased by 50% to compensate for elevated metabolic rate.

Fluid therapy for maintenance of this 3½-year-old child is as follows: IWL = 40 − [(3.5/16)(20)] + (15% × calc. IWL) = 41 ml/kg/day; renal = 50 − [(3.5/16)(25)] = 44.5 ml/kg/day; gastrointestinal = 5 − [(3.5/16) (2.5)] = 4.5 ml/kg/day; total maintenance = 91 ml/kg/day. Since the increased metabolic rate is 50%, maintenance fluids × 0.5 = 45 ml/kg/day. Repair fluid for 10% dehydration should replace two-thirds in 24 hr = 66 ml/kg/day. Thus total fluid = 91 + 45 + 66 = 202 ml/kg/day.

The dehydration appears to be isotonic which a change in the concentration of the anion component. The repair fluids are isotonic to plasma and contain Na^+ = 150 mEq/liter, Cl^- = 110 mEq/liter, and HCO_3^- = 40 mEq/liter in 890 ml/day (66 ml/kg/day × 13.5 kg). The 1836 ml/day (136 ml/kg/day × 13.5 kg) of maintenance fluid contains 5% glucose. The final 2726 ml/day (890 + 1836) contains Na^+ = 49 mEq/liter [(890/2726)(150)], Cl^- = 36 mEq/liter, HCO_3^- = 13 mEq/liter, and glucose = 5 g/dl.

Plan. Administer intravenous fluids at 170 ml/hr (2.8 ml/min) for first 8 hr; repeat electrolytes in 2 hr, then give 85 ml/hr (1.4 ml/min) for the next 16 hr.

Problem 3: Acid–Base Disorder

Assessment. The initial acid–base event in salicylism is respiratory alkalosis. However, the elevation in the [H^+] indicates an acidemia. Although the low Pco_2 is compatible with respiratory alkalosis, and a reduction in [HCO_3^-] may occur as compensation for respiratory alkalosis, such compensation by itself never proceeds quite to the point of returning the [H^+] toward normal. If this were compensated respiratory alkalosis, the [H^+] would still be less than 40 nEq/liter. Since the [H^+] is 58 nEq/liter, this can no longer be just compensation for respiratory alkalosis, and therefore metabolic acidosis seems to have been superimposed on the original respiratory alkalosis.

It has been recommended in other texts that $NaHCO_3$ be used in the treatment of metabolic acidosis. However, in the management of the metabolic acidosis seen in salicylism, it is riskier than usual to administer $NaHCO_3$ therapeutically. Although an electrolyte mixture containing balanced amounts of Na^+, K^+, Cl^-, and HCO_3^- has the potential disadvantage of creating further intracellular acidosis, the use of a balanced mixture (rather than larger amounts of $NaHCO_3$) ordinarily should not produce this difficulty. In the case of salicylism there is an added problem: should one return the [HCO_3^-] to normal too rapidly, before the salicylate effect on the respiratory center has disappeared, severe respiratory alkalosis can reappear.

On occasion, when respiratory effort is extreme and respiratory failure seems imminent, judicious use of sufficient HCO_3^- to raise the [HCO_3^-] to 15 mEq/liter may be indicated. Such a procedure will reduce part of the stimulus to hyperventilation and conceivably could reduce the likelihood of respiratory failure.

Plan

1. Vital signs should be monitored as described in problem 1, every 30 min. Particularly, rate, depth, and regularity of respiration should be noted.
2. Blood gases should be monitored every 12 hr.

CASE 5: RENAL FAILURE IN MERCURY POISONING

Seventy-two hours prior to hospital admission, an 11-year-old white boy attempted suicide by swallowing an unknown number of mercuric bichloride tablets. He was taken to the emergency room where his stomach was lavaged. No further treatment was given, and he was sent home.

The boy returned later the day of admission because his mother had noted that he had not urinated for 24 hr. On physical examination he appeared moderately ill. His vital signs were blood pressure 130/76 mm Hg, pulse 104/min, respirations 36/min and deep, temperature 37°C. He appeared slightly dehydrated, but his sensorium was clear. He weighed 36.7 kg and was 141 cm tall. The laboratory values were as follows: hemoglobin = 11.5/dl; WBC count = 8600/mm^3; Na$^+$ = 133 mEq/liter; K$^+$ = 7.1 mEq/liter; Cl$^-$ = 94 mEq/liter; Ca^{++} = 4.9 mEq/liter (9.8 mg/dl); PO$_4^{--}$ = 7.0 mg/dl; BUN = 67 mg/dl; creatinine = 2.0 mg/dl; CO$_2$ content = 14 mEq/liter; Pco$_2$ = 35 mm Hg; H$^+$ = 60 nEq/liter. No urine was present in the bladder when he was catheterized.

Problem List

1. Anuria
2. Metabolic acidosis
3. Intentional poison ingestion

Problem 1: Anuria

Assessment. Acute poisoning from ingestion of mercuric chloride first causes cell destruction in the mucous membranes by protein precipitation. The mouth and pharynx appear ash gray and are painful. Edema of the pharynx and fauces may also occur and may occlude the airway, resulting in asphyxia. Vomiting is a protective measure and is to be encouraged, but stomach lavage is also appropriate. If the poison reaches the small intestine, a severe bloody diarrhea will result. The local effects usually subside after 1–2 days, but systemic effects start in the first few hours and may last for days. These include effects on capillaries, kidneys, the colon, and the mouth. The kidney may be affected soon after the metal reaches the blood: diuresis due to impairment of reabsorption may be present, and later when more extensive damage occurs oliguria may result. Fluid losses due to vomiting, diarrhea, and renal losses result in hypovolemia. Capillary dilatation may result in shock as a result of expansion of the vascular space and loss of protein and fluids through the vessel walls producing absolute as well as relative hypovolemia. After stomach lavage and use of metal-chelating agents (dimercaprol) in the first few hours, the fluid and electrolyte problems or potential problems must be addressed.

The anuria present in this boy probably is the result of the hypovolemia combined with 10% dehydration and direct toxic damage to the kidney. The kidneys may have been damaged by the mercury, and their status should be checked after any dehydration has been repaired. Hypotension and shock are complications that can occur. It is likely that this patient has acute renal failure (ARF).

The fluid therapy calculation is as follows: Maintenance fluids for 11-year-old boy: $IWL = 40 - [(11/16)(20)] = 26$ ml/kg/day; renal $= 50 - [(11/16)(25)] = 36$ ml/kg/day; gastrointestinal $= 5 - [(11/16)(2.5) = 3$ ml/kg/day; total maintenance fluids $= 65$ ml/kg/day. Repair fluids: 10% dehydration $= 100$ ml/kg/day; replace two-thirds in 24 hr $= 66$ ml/kg/day; total fluids in first day $= 131$ ml/kg $(65 + 66)$; 131×37 kg $= 4845$ ml/day.

This solution should contain Na^+, Cl^-, and HCO_3^- at about half their effective extracellular concentration, since about half is for repair and half for nonelectrolyte maintenance (see problem 2): $Na^+ = 75$ mEq/liter, $Cl^- = 55$ mEq/liter, $HCO_3^- = 20$ mEq/liter, and glucose $= 2.5\%$. Thus one-third of fluids in first 6 hr $= 1788$ ml; one-half of fluids in next 8 hr $= 2683$ ml; rest of fluids in last 10 hr $= 894$ ml. Unless patient begins to void, no K^+ will be given.

If the boy fails to void during this 24-hr period, theoretically he will have a fluid overload equivalent to the amount of fluid recommended for renal function. For this patient the overload would be about 36 ml/kg (3–4%), and this is well within the acceptable limits of hydration.

Plan. Fluid is needed to repair the dehydration and to maintain water balance. When hydration is completed, electrolytes, BUN, creatinine, calcium, and phosphorus must be rechecked.

1. Fluid therapy should be as follows: rate for first 6 hr $= 298$ ml/hr; rate for next 8 hr $= 335$ ml/hr; rate for final 10 hr $= 90$ ml/hr. Composition: $Na^+ = 75$ mEq/liter, $Cl^- = 55$ mEq/liter, $HCO_3^- = 20$ mEq/liter, and glucose $= 2.5\%$.
2. The patient should be weighed every 12 hr to assess repair of dehydration; then the slow weight loss of 0.5%–1.0% each day should be checked.
3. The patient should have an EKG stat; then lead 2 should be rechecked every 8 hr.
4. Although an indwelling catheter to monitor urine flow has been suggested, it is our view that the risk is greater than the benefit. If this boy has a significant urine flow, spontaneous voiding will usually occur. The patient's overall status requires close observation.

Problem 2: Metabolic Acidosis

Assessment. The increase in hydrogen ion concentration, the decrease in Pco_2, and the increase in respiratory rate indicate metabolic acidosis with some compensation. To find what the hydrogen ion concentration would have been if there had been no respiratory compensation, insert a normal H_2CO_3 (P_{CO_2}) value and the measured total CO_2 value into the equation $([H^+][HCO_3^-])/[P_{CO_2}] = 24$:

$$\frac{[H^+][14]}{40} = 24$$

$$[H^+] = 69 \text{ mEq/liter}$$

The result indicates the [H^+] in the absence of significant hyperventilation; it reveals a slight amount of compensation due to the hyperventilation. Addition of bicarbonate will decrease the hydrogen ion concentration, and the buffer anion will increase. The administration of too much H^+ acceptor will decrease the stimulus to hyperventilation and result in an increase in P_{CO_2}. The increased H_2CO_3 diffuses easily into the cells of the body and will result in a rise in cellular H^+. To avoid a rise in intracellular hydrogen, use of smaller amounts of bicarbonate (⅓ to ¼ of the total anion infused) will help reduce the ECF [H^+] while not creating further ICF acidosis, thus avoiding adverse intracellular effects.

Plan.   See the plan outlined for problem 1.

Problem 3: Intentional Poison Ingestion

Assessment.   Suicide attempts during childhood are complex behavioral problems; they require serious consideration and treatment. Psychiatric assistance is almost mandatory.

Plan.   It is necessary to question this boy about the incident to determine the circumstances and the background for taking the pills. His parents may be helpful in determining what problems he has. The services of a social worker should be obtained to assist in appropriate psychiatric consultation.

Progress Notes (24 hr)

PROBLEM 1: ANURIA (RETITLE: ACUTE RENAL FAILURE)

Assessment.   The boy remained alert and in no pain. He did not void. Catheterization was done; it revealed no urine in the bladder. Tissue turgor was firm. Repeat serum values were as follows: $Na^+ = 130$ mEq/liter; $K^+ = 7.4$ mEq/liter; $Cl^- = 90$ mEq/liter; $Ca^{++} = 4.8$ mEq/liter (9.6 mg/dl); $PO_4^{--} = 7.2$ mg/dl; BUN = 80 mg/dl; creatinine = 2.3 mg/dl; CO_2

content = 16 mEq/liter; Pco_2 = 35 mm Hg; H^+ = 53 nEq/liter (pH = 7.28); weight = 40.4 kg. The EKG showed evidence of hyperkalemia, with elevated and peaked T waves, but no further EKG signs of this disorder were present.

At 24 hr acute renal failure was apparent. There was no evidence of renal function, and the boy was well hydrated. His weight had increased by an amount equal to the sum of the fluid provided for rehydration and that given for possible urine excretion. Although he might begin to void even later that 24 hr, the rising $[K^+]$ in the serum and the EKG effects suggested that peritoneal dialysis was indicated at that time.

Plan

1. Peritoneal dialysis should be performed.
2. Monitoring of serum values, EKG, and weight should be continued.
3. Oral intake of high-carbohydrate, high-fat, low-protein, low-K^+ diet should be planned.
4. Fluids should be limited to 950 ml/day (IWL 26 ml/kg × 37 kg) plus or minus the balance from peritoneal dialysis (the amount introduced minus the amount removed; a positive balance on peritoneal dialysis would be subtracted from the planned fluids).

PROBLEM 2: METABOLIC ACIDOSIS

Assessment. There were no changes in symptoms. The CO_2 content increased, and $[H^+]$ decreased slightly. Some improvement occurred, and this should be enhanced by peritoneal dialysis.

Plan. See the plan outlined for problem 1.

PROBLEM 3: INTENTIONAL POISON INGESTION

Plan. The social worker will begin to talk with the family regarding psychiatric consultation.

CASE 6: HYPERTONIC DEHYDRATION

A 4-month-old white female infant was stated to be in good health until 4 days prior to her hospital admission. Her illness began with low-grade fever, vomiting, and diarrhea. Her mother called a physician 2 days later because the diarrhea and vomiting had continued. The physician recommended that the mother stop trying to feed the infant her usual formula and offer a salt and sugar solution instead. This solution was to contain 1 teaspoon of salt and 3 tablespoons of sugar in 1 quart of water. The mother was able to get the infant to take about 8 ounces of this solution for each of the next 2 days. The vomiting subsided slightly, but the diarrhea continued. When the infant's rectal temperature rose to 103°F, she was brought to the emergency room. The infant was last known to void about 12 hr prior to admission. When questioned, the mother stated that she had not noticed any tearing when the infant cried, for at least 1 day. The stools had been liquid and green in color for 3 days. No blood had been noted in the stools or vomitus. The last recorded weight of the infant had been 10 lb 14 ounces (5.4 kg) 10 days previously on a well-child examination.

The infant was the product of a term pregnancy, the third for this mother, and was delivered spontaneously, weighing 3.0 kg. Since birth she had been on an iron-enriched commercial formula, and 1 month earlier she had begun to take solid food prepared by the mother. There had been no other illnesses.

On physical examination the infant appeared very lethargic and only moderately dehydrated, as judged by depression of the anterior fontanelle and turgor of the skin. There was no cyanosis and no jaundice. Weight was 4800 g and length 59 cm. Her rectal temperature was 39.4°C. Pulse was 120/min, respirations 24/min, and blood pressure 80/50 mm Hg. There was occasional twitching of the right hand and arm, but no other neurologic findings. There were no significant findings in the remainder of the physical examination.

The initial laboratory findings included urine specific gravity of 1.019, pH of 5.0, and no albumin, sugar, ketones, or unusual sediment. The hemoglobin was 14.5 g/dl; the hematocrit was 42 vol%, WBC count was 20,700/mm^3 (27% neutrophils, 70% lymphocytes, 1% eosinophils, 2% monocytes).

A lumbar puncture was done in the emergency room; spinal fluid pressure was not elevated, the fluid was clear and colorless, the sugar level was 50 mg/dl (simultaneous blood sugar = 65 mg/dl), and the protein was 60 mg/dl.

Problem List

1. Dehydration, secondary to vomiting and diarrhea
2. CNS irritation
3. Diarrhea and vomiting
4. Metabolic acidosis

Problem 1: Dehydration, Secondary to Vomiting and Diarrhea

Assessment. From the evidence of weight loss (5.4 to 4.8 kg), poor skin turgor, depressed fontanelle, lack of tears, recent anuria (12 hr), and high hemoglobin and hematocrit, acute dehydration of at least 10% of body weight is likely. The fever may be a result of dehydration because of reduced peripheral circulation and consequent reduced heat loss.

There appears to be some discrepancy between the measured weight loss of at least 10% and the state of the skin turgor, which is only moderately reduced. This discrepancy, combined with the lethargy, the twitching of the upper extremity, and the somewhat elevated spinal fluid protein, would suggest a hypernatremic type of dehydration. Alternatively, these findings could be interpreted on another basis (see problem 2). The urine specific gravity of 1.019 is not as high as one might expect in acute dehydration; this may be the result of some renal impairment from the dehydration, and it is consistent with hypernatremic dehydration.

The fluid therapy calculation is as follows: Maintenance fluids: IWL = 48 ml/kg/day (40 + 20% for fever); renal = 50 ml/kg/day; gastrointestinal = 30 ml/kg/day; total maintenance fluid = 128 ml/kg/day. Repair fluids: 100 ml/kg; provide 75% of this in the first 24 hr (75 ml/kg/day). Total fluids: 200 ml/kg/day; 4.8 kg × 200 ml/kg/day = 960 ml/day.

To provide rapid rehydration initially, plan for 50% of the fluid during the first 8 hr (480 ml or 60 ml/hr). The remaining 480 ml will be given over the next 16 hr (30 ml/hr × 16 hr).

The composition of the fluid should be as follows: Fluid for IWL and urine formation to be given as 5% dextrose in water: 48 + 50 = 98 ml/kg. Fluid for gastrointestinal loss and for repair to be given as an isotonic salt solution: 30 + 75 = 105 ml/kg. Of the total fluid, approximately half is a glucose solution and half is an isotonic salt solution; therefore, when combined, the total fluid can be a half-isotonic salt solution with 2.5% glucose. Initially, since the K^+ is unknown, and it is not known how long the anuria may persist, no K^+ will be ordered until these issues are clear. To provide a half-isotonic salt solution without K^+ but appropriately buffered to provide a physiologic mixture, the ionic concentrations are $Na^+ = 75$ mEq/liter, $Cl^- = 50$ mEq/liter, $HCO_3^- = 25$ mEq/liter, and glucose = 2.5%.

Plan

1. Blood should be obtained for Na^+, K^+, Cl^-, CO_2, pH, BUN, and Ca^{++} determinations.
2. Intravenous fluid therapy should be begun at the following rate: first 8 hr = 60 ml/hr × 8 hr; next 16 hr = 30 ml/hr × 16 hr. Composition: $Na^+ = 75$ mEq/liter, $Cl^- = 50$ mEq/liter, $HCO_3^- = 25$ mEq/liter, and glucose = 2.5%.

Problem 2: CNS Irritation

Assessment. The findings of CNS depression, twitching of the extremities, and elevated spinal fluid protein suggest some form of CNS irritation. Although these findings are compatible with hypernatremic dehydration, other causes should be considered. These include other metabolic problems such as hypocalcemia and hypoglycemia (which is ruled out by the normal value for blood sugar), as well as cerebral hemorrhage, subdural hematoma, and infectious processes. Of the infections, bacterial meningitis is unlikely because of the lack of cells in the spinal fluid and the normal level of spinal fluid sugar. Viral meningitis is also unlikely, in spite of the elevated spinal fluid protein, because of the absence of cells in the fluid. An encephalitic process is possible and cannot be excluded at this time.

Cerebral bleeding is known to occur with hypernatremia, and if CNS symptoms persist, subdural taps and repeat lumbar puncture should be considered.

Plan

1. The patient should be monitored carefully for changes in vital signs, pupillary reactions, changes in the fundi, and seizures.
2. Further plans should await the results of serum Ca determination and spinal fluid culture.

Problem 3: Diarrhea and Vomiting

Assessment.   Most gastroenteritis in infancy is due to nonspecific viral agents; the other major cause is nonenteric infection. Specific enteric infections occur, but they are less likely.

Plan.   Blood cultures, spinal fluid culture, urine culture, stool culture, and chest x-ray should be performed.

Progress Notes (4 hr)

PROBLEM 1: DEHYDRATION SECONDARY
TO VOMITING AND DIARRHEA

Assessment.   The infant is more alert; there has been no twitching of extremities since admission. Subcutaneous tissue seems doughy. Laboratory values are as follows: $Na^+ = 165$ mEq/liter; $K^+ = 5$ mEq/liter; $Cl^- = 138$ mEq/liter; CO_2 content $= 9$ mEq/liter; pH $= 7.10$ mEq/liter; BUN $= 24$ mg/dl; $Ca^{++} = 4.9$ mEq/liter (9.8 mg/dl). The infant has just begun to void and has a total urinary output of 25 ml for the first 4 hr. Intake has been 240 ml. There has been one liquid stool since admission. Her weight has risen to 4925 g.

An intake of 240 ml, minus an estimated IWL of 44 ml, urine loss of 25 ml, and an estimated stool loss of 30 ml, gives a net positive fluid balance of 140 ml, which correlates well with the weight gain of 125 g. The child has voided, and serum K^+ is normal; so K^+ can be added to the intravenous fluids. BUN elevation is consistent with hydration and pre-renal azotemia.

The composition should be changed to include K^+, which can be given safely up to a concentration of 30 mEq/liter if this is no more than 3–4 mEq/kg/day.

The new fluid composition proposed is as follows: $Na^+ = 45$ mEq/liter, $K^+ = 30$ mEq/liter, $Cl^- = 50$ mEq/liter, $HCO_3^- = 25$ mEq/liter.

There are 960 ml of fluid ordered; 240 ml have been given, and 720 ml remain. Thus $0.720 \times 30 = 21.6$ mEq, and $21.6 \div 4.9$ kg = 4.4 mEq/kg. This is more K^+ per kilogram than is desired; thus the fluid composition should be changed: $Na^+ = 50$ mEq/liter, $K^+ = 25$ mEq/liter, $Cl^- = 50$ mEq/liter, and $HCO_3^- = 25$ mEq/liter. Thus 0.720 liter $\times 25$ mEq/liter = 18.0 mEq; 18.0 mEq $\div 4.7$ kg = 3.7 mEq/kg, a value within safe limits.

Plan

1. Fluid therapy should be as follows: Rate: first 8 hr = 60 ml/hr × 8 hr; next 16 hr = 30 ml/hr × 16 hr. Composition: $Na^+ =$ mEq/liter, $K^+ = 25$ mEq/liter, $Cl^- = 50$ mEq/liter, $HCO_3^- = 25$ mEq/liter, and glucose = 2.5%.
2. Repeat serum determinations of Na^+, K^+, Cl^-, CO_2, and pH should be made in 12 hr.

PROBLEM 2: CNS IRRITATION

Assessment. There have been no changes in symptoms and no new findings. Vital signs are stable; $[Ca^{++}] = 4.9$ mEq/liter. Symptomatology may be subsiding.

Plan. No change in plan.

PROBLEM 4: METABOLIC ACIDOSIS

Assessment. There is no evidence of unusual respiration; pH = 7.10; $[H^+] = 80$ nEq/liter; $CO_2 = 9$ mEq/liter. Using the formula $[H^+][HCO_3^-]/P_{CO_2} = 24$, one can obtain a value of 30 mm Hg for the P_{CO_2}:

$$\frac{(80)(9)}{P_{CO_2}} = 24; \qquad P_{CO_2} = \frac{(80)(9)}{24} = \frac{720}{24} = 30$$

This represents a moderate degree of hyperventilation, but not a maximum compensatory response. Thus it appears that this infant is acidemic, and the primary cause is metabolic, since the $[HCO_3^-]$ is low and some degree of secondary hyperventilation has taken place. The absence of a more marked response suggests either that there is some depression of respiratory function by the CNS state or that a pulmonary process could be interfering with gaseous exchange. Acidosis may be complicated by decreased ability of the kidney to excrete H^+ because of decreased GFR, and diarrhea may have caused the acidosis as a result of bicarbonate loss from the body. In severe diarrhea, which is often accompanied by anorexia, the intake of calories may be insufficient, and thus increased metabolism of fats can lead to increased production of acids.

Plan

1. Examine chest x-ray.
2. Draw blood for determination of blood gases, including P_{O_2}.
3. Parenteral fluids are appropriately buffered as originally ordered, and there is no evidence of renal impairment. Unless later values suggest lack of correction of the metabolic acidosis, composition of intravenous fluids should not be changed.

CASE 7: RESPIRATORY DISTRESS AND HYPOGLYCEMIA

A 26-year-old primigravida with diabetes of 12 years duration gave birth by cesarean section after a 37-week gestation. The indication for this procedure was cephalopelvic disproportion. Spinal anesthesia was the only analgesic agent employed. Twenty units of NPH insulin were administered 1 hr before the procedure. The morning urine showed a trace of sugar and a negative test for acetone. An infusion of 5% dextrose in water was started prior to induction of spinal anesthesia; it was set to run at the rate of 80 ml/hr. A 4.8-kg (10.5-lb) male infant was delivered; he breathed and cried at once. The infant appeared plethoric and puffy, but no true pitting edema was observed. The physical examination revealed a liver edge palpable 3 cm below the right costal margin in the midclavicular line; otherwise the examination revealed nothing unusual. The infant was left unclothed and head down in a heated incubator; every 15 min his respiratory rate was checked. During the next 6 hr his respiratory rate progressively increased; at the end of that period the rate was noted to be 48/min. Observation at that time showed the infant to be in mild respiratory distress, with grunting expirations, poor aeration at the right lung base, and pitting edema of the feet. There was no cyanosis. The cord blood sugar level taken at the time of delivery was reported as 120 mg/dl. The blood sugar determination was repeated on heel-stick blood 7 hr after delivery and was found to be 20 mg/dl. (Smogyi). No other blood determinations were done.

Problem List

1. Respiratory distress
2. Hypoglycemia
3. Pitting edema of feet

Problem 1: Respiratory Distress

Assessment.   Infants of diabetic mothers are often large and plump; others, particularly when diabetic control is poor in the mother, may be small for gestational age. These infants show greater decreases in blood glucose levels after birth than do other infants. A higher incidence of neonatal complications is seen in infants of diabetic mothers, including congenital malformations, respiratory distress, apneic spells, hypoglycemia, hyperbilirubinemia, increased muscular excitability, sepsis, and respiratory and metabolic acidosis.

Maternal diabetes is associated with an increased frequency of hyaline membrane disease (HMD) in offspring; this may result from delayed maturation or from the increased incidence of prematurity. The respiratory distress is usually evident by a few hours of age. Most infants with HMD will have elevated respiratory rates and will show flaring of the alae nasi, as well as intercostal or xiphoid retractions. Systemic hypotension and hypothermia are usually present. Cyanosis is present in severely affected infants, and grunting or crying on expiration is a sign of moderate severity. The expiratory grunting may serve the purpose of increasing alveolar pressure and helping prevent collapse of alveoli, thus increasing alveolar ventilation. The respiratory rate in HMD is commonly higher than 60/min, compared to a normal value of 20–40/min in normal infants. An increase in respiratory rate, as in this infant, is important, although it is still in the "normal" range. A chest radiograph is necessary to rule out other causes of respiratory distress, i.e., pneumothorax, diaphragmatic hernia or cardiac failure, and type II respiratory distress syndrome. Serum glucose, K^+, Cl^-, Na^+, and total proteins are usually within normal limits, but bilirubin and lactic acid are often elevated. In severe acidosis the [K^+] may be elevated. The arterial blood gases often show oxygen unsaturation combined with respiratory and metabolic acidosis. Infants at birth normally have P_{CO_2} of 45–50 mm Hg and HCO_3^- levels of 18–22 mEq/liter. The newborn infant depends on the pulmonary system to blow off the CO_2. Many infants of diabetic mothers develop tachypnea in the first few days after birth. This infant's increased respiratory rate may not be the result of HMD, but the presence of expiratory grunting necessitates its consideration.

Plan

1. An arterial blood sample should be taken to determine hemoglobin, hematocrit, P_{O_2}, P_{CO_2}, pH, HCO_3^-, K^+, Cl^-, and Na^+ and serum albumin if jaundice is clinically evident.
2. Respiratory rate, pulse rate, and blood pressure should be monitored every 30 min.
3. A chest x-ray should be taken.

Problem 2: Hypoglycemia

Assessment.   Although the blood glucose level may be normal or elevated at birth, low levels are more apt to develop in infants of diabetic mothers than in normal infants, and hypoglycemia is often a problem, presumably because of hypertrophy of the pancreatic islets. Infants who are hypoglycemic tend to be jittery or trembly; they are often apathetic and may be cyanotic. If these symptoms disappear with glucose administration, hypoglycemia may be considered to be the cause. This infant's blood glucose level is dangerously low and may be involved in a "starvation acidosis." An evolving acidosis would explain the increasing respiratory rate.

Although maintenance fluids given to infants may be 120 ml/kg/day in the first 24–48 hr of life, this value can be reduced by 50% because of the extra fluid present in the newborn. Thus 4.8 kg × 60 ml/kg/day = 288 ml/day or 12 ml/hr. After 48–72 hr the maintenance fluids can be given at a rate comparable to that for young infants (120 ml/kg/day).

Composition

An initial infusion of 25% glucose (1–2 ml/kg) should be followed by a 10% glucose solution until the infant is stabilized. Blood sugars can be monitored by use of Dextrostix.

Plan

1. The laboratory values listed for problem 1, plus blood sugar, should be determined.

2. Intravenous fluids should be given at an initial infusion 9.6 ml of 25% glucose, followed by 10% glucose solution.

Problem 3: Pitting Edema of Feet

Assessment. Although pitting edema has been reported in infants with hyaline membrane disease, these cases commonly involved infants with metabolic and/or respiratory acidosis who often were given relatively large amounts of sodium bicarbonate. This does not appear to have happened with this infant; so other causes of edema (heart failure, kidney failure, decreased plasma oncotic pressure) must be considered.

Plan

1. Clinical evaluation of cardiac status should be made.
2. The plan outlined for problem 1 should be followed.

8

Primary Surgical Problems

CASE 8: BURNS

A 3-year-old male child was admitted directly to the intensive care unit from the emergency room because of severe burns. While trying to light a gas heater, his clothes had caught fire. It appeared that he had burned his face, neck, both upper arms, and entire anterior and posterior thorax with second- and third-degree burns. A rapid physical examination, in addition to assessing the extent and degree of external burned tissue, revealed burns in the mouth and nose, weight of 15 kg, blood pressure of 50/30 mm Hg in the right leg, and pulse rate of 160/min, with sinus rhythm and no cardiac murmurs. The lungs were clear and the abdomen soft; no masses were palpable.

Problem List

1. Shock
2. Severe burns of surface
3. Respiratory tract burns

251

Problem 1: Shock

Assessment.   Hypotension and tachycardia are indicative of shock, which is probably hypovolemic because of fluid losses into the burned tissue and evaporation of water from the burned surfaces.

This is an emergency situation, and the amount of fluid given initially must be based on the amount of fluid lost from the vascular volume. Shock may occur with 25%–40% loss of vascular volume. Since the vascular volume amounts to about 10% of body weight, a 25%–40% reduction in vascular volume is equivalent to a 2.5%–4% loss in body weight. This translates to 25–40 ml/kg body weight. If the child remains in shock after administration of 20 ml/kg another 20 ml/kg may be given. This second push of fluids should be done with greater caution because of the potential for temporary overload on the right side of the heart.

Plan.   Either lactated Ringer's solution (20 mg/kg) or an equivalent mixture of NaCl and $NaHCO_3$* should be given intravenously as rapidly as possible.

Problem 2: Surface Burns

Assessment.   The immediate problem with a severe burn is fluid therapy. Many formulas have been proposed for fluid replacement in burned people; most of these formulations have been based on the degree and extent of the burn and have been derived empirically for adults. Modifications of these formulas for infants and children have not been particularly satisfactory, primarily because of the variations in size and metabolic rate for children of different ages.

The fluid lost from the circulation is either translocated into the burned tissue or lost by evaporation from the burned surfaces after seeping onto the surface from injured capillaries. In both situations the fluid tends to be similar to plasma in its electrolyte composition and tends to have a protein concentration approaching that of the plasma. Therefore, replacement of such fluid should be with a solution containing about 140 mEq/liter Na^+, 110 mEq/liter Cl^-, and about 30 mEq/liter HCO_3^-. In general, no K^+ is given initially because the damaged tissues may leak a large amount of intracellular K^+ into the extracellular (and vascular) fluid. The protein content of the translocated fluid is variable. If there are 1–2 g of albumin per deciliter of repair fluid, serum protein concentrations are usually well maintained. There is some controversy about the use of colloid (albumin) in the management of thermal burns. Some authors recommend no colloid at all; some recommend the use of colloid on the second

---

* NaCl (110 mEq/liter) plus $NaHCO_3$ (35 mEq/liter).

Table 8-1
"Rule of 6's" for Burns

Location	Infant	Adult
Head and neck		
Anterior	6% ⎞	9%
Posterior	6% ⎠	
Upper extremities		
Left	(6 + 3) 9%	9%
Right	(6 + 3) 9%	9%
Trunk		
Thorax		
Anterior	12%	9%
Posterior	12%	9%
Abdomen		
Anterior	12%	9%
Posterior	12%	9%
Lower extremities		
Left		
Anterior	6%	9%
Posterior	6%	9%
Right		
Anterior	6%	9%
Posterior	6%	9%

day; others suggest the approach used here i.e., use of colloid with the repair fluids on both the first and second days.

The amount of loss will be proportionate to the extent of the burn. Therefore it is of some value to estimate the area burned. In adults a useful method has been based on the "rule of 9's," which must be modified for infants and children because of their relatively larger surface areas on the head and upper extremities and smaller relative surface areas on the lower extremities. A "rule of 6's" has been proposed for infants. These two rules are illustrated in Table 8-1; they represent approximations only. Values for children of intermediate ages must be interpolated.

This particular child had burns covering 39% of his body (6% for anterior surface of head and neck, 9% for both upper arms, 24% for thorax, anterior and posterior) based on the infant formula. This would have been about 32% in an adult. Interpolation for a 3-year-old child produces a value somewhere between 35% and 39%.

The purposes of providing fluids to the person who has been burned are the same as those for any other person requiring fluid therapy: replacement of deficits and maintenance fluids for continuing losses. In the burned patient, the fluid that has shifted prior to initiation of treatment and

Table 8-2
Translocation of Fluid

	Amount in 1st 24 hr (ml/kg)	
Area Burned (% of Surface Area)	*Infant*	*Adult*
1%	2–4	1–2
10%	20–40	10–20
25%	50–100	25–50
50%	100–200	50–100

the fluid that translocates while fluid therapy is being provided can be considered as part of the repair problem and also as part of the maintenance needs. The major differences in cases of burns are that the translocated fluid contains protein and that some of the translocated fluid will return to the functional ECF and vascular volume after 72 hr.

The volume of fluid that is involved in translocation varies with the area of the burn. In the small infant the area-to-weight ratio is greater than the area-to-weight ratio in the adult. Therefore a burn involving 25% of the infant's surface area will cause a higher percentage of translocation than would a 25% surface burn in the adult. In general, for second- and third-degree burns in the adult, most formulas suggest about 2 ml/kg body weight for each 1% of burned surface. The values for an infant are double this amount on a per kilogram basis. Table 8-2 illustrates these relationships; the values given in the Table are ranges. The larger number is for essentially second- and third-degree burns; the smaller number is for burns that are mixtures of first-, second-, and third-degree burns. The values for older children are intermediate between those for the infant and those for the adult. The amount of fluid that undergoes translocation in the second 24 hr after a burn is about half the amount that shifts in the initial 24-hr period. By the third day there usually is no further translocation, and fluid may begin to move back into the active ECF.

The fluid therapy calculation is as follows: For translocation repair, assume a burn of 36% and a value of 3 ml/%/kg for translocation = $3 \times 36 = 108$ ml/kg. The child weighs 15 kg; $15 \times 108 = 1620$ ml total. Maintenance = $95 - (3 \times age) = 95 - 9 = 86$ ml/kg. IWL = $40 - [(3/15)(20)] = 36$ ml/kg; renal = $50 - [(3/15)(25)] = 45$ ml/kg; gastrointestinal = $5 - [(3/15)(2.5)] = 4.5$ ml/kg; therefore total losses = 85.5 ml/kg. Total fluid = $1620 + 1290 = 2910$ ml.

The composition of fluids is as follows: Isotonic balanced salt solution = $1620 + (4.5 \times 15) = 1688$ ml; 5% dextrose = $(36 + 45) \times 15$ kg = 1215 ml. $Na^+ = 140 \times (1688/2910) = 81$ mEq/liter, $Cl^- = 110 \times$

($1688/2910 = 64$ mEq/liter, $HCO_3^- = 30 \times (1688/2910) = 17$ mEq/liter, and albumin $= 2$ g/dl $\times (1620^*/2910) = 1.1$ g/dl.

The fluid is to be administered at a rate such that one-half will be given in the first 8 hr and the second half in the remaining 16 hr. Thus $2910 \times 0.5 = 1455$ ml; $1455 \div 8 = 182$ ml/hr $\times$ 8 hr. And then, $1455 \div 16 = 91$ ml/hr $\times$ 16 hr.

Plan

1. Laboratory studies: the initial studies, before treatment is begun, should include the following: complete blood count; urinalysis; serum values for Na^+, K^+, Cl^-, H^+, pH, Pco_2, total CO_2 (HCO_3^-), and Po_2; serum proteins and albumin and globulin concentrations; BUN and creatinine.
2. Monitoring: A flow sheet should be constructed that includes all the variables that need to be considered in monitoring the progress of the child. These include the following: initial weight and weight after all connections, dressings, etc., are in place; vital signs (pulse, temperature, respiratory rate, and blood pressure); initial laboratory values, with space for those that may be needed later, including cultures of skin, throat, blood, and urine; fluid balance, including oral intake and intravenous intake of fluid, Na^+, K^+, HCO_3^-, and albumin; urine output, gastric suction losses, stool losses, and any other losses; calorie intake; medications. The time or frequency for each variable should be noted.
3. Medications: Medical and surgical management of burns involves the use of many therapies and will not be discussed. Mafenide acetate and silver sulfadiazine creams as currently used produce the least disturbance of fluid balance. In addition to close observation for an early hemolytic process and for any evidence of infection, major attention needs to be directed to meeting the child's nutritional needs. Calorie requirements may be increased by 25% because of increased heat losses occurring from the burned areas.
4. Fluid therapy should be instituted after initial shock fluids. Rate: first 8 hr = 182 ml/hr; next 16 hr = 91 ml/hr. Composition (depends on laboratory tests): $Na^+ = 81$ mEq/liter, $Cl^- = 64$ mEq/liter, $HCO_3^- = 17$ mEq/liter, albumin = 1.1 g/dl, and glucose = 2.1%.

Problem 3: Respiratory Tract Burns

This problem will not be discussed because it does not appreciably alter the fluid problems.

---

* Note that the volume for repair fluid (1620 ml) rather than the total salt-containing fluid (1688 ml) is used for this calculation.

CASE 9: BOWEL OBSTRUCTION

A 2.73-kg infant was born after gestation of 8 months. He vomited most of every feeding from the first day of life, and this continued for the 8 days preceding his admission to the hospital. He had only one bowel movement (meconium), on the third day of life. His vomitus appeared fecal in nature.

Physical examination showed a small, afebrile infant with marked dehydration. He was "arousable" and had a good cry. Pulse was 120/min, respirations 30/min, weight 2.20 kg, and length 43 cm. The abdomen was scaphoid. The remainder of the examination was unremarkable.

The laboratory values were as follows: hematocrit = 50 vol%; WBC count = 22,000/mm^3; total CO_2 = 10 mEq/liter; Na^+ = 140 mEq/liter; K^+ = 9.3 mEq/liter; Cl^- = 111 mEq/liter; BUN = 60 mg/dl. Urinalysis revealed these values: specific gravity = 1.015; protein = 1+; WBC count = 2–3/hpf.

Problem List

1. Dehydration
2. Hyperkalemia
3. Vomiting
4. Metabolic acidosis

Problem 1: Dehydration

Assessment. Dehydration has resulted from an apparent total lack of intake plus loss of gastric (and possibly intestinal) secretions in the vomitus. The lack of renal function, the tachycardia, and hemoconcentration may be the result of the dehydration.

The weight loss (0.53 kg) represents a 19.4% weight loss and does not include any fluid that might be sequestered in the intestine. The actual dehydration is probably less than 15% because newborns may be approximately 5% overhydrated at birth. This child's fluid loss is severe and life-threatening.

The fluid therapy calculation is as follows: Maintenance: IWL = 45 ml/kg/day; renal = 50 ml/kg/day; gastrointestinal = 0 ml/kg/day; total = 95 ml/kg/day. Repair: 120 ml/kg; 75% in first 24 hr = 90 ml/kg on the first day, with an additional 30 ml/kg on the second day. Total fluids: maintenance (95 ml/kg) + repair (90 ml/kg) = 185 ml/kg; 2.20 kg × 185 ml/kg/day = 407 ml/day. Plan for 50% in the first 8 hr (205 ml or 25.5 ml/hr); the remaining 205 ml will be given in 16 hr (12.8 ml/hr).

Composition: IWL and renal losses are given as 5% dextrose in water: $45 + 50 = 95$ ml/kg; gastrointestinal and repair losses are replaced by an isotonic "salt" solution (90 ml/kg) with these ionic concentrations: $Na^+ = 150$ mEq/liter, $Cl^- = 100$ mEq/liter, and $HCO_3^- = 50$ mEq/liter. The final solution will be essentially the following: $Na^+ = 75$ mEq/liter, $Cl^- = 50$ mEq/liter, $HCO_3^- = 25$ mEq/liter, and glucose = 2.5%.

Plan. Begin intravenous fluids and monitor fluid output. Rate: first 8 hr = 25.5 ml/hr; next 16 hr = 12.8 ml/hr. Composition: $Na^+ = 75$ mEq/liter, $Cl^- = 50$ mEq/liter, $HCO_3^- = 25$ mEq/liter, and glucose = 2.5%.

Problem 2: Hyperkalemia

Assessment. Decreased renal function secondary to the dehydration may have produced the BUN of 60 mg/dl and the $[K^+]$ of 9.3 mEq/liter. Alternatively, there may be congenital disease of the excretory system, such as renal dysplasia, obstruction of the urethra, or renal vein thrombosis. However, the urine values obtained on admission tend to indicate that this is less likely. If vigorous fluid therapy fails to increase urine output, the excretory system should be investigated further. The increased potassium may also be the result of tissue destruction in combination with decreased renal function. Hyperkalemia of this magnitude is dangerous, and cardiac function is probably impaired. Immediate measures are necessary.

Plan

1. An initial EKG should be taken, which should be followed with monitoring.
2. Calcium gluconate (10%) should be given: 2 ml/kg intravenously by slow push.
3. Intravenous fluids (see problem 1) containing no potassium should be given.
4. Na^+, K^+, Cl^-, HCO_3^-, Pco_2, pH, BUN, and CBC should be determined 2 hr after intravenous fluid is started (arterial sample).

Problem 3: Vomiting

Assessment. The persistent vomiting since birth, the scaphoid abdomen, and the lack of bowel movements suggest that this infant has complete high intestinal obstruction. Fecal vomiting (the fecal appearance is the result of bacterial colonization of the small intestine and is not feces) is related to the length of time the intestine has been obstructed and is observed in complete obstruction. Vomiting is a sign of duodenal or proximal jejunal obstruction when it precedes abdominal distension. In obstruction of the lower jejunum or ileum, marked abdominal distension often occurs before vomiting. Air and gas begin to accumulate 3 hr after obstruction. Distension of the small bowel inhibits the absorption process and results in increased secretion, with pooling of Na^+, K^+, and fluids in the intestinal lumen.

"Marked dehydration" occurs in intestinal obstrucfion as a result of vomiting and no fluid intake. Dehydration and electrolyte disturbances are seen in high and low obstruction and are exacerbated by the loss of vomitus.

Obstruction of the small intestine in newborn infants may be the result of atresia, stenosis, webs, malrotation, or meconium ileus. Pyloric stenosis does not produce obstruction from birth. Intussusception, volvulus, duplication, and foreign bodies are causes of obstruction at a later age.

Strangulation obstruction is an indication for prompt surgical intervention; it is suggested by the presence of fever, tachycardia, and tachypnea. The vital signs are essentially normal for patients with uncomplicated (simple) obstruction. The WBC count is usually normal, but in strangulation obstruction the leukocyte count may increase quickly to 15,000–20,000/mm^3.

After 12 hr of decompression by suction and fluid replacement, operative intervention is indicated if the patient's condition has not changed or has become worse, if the WBC count has increased, or if fever has developed. If surgery is indicated, preoperative correction of fluid and electrolyte disturbances is necessary. The body's homeostatic mechanisms will not be capable of maintaining an adequate degree of compensation for existing imbalances under the influence of surgery and an anesthetic.

Plan

1. Nasogastric suction should be employed.
2. Plain films of the abdomen, upright and supine, and chest x-ray should be obtained.
3. Vital signs should be monitored.
4. Laboratory values should be determined as in problem 2.

Problem 4: Metabolic Acidosis

Assessment. The increased respiratory rate and the decreased $[HCO_3^-]$ suggest metabolic acidosis. Starvation, ketosis, loss of alkaline secretions, and decreased renal function contribute to the genesis of metabolic acidosis. The respiratory rate of 30/min may be compensatory for the decreased total CO_2 content. If strangulation obstruction has occurred, the metabolic acidosis may be worsened by lactic acid elevation.

Plan

1. Fluid therapy should be employed as in problem 1.
2. Laboratory values should be determined as in problem 2.

Progress Note

The infant had an abdominal laparotomy 48 hr after admission showing jejunal obstruction in two areas. His BUN had dropped to 39 mg/dl, his K^+ was 6 mEq/liter, and his CO_2 was normal. The infant had a stormy post-operative course, with delayed functioning of the anastomosis. Five days postoperatively his serum Na^+ dropped to 125 mEq/liter, and his CO_2 dropped to 14 mEq/liter. On the 10th postoperative day he was finally able to be fed orally, and 17 days after surgery he had a *Proteus* sepsis that was treated with appropriate antibiotics. He was finally discharged 2½ months after admission weighing 2.9 kg.

CASE 10: POSTOPERATIVE WATER INTOXICATION

A 6-year-old black boy was admitted to the surgical service for an appendectomy after 36 hr of acute abdominal pain with vomiting; 48 hr after removal of his ruptured appendix, he was transferred to the medical service because he became quite ill and had diminishing urine volume. He had been receiving 5% glucose in water parenterally.

The physical examination revealed an acutely ill child with temperature of 37.5°C, blood pressure 105/70 mm Hg, and pulse 136/min and weak. He weighed 21.6 kg and was 115 cm tall. His sensorium was depressed, and his hydration appeared unremarkable (skin turgor was not decreased, mucous membranes were not dry, and there was no edema).

The laboratory values were as follows: hemoglobin = 8.6 g/dl; WBC count = 12,300/mm³; Na^+ = 118 mEq/liter; K^+ = 4.1 mEq/liter; Cl^- = 80 mEq/liter; total CO_2 = 20 mEq/liter; Pco_2 = 36 mm Hg; H^+ = 43 nEq/liter. No urine specimen was available.

Problem List

1. Hyponatremia secondary to water intoxication
2. Appendectomy sequelae
3. Low hemoglobin

Problem 1: Hyponatremia Secondary to Water Intoxication

Assessment. A patient with postoperative water intoxication will show signs of weakness, mental confusion, lethargy, headache, and nausea leading to vomiting. However, the symptoms are dependent on the speed of development and the extent of the water intoxication and the subsequent sodium dilution. Patients who develop symptoms within 48 hr after the onset of a series of events leading to water intoxication may show CNS symptoms, which may in turn lead to coma. The absolute value of the plasma sodium concentration does not appear to be as important in relationship to the symptoms as is the rate at which the hyponatremia develops. The usual patient is not edematous, as the excess water is distributed throughout the ECF and ICF compartments. The major factors leading to clinical water intoxication are decreased urine flow and administration of hypotonic fluids. Because the volumes of urine excreted and the volumes of infused solutions used in managing small children are small, detection of major discrepancies is more difficult; therefore small children are more prone to develop serious postoperative water intoxication than are older children and adults.

Hypotonic dehydration must be differentiated from water intoxication on the basis of clinical signs of dehydration and a history of negative water and sodium balances.

Surgery, preoperative medication, fluid restriction, and anesthesia may contribute to excess secretion of antidiuretic hormone (ADH), which begins the process by reducing urine volume and free water clearance. The diminished urine volume may lead the physician to diagnose dehydration and increase the volume of parenteral infusions. If these solutions are devoid of significant amounts of sodium, water intoxication may ensue. The hyponatremia and the low hemoglobin (see problem 3) are probably secondary to increased total body water and ECF volume. Although the patient is oliguric, there are no other signs of dehydration; thus hypotonic dehydration seems unlikely. Acute hyponatremia usually becomes a therapeutic problem when the concentration of sodium is less than 125 mEq/liter.

The fluid therapy calculation is as follows: IWL = 40 − [(6/16)(20)] = 32.5 ml/kg; renal = 50 − [(6/16)(25)] = 40.6 ml/kg; gastrointestinal = 5 − [(6/16)(2.5)] = 4.1 ml/kg; total = 77.2 ml/kg, or 21.6 kg × 77.2 ml/kg/day = 1668 ml/day.

There are two approaches that could be appropriate for this child. The first is to use hypertonic NaCl (3% = 0.5 mEq/ml) and then provide the remaining maintenance fluids as would be done under ordinary circumstances. This method will be explained first.

Fluid composition: The amount of sodium needed to correct the deficiency is 140 − 118 = 22 mEq/liter. The total amount of sodium needed to repair the deficit is calculated by multiplying the body water (which is 60% of the whole body weight) times the sodium deficiency: 0.6 × 21.6 kg × 22 mEq/liter = 285 mEq. One-half of the total sodium deficit (143 mEq) should be given in three parts. The first third should be given over a 2-hr period. Then, after waiting for 2 hr, and provided the patient is not worse or is improving, the next third should be started. This procedure is repeated a third time to complete the initial program. All oral intake and other intravenous fluids must be stopped, as congestive heart failure and/or pulmonary edema may complicate the problem.

One-third of the 143 mEq, or 48 mEq, should be given in the first 2 hr by using a 3% NaCl solution (513 mEq/liter); 93 ml of this salt solution will provide the 48 mEq. At the end of 12 hr all the sodium in the first half should have been given; 1389 ml (1668 ml − 279 ml) of fluid will remain to be given at a rate of 116 ml/hr. Reevaluation of the fluid composition should be made at that time.

The problem with this procedure is that if the patient continues to have increased ADH activity, infusion of the remaining maintenance fluids without significant amounts of Na^+ may lead to repeated hyponatremia. If this is a potential problem, the fluids for that 24-hr period should be reduced significantly or should be given with enough Na^+ to provide a concentration of 60–80 mEq/liter.

The other basic approach is to give the calculated maintenance (1668 ml) with the total Na^+ (285 mEq) distributed evenly, i.e., 1668 ml at a $[Na^+]$ of 170 mEq/liter.

Acid–base equilibrium: The $[H^+]$ is near normal and need not be considered at this time. If hypertonic NaCl is to be used, the lack of buffer in the solution, combined with diminished renal function, could lead to metabolic acidosis.

Plan

1. Intake and output should be monitored.
2. A urinalysis should be performed.
3. The rate of fluid therapy should be as follows: first 2 hr = 46.5 ml/ hr × 2 hr; wait 2 hr; administer the second third (46.5 ml/hr × 2 hr); wait 2 hr; administer the last third (46.5 ml/hr × 2 hr); wait 2 hr, then reevaluate. Composition: 3% NaCl.

Problem 2: Appendectomy Sequelae

Assessment. Complications of appendectomy include infection of the wound, intraabdominal abscess, obstruction of the small bowel, fecal fistulas, and intraperitoneal hemorrhage. These should be considered if there is fever, prolonged absence of bowel sounds, increasing distension, marked pain, or increasing anemia.

Problem 3: Low Hemoglobin

Assessment. After correction of the hypotonicity, the hemoglobin and hematocrit values should be reassessed and appropriate therapy planned, as the values could fall if the ECF were contracted, or they could rise if the ECF were expanded.

CASE 11: TOTAL PARENTERAL THERAPY

A 6-week-old white female infant was admitted to the hospital for evaluation of diarrhea occurring over the previous week. She was born prematurely and weighed 4 lb 6 ounces. On admission her weight was 4 lb 8 ounces. She had not been taking her formula well.

On physical examination she appeared dehydrated (decreased skin turgor, fontanelle depression, and dry mouth), and a decreased amount of subcutaneous tissue was noted. She was afebrile; she had a pulse rate of 110/min and respirations of 45/min.

The laboratory values were as follows: $Na^+ = 125$ mEq/liter; $K^+ = 4.3$ mEq/liter; $Cl^- = 98$ mEq/liter; total $CO_2 = 16$ mEq/liter; $pCO_2 = 38$ mm Hg; $H^+ = 60$ nEq/liter; glucose = 50 mg/dl; protein = 5.4 g/dl; RBC count = $4.0 \times 10^6/cc^3$; WBC count = 8000/mm^3, with normal differential.

Problem List

1. Dehydration and electrolyte imbalance secondary to diarrhea
2. Diarrhea
3. Acidosis

Problem 1: Dehydration and Electrolyte Imbalance Secondary to Diarrhea

Assessment. The infant's dehydration is moderately severe, and repair fluids at 100 ml/kg should be started. The hyponatremia should be corrected by giving an intravenous solution equal to the amount of sodium lost plus the maintenance requirements. The hypoglycemia should be further evaluated after the intravenous solution has been started. The hypoglycemia appears to be secondary to diarrhea.

The maintenance fluid requirements are as follows: IWL = 40 ml/kg;

renal = 50 ml/kg; gastrointestinal = 35 ml/kg; total maintenance fluid requirements = 125 ml/kg. Repair fluids: 100 ml/kg; two-thirds on the first day (65 ml/kg). One-third of these fluids will be given in the first 6 hr; the remaining two-thirds will be given in the next 18 hr.

The fluid composition is as follows: IWL and renal = 40 + 50 (5% dextrose in water); gastrointestinal and repair = 35 + 65 (isotonic salt); additional Na^+ = 67% × 2.05 kg = 1.37 liters; the deficit is 140 − 125 = 15 mEq/liter. First day repair (one-half of deficit): total = 7.5 mEq/liter; total Na^+ needed = 1.37 × 7.5 = 10 mEq. Thus intravenous fluid requirements are as follows: total fluids (190 ml/kg × 2.05 kg) = 390 ml/day; Na^+ = 75 mEq/liter; additional Na^+ = 25 mEq/liter (10 mEq ÷ 0.390 liter); Cl^- = 70 mEq/liter; HCO_3^- = 30 mEq/liter; glucose = 2.5%.

Plan

1. Intravenous fluids should be started at a rate of 22 ml/hr for the first 6 hr (132 ml). The patient's status should be evaluated at that time before administering the remaining fluids at 16 ml/hr (258 ml).
2. In the 6 hr after intravenous fluid is begun, H^+, Na^+, K^+, Cl^-, HCO_3^-, glucose, total CO_2, hemoglobin, hematocrit, RBC, and WBC should be monitored.
3. Weight should be monitored daily, as well as fluid intake and output.

Problem 2: Diarrhea

Assessment. This infant's diarrhea is probably responsible for the dehydration and could account for the electrolyte disturbance. This infant should weigh at least 2 lb more than she does, and she appears malnourished. The circulation must be restored (see problem 1) and the electrolyte imbalance corrected. Cultures should be taken in an attempt to isolate bacterial organisms, and viral gastroenteritis is also possible. The hypoglycemia may be secondary to malabsorption.

Plan

1. Abdominal x-ray should be performed.
2. Stool pH and culture should be determined.
3. Tests for stool-reducing substances should be performed.
4. Supportive treatment should be provided as detailed for problem 1.

Problem 3: Acidosis

The acidosis is not severe, but it should be reevaluated after the intravenous fluid has been started (see problem 1).

Progress Notes

Repeated stool cultures did not show any growth. The infant's diarrhea subsided over the next 2 days; her electrolyte values approached normal, as did glucose and pH values. At that time oral feedings were started, and the diarrhea began again. A gastrointestinal series showed losses of intestinal mucosa and inflammatory infiltration of the intestinal wall. An IVP was normal, as was a barium enema. The stool pH was < 6.0, and reducing substances were present. Five days after admission, the infant weighed 4 lb 9 ounces and could not tolerate oral feedings.

The laboratory values were as follows: $Na^+ = 135$ mEq/liter; $K^+ = 4.5$ mEq/liter; $Cl^- = 100$ mEq/liter; total $CO_2 = 16$ mEq/liter; $Pco_2 = 38$ mm Hg; $H^+ = 45$ nEq/liter; glucose = 85 mg/dl; protein = 5.3 mg/dl; RBC count = $4.2 \times 10^6/cc^3$; WBC count = 7800/mm^3, with normal differential. Urine catecholamines.

PROBLEM 1: DEHYDRATION AND
ELECTROLYTE IMBALANCE

Assessment.   The patient's hydration and electrolyte balance were much improved. Fluid therapy should be as outlined in problem 2. The diarrhea must be treated in order to prove the cause of the fluid problems.

Plan.   Fluid therapy should be instituted as outlined for problem 2.

PROBLEM 2: INTRACTABLE DIARRHEA

Assessment.   Diarrhea in the infant is usually self-limiting and will respond to support measures or antibiotics, if indicated. In some infants the diarrhea is not helped by these treatments. The diarrhea may be secondary to disaccharide deficiency, monosaccharide intolerance, cystic fibrosis, *Salmonella* infection, ulcerative colitis, ileal stenosis, or other causes that may not seem significant enough to result in such severe stool losses. A mechanism that has been proposed suggests that the diarrhea perpetuates itself by introducing malabsorption followed by malnutrition, which may have deleterious effects on gastrointestinal structure and function. The prognosis for infants with intractable diarrhea has improved since the institution of total parenteral therapy. The state of malnutrition should be corrected in the hope of avoiding adverse effects on the CNS. Fluids for this infant should contain calories, $\sim$ 580 kcal/day (100 kcal/kg), and protein, $\sim$ 11 g/day (2/kg). The fluids should contain the following fat-soluble vitamins: vitamin A = 420 retinol equivalents or 1400 international units (IU), vitamin D = 400 IU, vitamin E = 4 IU. The fluids should contain these water-soluble vitamins: ascorbic acid = 35 mg; folacin = 50 μg; niacin = 5 mg; riboflavin = 0.4 mg; thiamine = 0.3 mg;

vitamin B_6 = 0.3 mg; vitamin B_{12} = 0.3 μg. The fluids should contain these minerals: calcium = 360 mg; phosphorus = 240 mg; iodine = 35 μg; iron = 10 mg; magnesium = 60 mg; zinc = 3 mg. These are the daily dietary allowances recommended by the Food and Nutrition Board of the National Academy of Sciences–National Research Council.

The maintenance fluid volume calculation is as follows: IWL = 40 ml/kg/day; renal = 50 ml/kg/day; gastrointestinal = 35 ml/kg/day; total fluids = 125 ml/kg/day.

Plan

1. A catheter should be placed into the superior vena cava via scalp vein.
2. Sterile parenteral solution should be infused.
3. Electrolytes, total CO_2, Pco_2, and glucose should be monitored daily.
4. Fluid intake and output should be measured.
5. Urinalysis should be performed (glucose and specific gravity); measure four times daily.

PROBLEM 3: ACIDOSIS

The patient's acid–base status must be carefully monitored as described earlier (problem 2).

Follow-up

This infant was maintained on parenteral fluids for 3 weeks. At that time she had gained 2.5 lb and was stabilized. A trial of Pregestimil (contains monosaccharide, amino acids, and medium-chain triglycerides) was given orally and was tolerated. The oral feedings were increased during the week, and at the end of 4 weeks the catheter was removed. She remained in the hospital for observation for 1 week more, and no relapse to diarrhea occurred.

APPENDICES

Appendix 1
Acid–Base Figures

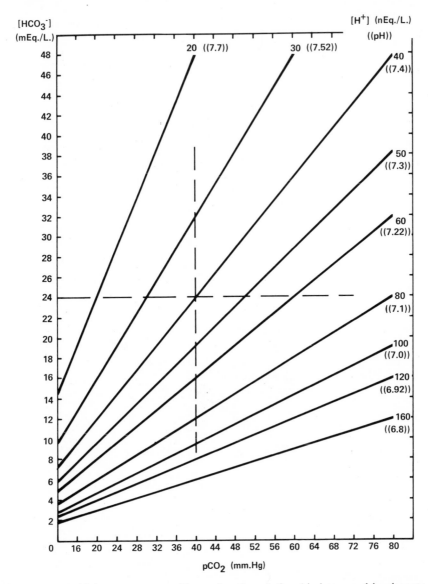

Fig. A-1.   Acid–base nomogram illustrating the relationship between bicarbonate concentration, hydrogen ion concentration, and Pco₂. Each diagonal line represents a specific hydrogen ion concentration. Values for pH are given in double parentheses.

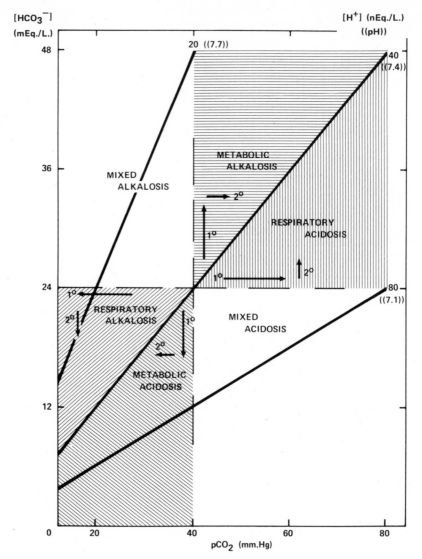

Fig. A-2. Acid–base nomogram and acid–base disorders. The areas involved in the primary acid–base disorders are shaded diagonally, horizontally, or vertically: the areas of mixed alkalosis and mixed acidosis are shown as clear areas.

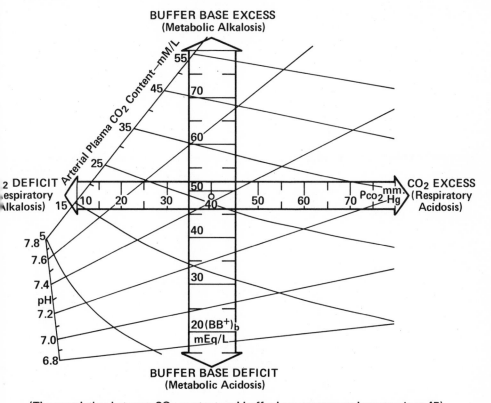

(The correlation between CO_2 content and buffer base assumes an hematocrit at 45)

Fig. A-3.   Acid–base equilibria involving buffer base values. Consideration of buffer base concentrations alters the traditional nomogram for acid–base relationships. Assuming a hematocrit of 45 mEq/liter, the average "normal" value for buffer base in older children and adults would be 4–8 mEq/liter. Using alternate terminology, one could equate a value of 45 mEq/liter with a "negative base excess" of 3 mEq/liter.

Appendix 2
Surface–Area Figures

Nomogram *For estimating surface area of infants and young children**

HEIGHT		SURFACE AREA	WEIGHT	
feet	centimeters	in square meters	pounds	kilograms

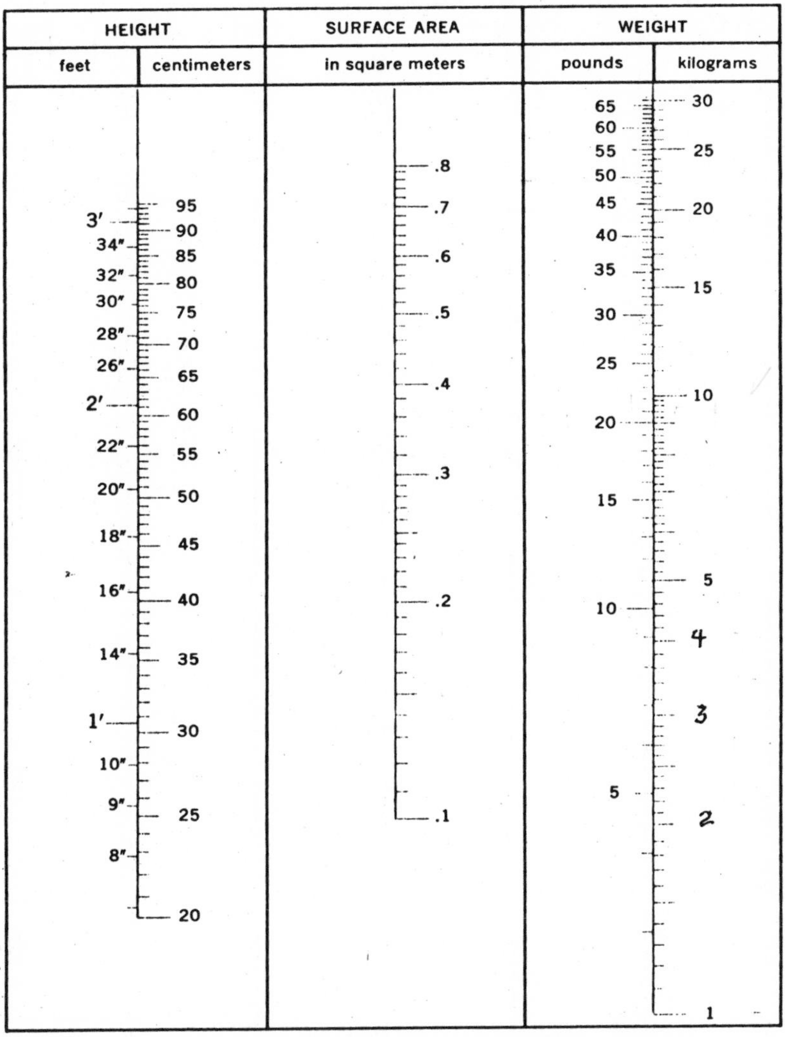

To determine the surface area of the patient draw a straight line between the point representing his height on the left vertical scale to the point representing his weight on the right vertical scale. The point at which this line intersects the middle vertical scale represents the patient's surface area in square meters.

*From Talbot, N. B., Sobel, E. H., McArthur, J. W. and Crawford, J. D., *Functional Endocrinology From Birth Through Adolescence*, Cambridge, Mass., Harvard University Press, 1952.

Fig. A-4.   Surface areas of infants and young children.

Nomogram *For estimating surface area of older children and adults*

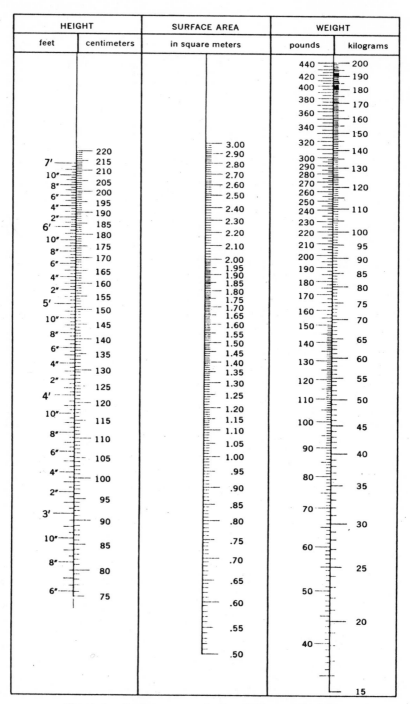

Fig. A-5.   Surface areas of older children and adults.

Appendix 3
Height–Weight Table and Figures

Table A-1
Surface Area as a Function of Height and Weight

Age	Median Weight (kg)	Height (Percentile)			Surface Area (Based on Median Weight and Height by Percentage)		
		10	50	90	10%	50%	90%
Premature	1.0	31	36	40	0.08	0.09	0.10
Premature	1.5	37	42	46	0.12	0.13	0.14
Premature	2.0	40	45	49	0.14	0.15	0.16
Premature	2.5	42	47	50	0.16	0.17	0.18
Premature	3.0	45	49	52	0.18	0.19	0.20
Birth	3.5	48	50	54	0.20	0.21	0.22
1 month	4.3	51	54	58	0.23	0.24	0.26
3 months	6.0	58	61	64	0.29	0.30	0.31
6 months	8.0	64	68	71	0.35	0.37	0.38
9 months	9.0	69	72	76	0.39	0.41	0.42
12 months	10	73	76	80	0.41	0.44	0.46
18 months	11.5	79	82	86	0.48	0.50	0.52
24 months	13	84	88	92	0.54	0.56	0.58
3 years	15	92	96	102	0.60	0.62	0.64
4 years	17	97	103	108	0.66	0.68	0.71
5 years	19	104	110	115	0.72	0.76	0.78
6 years	21	110	116	122	0.78	0.82	0.85
7 years	23	115	122	128	0.85	0.88	0.92
8 years	25	120	127	133	0.90	0.93	0.97
9 years	28	125	132	139	0.98	1.01	1.05
10 years	32	130	137	145	1.06	1.11	1.16
11 years	35	135	143	152	1.13	1.19	1.25
12 years	40	140	150	159	1.25	1.30	1.35
13 years	45	146	156	167	1.34	1.40	1.48
14 years	50	152	163	173	1.44	1.51	1.59
15 years	57	158	169	179	1.57	1.64	1.71
16 years	62	164	173	182	1.67	1.73	1.80
17 years	67	168	176	184	1.75	1.81	1.86

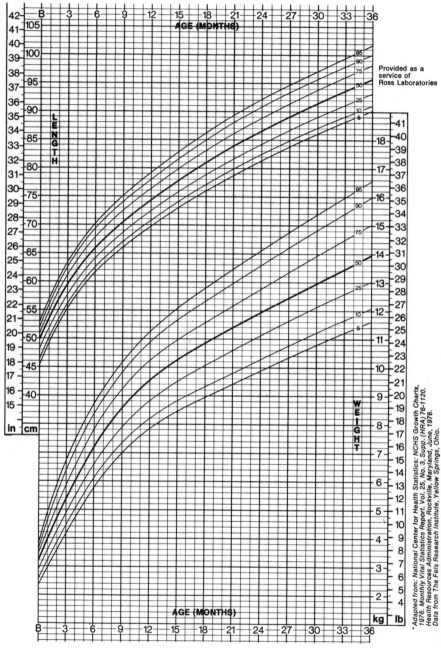

**GIRLS: BIRTH TO 36 MONTHS
PHYSICAL GROWTH
NCHS PERCENTILES***

Fig. A-6.   Girls: age for length, weight for age: birth to 36 months.

GIRLS: BIRTH TO 36 MONTHS
PHYSICAL GROWTH
NCHS PERCENTILES*

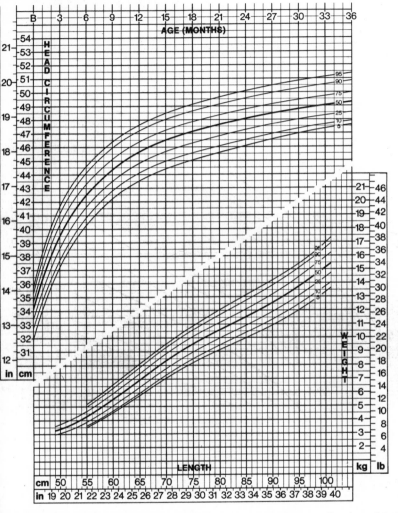

*Adapted from: National Center for Health Statistics: NCHS Growth Charts, 1976. Monthly Vital Statistics Report. Vol. 25, No. 3, Supp. (HRA) 76-1120. Health Resources Administration, Rockville, Maryland, June, 1976. Data from The Fels Research Institute, Yellow Springs, Ohio.
© 1976 ROSS LABORATORIES

Fig. A-7. Girls: weight for length, head circumference for age; birth to 36 months.

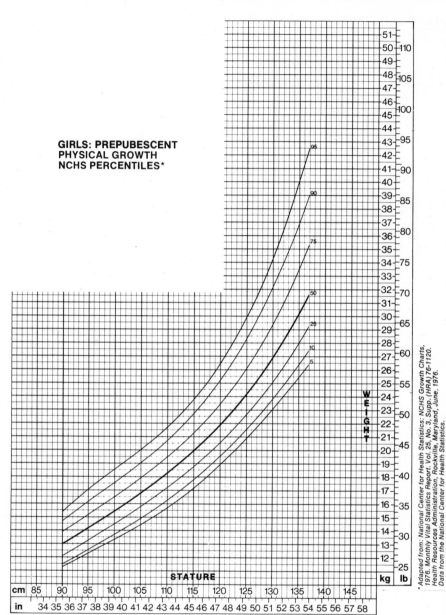

GIRLS: PREPUBESCENT PHYSICAL GROWTH NCHS PERCENTILES*

*Adapted from: National Center for Health Statistics: NCHS Growth Charts, 1976. Monthly Vital Statistics Report. Vol. 25, No. 3, Supp. (HRA) 76-1120. Health Resources Administration, Rockville, Maryland, June, 1976. Data from the National Center for Health Statistics.

Fig. A-8.   Girls: weight for stature; prepubescent.

**GIRLS: 2 TO 18 YEARS
PHYSICAL GROWTH
NCHS PERCENTILES***

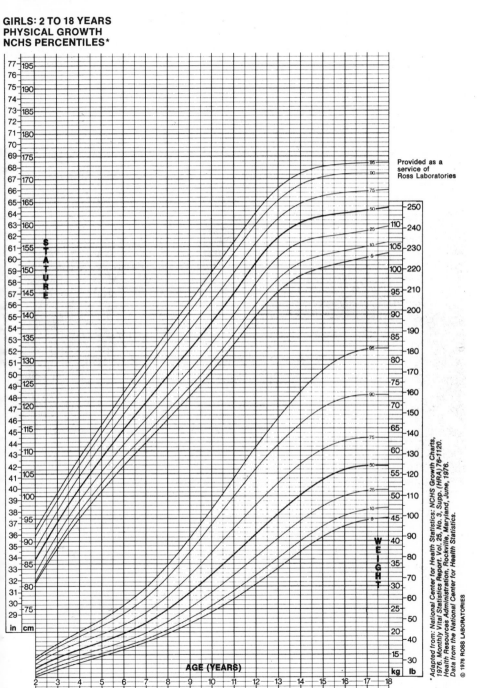

Fig. A-9. Girls: stature for age, weight for age; 2 to 18 years.

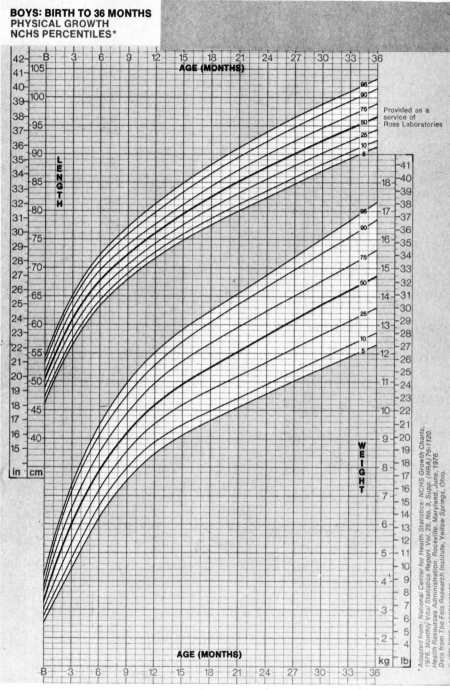

Fig. A-10.   Boys: age for length, weight for age; birth to 36 months.

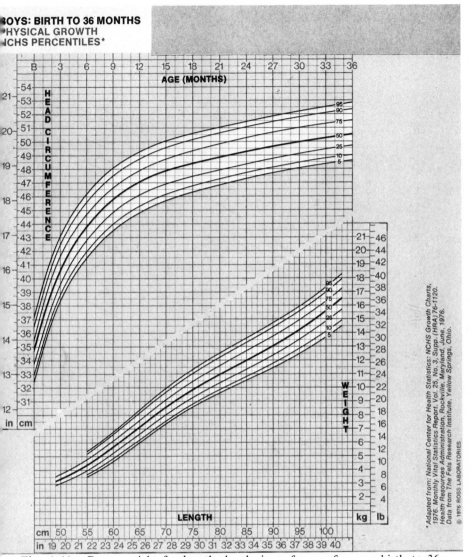

Fig. A-11. Boys: weight for length, head circumference for age; birth to 36 months.

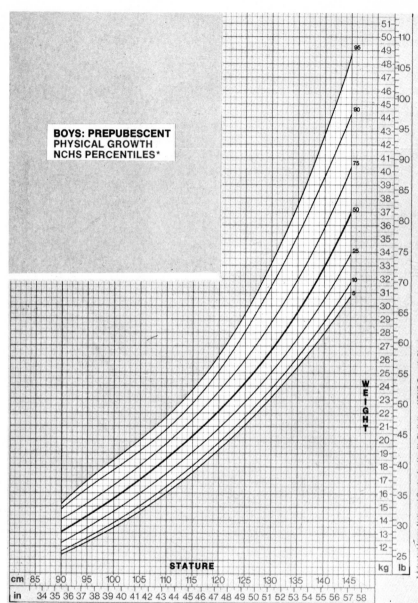

Fig. A-12. Boys: weight for stature; prepubescent.

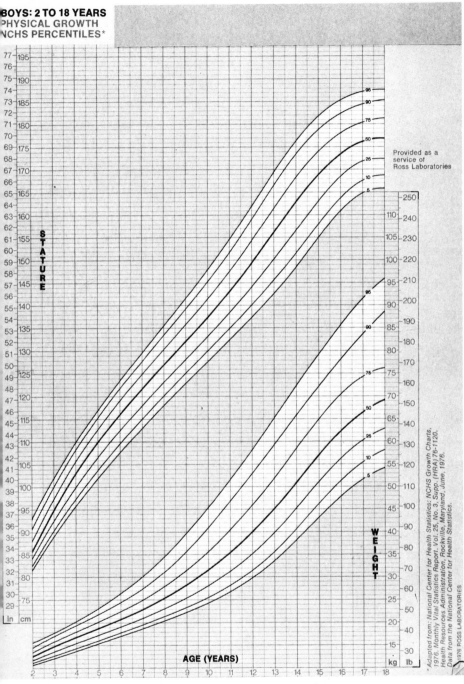

Provided as a
service of
Ross Laboratories

AGE (YEARS)

*Adapted from: National Center for Health Statistics: NCHS Growth Charts, 1976. Monthly Vital Statistics Report, Vol. 25, No. 3, Supp. (HRA) 76-1120. Health Resources Administration, Rockville, Maryland, June, 1976. Data from the National Center for Health Statistics.

1976 ROSS LABORATORIES

Fig. A-13.   Boys: stature for age, weight for age; 2 to 18 years.

Appendix 4

Laboratory Normal Values

	Mean		Range*
Serum			
Na$^+$	140	mEq/liter	130–150
K$^+$	5.0	mEq/liter	4.0–6.0
Ca^{++}	5	mEq/liter	4–5.5
Mg^{++}	2.0	mEq/liter	1.0–3.0
Cl$^-$	100	mEq/liter	95–105
PO$_4^{--}$†	3	mEq/liter	2.0–4.0
HCO$_3^-$	24	mEq/liter	18–26
H$^+$	40	nEq/liter	35–50
pH	7.40		7.3–7.45
Pco$_2$	40	mm Hg	35–45
Proteins	6.5	g/dl	6.0–7.5
Albumin	5.0	g/dl	4.5–6.0
Globulin	1.5	g/dl	1.0–2.0
Whole blood NH$^+$	100	μg/dl	20–150
Urea nitrogen‡	15	mg/dl	5–20
Urine creatinine	20	mg/kg/24 hr	10–30

* A range that encompasses values that are within reasonable normophysiologic limits.

† Assuming a net negative charge of 1.8 (values in mg/dl: mean = 5, range = 3–7).

‡ Values in blood, plasma, and serum are approximately the same.

Appendix 5
Fluid requirements

	Maintenance Requirements (24 hr)	
Loss	*0.5 Year*	*16 Years*
IWL	40 ml/kg	20 ml/kg
Renal	50 ml/kg	25 ml/kg
Gastrointestinal	5 ml/kg	2.5 ml/kg

* Maintenance (ml/kg) = 95 − (3 × age in years) for ages 1 month to 16 years.

Skin and Lung Losses

Insensible water loss increases with activity and fever. Values are reduced in sleep and coma, but may be doubled with activity. Values increase 10% for 1°C of fever.

Sweating begins with environmental temperatures above 80°F. Losses may vary from zero to 14,000 ml/m²/day (adult, up to 1 liter/hr). Usual range = 140–1400 ml/m²/day; infant = 7–70 ml/m²/day; adult = 3.5–35 ml/m²/day. The mean value for children is 20 ml/m²/day and for adults, 10 ml/m²/day.

Gastrointestinal Losses

Diarrhea losses are as follows: infant = 35 ml/kg/day (range, 0–70); adult = 20 ml/kg/day (range, 0–35).

Suction losses must be measured; as a guide, digestive fluids produced each day (adult): saliva = 1500 ml/day; bile = 500 ml/day; gastric = 2400 ml/day; pancreatic = 700 ml/day; small bowel = 3000 ml/day.

Renal Water Requirements

		Solute Load			Ill infant
Concentration		$300\ mOsm/m^2$ (CHO: 100 g			(7 kg, 0.36 m^2)
Specific Gravity	Osmo-larity	adult, 3 g/kg infant)	$500\ mOsm/m^2$ (Fasting)	$750\ mOsm/m^2$ (Average Diet)	Receiving CHO
1.005	150	2000*	3200*	5000*	160†
1.010	300	1000	1600	2500	80
1.020	650	450	750	1150	40
1.030	1000	300	500	750	25
1.040	1400	200	350	500	18

* Volume of urine (ml/m²/day).
† Volume of urine (ml/kg/day).

URINE VOLUME

The absolute minimum for fliuds with maximum urinary concentration, without azotemia, is about 200 ml/m²/day. The absolute maximum may be up to 10,000 ml/m²/day, as in diabetes insipidus. Infant minimum = 10 ml/kg/day; infant maximum = 500 ml/kg/day; adult minimum = 5 ml/kg/day; adult maximum = 250 ml/kg/day.

SOLUTE LOADS

The solute loads are as follows: 40 mOsm/100 kcal (ordinary diet); 660 mOsm/100 g protein; 1650 mOsm/kg meat; 1200 mOsm/day in adult male; 800 mOsm/day in fasting normal adult (caloric expenditure is two-thirds normal)

WATER REQUIREMENTS

Water requirements are 40–50 ml/100 kcal in the "average" diet; 10 ml/100 kcal is the water of oxidation.

CALORIES REQUIRED

The calories required are as follows: newborns = 110 kcal/kg; 3–6 months = 100 kcal/kg; kcal/kg = 95 − (3 × age in years) for children weighing less than 40 kg and those who are younger than 16 years.

RENAL FUNCTION

GFR = $30 + (5 \times$ age in years) (for years 2–13); creatinine clearance (ml/min = (urine creatinine $\times$ urine volume)/plasma creatinine; transport maximum (t_m) glucose = 375 mg/min; excreted urea = 80% of excreted nitrogen.

SURFACE AREA AND AVERAGE DAILY MAINTENANCE

Age	Surface Area (m^2)	Average Daily Maintenance (ml/kg/day)	Total Maintenance
Premature (2 kg)	0.15	135	270
1 month	0.25	100	450
3 months	0.30	95	540
18 months	0.50	80	900
5 years	0.75	75	1350
9 years	1.00	65	1800
14 years	1.50	55	2700
Adult	1.75	45	3100

Maintenance fluid requirements in the first days of life are greatly reduced and may approach zero.

FLUID COMPOSITION FOR REPLACEMENT SOLUTIONS

Fluid Losses	Electrolytes in Replacement Fluid
IWL	Electrolyte-free
Renal	Electrolyte-free
Gastrointestinal	Isotonic to ECF
Maintenance electrolytes	1 mEq/kg/day of each Na^+, K^+, Cl^- in infant; adult values are half these
Diarrhea	Isotonic to ECF
Dehydration repair	Isotonic to ECF

Maintenance fluids administered for IWL and renal losses are best given as CHO-water solutions. For gastrointestinal losses, isotonic salt solutions are usually appropriate. In general, under average conditions requiring parenteral fluids, when hydration and renal function are normal, total maintenance fluids can usually be given as a solution containing cation at 40–50 mEq/liter, about equally divided between Na^+ and K^+.

REPAIR OF ABNORMAL HYDRATION

Weight is the best single measurement for determination of hydration level. Weigh patients frequently. With prolonged periods of inadequate calories, weight should decrease 0.5%–1.0%/day.

Estimation of dehydration: 5% weight loss (50 ml/kg) = first clinical signs; 10% weight loss (100 ml/kg) = severe, requiring hospitalization; 15% weight loss (150 ml/kg) = usually in shock; 20% weight loss (200 ml/kg) = death. Replace existing dehydration with isotonic salt solutions over a period of 24–72 hr.

Summary: Common commercial intravenous fluids for an infant with diarrhea: first 12 hr = 95 ml/kg one-half Ringer's lactate; second 12 hr = 80 ml/kg Electrolyte 75 (Talbot's); third 12 hr = 65 ml/kg Electrolyte 75 or Electrolyte 48; fourth 12 hr = 50 ml/kg Electrolyte 48 (modified Butler).

TONICITY OF BODY FLUIDS

The $[Na^+]_s = [Cl^-]_s + [HCO_3^-]$ a (12 ± 3). ECF $[Cl^-] = [Cl^-]_s \times 110\%$ ECF $[Na^+] = [Na^+]_s$. Osmolarity = $(2 \times [Na^+]) +$ nonionic solute (in mOsm/liter). $Protein^-$ (g/dl) $\times 2.43$ = mEq/liter (average 16 mEq/liter); mEq = (mg $\times$ charge)/molecular weight; mOsm = mg/molecular weight.

Molecular weights: glucose = 180, BUN = 28, urea = 60.

Altered tonicity: Acute reduction of serum Na^+ associated with symptoms should be treated with an appropriate salt solution. The quantity of Na^+ required (mEq) equals desired $[Na^+]_s$ – measured $[Na^+]_s$ $\times$ 0.6 $\times$ weight (kg). Serum Na^+ may be reduced secondary to hyperglycemia or uremia.

Glucose or (mg/dl)	Urea	= mOsm/liter	Expected $[Na^+]_s$ (mEq/liter)
180	60	10	140
360	120	20	130
720	240	40	120
1080	360	60	110

Hypernatremia should be corrected slowly—over a period of 72 hr or more.

POTASSIUM ADMINISTRATION

Do not give potassium until patient is voiding well and serum $[K^+]$ is known or EKG has been evaluated. Maximum rates: 3 mEq/kg-day or 30 mEq/liter intravenous fluid.

BODY WATER

WBW = whole body weight
TBW = total body water
LBM = lean body mass
ECF/ICF = extra cellular/intracellular fluid
WBW = LBM + body fat
TBW = ICF + ECF
TBW = 75% × LBM
TBW = 67% × WBW (infant)
TBW = 60% × WBW (child/adult)
ICF = 45% × LBM
ICF = 40% × WBW
ECF = 25% × WBW (infant)
ECF = 20% × WBW (child/adult)

MISCELLANEOUS

$([H^+] [HCO_3^-])/[P_{CO_2}] = 24$
Primary change in numerator = metabolic.
Primary change in denominator = respiratory.
$CO_2 + H_2O \rightleftharpoons H_2CO_3 \rightleftharpoons H_2CO_3^- + H^+$
Total $CO_2 = [HCO_3^+] + [H_2CO_3 + CO_2]$
Total $CO_2 = \sim[HCO_3^-]$
Total $CO_2 = 24$ mEq/liter (adult)
Total $CO_2 = 20$ mEq/liter (infant)
$P_{CO_2} = 40$ mm Hg (adult)
$P_{CO_2} = 33$ mm Hg (infant)
H_2CO_3 (mM/liter) = P_{CO_2} (mm Hg) × 0.03
pH of 7.4 = $[H^+]$ of 40 nEq/liter
0.3 pH change = double/halve $[H^+]$
pH of 7.1 = $[H^+]$ of 80 nEq/liter

Appendix 6

Commercial Parenteral Solutions

Solution	Glu-cose*	Na$^+$	K$^+$	Ca^{++}	Mg^{++}	Cl$^-$	PO$_4^{--}$	HCO$_3^-$
5% dextrose	50							
0.85% NaCl		146				146		
0.45% NaCl		77				77		
0.2% NaCl		34				34		
3.0% NaCl		517				517		
KCl (2 mEq/ml)			2000			2000		
NaHCO$_3$ (8.4%)		1000						1000
Na lactate (1/6 M)		167						167§
Ca gluconate (10%)				464‡				
Ringer's lactate		130	4	3		109		28§
½ Ringer's lactate		65	2	1.5		54.5		14§
Isolyte E, Ionosol D		140	10	5	3	103		55
Isolyte G, Ionosol G,† Electrolyte 75		63	17			150		
Isolyte M, Ionosol T, Electrolyte 45		40	35			40	15	20
Isolyte P, Ionosol MB		25	20		3	22	3	23
Electrolyte 1, Ionosol DM		80	36	5	3	64		60
Electrolyte 2, Ionosol B		59	25		6	52	13	25

* Glucose in g/liter; all others in mEq/liter.

† Contains NH$_4$ = 70 mEq/liter (not recommended).

‡ 464 mEq/liter = 232 mM/liter.

§ Lactate.

Table A-2
Compositions of Milks and Milk-type Formulas*

Solution	Protein†	Na⁺	K⁺	Ca⁺⁺	Mg⁺⁺	Cl⁻	PO₄⁻⁻
				Solute Concentrations			
Cow's milk	3.3	25	35	65	10	30	60
Human's milk	1.2	7	14	16.5	3.2	12	8.7
Enfamil (20 kcal/oz)	1.5	11	19	27		13	27
Isomil (20 kcal/oz)	2.0	13	18	35		15	
Meat base	2.8	17	12	53			40
Mull-Soy	3.1	16	40	64			48
Nutramigen	2.2	20	27	54		22	42
Similac 13 (13 kcal/oz)	1.2	10	15	22.4	2.2		20.3
Similac 20 (20 kcal/oz)	1.8	11	19	35	3.4	15	32
Similac PM 60/40	1.6	7	14.8	17.5	3.3	13	10.5
SMA (20 kcal/oz)	1.5	6.4	14.1	22	4.3	10.3	19
Sobee	3.2	22	32	54			30
Soyalac liquid	2.1	14	23	21			18

* Adapted by permission from Committee on Nutrition, American Academy of Pediatrics: Commentary on breast-feeding and infant formulas including proposed standards for formulas. Pediatrics 57:278, 1976.

† Protein in g/dl; all others in mEq/liter.

References

CHAPTER 1: GENERAL REFERENCES

1. Bradbury MWB: Physiology of body fluids and electrolytes. Br J Anaesth 45:937, 1973
2. Christensen HN: in: Body Fliuds and the Acid-Base Balance. Philadelphia, WB Saunders, 1964
3. Darrow DC: in: A Giude to Learning Fliud Therapy. Springfield, Ill, Charles C Thomas, 1964
4. Lockwood APM: in: Animal Body Fliuds and Their Regulation. Cambridge, Cambridge University Press, 1964
5. Pitts RF: in: Physiology of the Kidney and Body Fliuds. Chicago, Year Book, 1966
6. Schrier R (guest ed): Water metabolism. Symp Kidney Int 10:1, 1976
7. Talbot NB, Richie RH, Crawford JD: in: Metabolic Homeostasis. A Syllabus for Those Concerned with the Care of Patients. The Commonwealth Fund, Cambridge, Harvard University Press, 1959
8. Winters RW (ed): in: The Body Fliuds in Pediatrics. Boston, Little, Brown, 1973
9. Winters RW: in: Principles of Pediatric Fliud Therapy. Chicago, Abbott Laboratories, 1975

CHAPTER 1: CLASSICAL PAPERS

1. Atchley DW, Loeb RE, Richards RF, et al: On diabetic acidosis: Detailed study of electrolyte balance following withdrawal and reestablishment of insulin therapy. J Clin Invest 12:297, 1933
2. Cotlove E, Holliday MA, Schwartz R, et al: Effects of electrolyte depletion and acid-base disturbance on muscle cations. Am J Physiol 167:665, 1951
3. Darrow DC, Hellerstein S: Interpretation of certain changes in body water and electrolytes. Physiol Rev 38:114, 1958

4. Darrow DC, Schwartz RC, Ianucci JF, et al: Relation of serum bicarbonate concentration to muscle composition. J Clin Invest 27:198, 1948

5. Gamble JL: in: Chemical Anatomy, Physiology and Pathology of Extracellular Fliud. A Lecture Syllabus. Cambridge, Harvard University Press, 1950

6. Gamble JL: in: Companionship of Water and Electrolyte in Organization of Body Fliuds. Stanford, Stanford University Press, 1951

7. Gamble JL, Fahey KR, Appleton J, et al: Congenital alkalosis with diarrhea. J Pediatr 26:509, 1945

8. Harrison HE, Finberg L, Fleischman E: Disturbances of ionic equilibrium of intracellular and extracellular electrolytes in patients with tuberculous meningitis. J Clin Invest 31:300, 1952

9. Kleiber M: in: The Fire of Life. An Introduction to Animal Energetics. New York, John Wiley, 1961

10. Mellanby E: An experimental investigation on rickets. Lancet 1:407, 1919

11. Nichols G, Nichols N, Weil WB, et al: The direct measurement of the extracellular phase of tissues. J Clin Invest 32:1299, 1953

12. Singer RB: The acid-base disturbance in salicylate intoxication. Medicine 33:1, 1954

13. Smith HW: in: Principles of Renal Physiology. New York, Oxford University Press, 1956

14. Wallace WM, Holliday M, Cushman M, et al: The application of the internal standard flame photometer to the analysis of biologic material. J Lab Clin Med 37:621, 1951

15. Wynn V, Rob CG: Water intoxication. Lancet 1:587, 1954

CHAPTER 2: GENERAL REFERENCES

1. Cohen LF, Farrel PM, Lundgren DW, et al: Electrolyte values of sweat obtained by local and whole body collection methods in cystic fibrosis patients. J Pediatr 89:430, 1976

2. Fomon SJ: in: Infant Nutrition. Philadelphia, WB Saunders, 1974

3. Ruch TC, Patton HC (ed): in: Physiology and Biophysics. Circulation, Respiration and Fliud Balance. Philadelphia, WB Saunders, 1974

CHAPTER 3: GENERAL REFERENCES

1. Bernstein LM, Allender JS, Elstein AS, et al: in: Renal Function and Renal Failure. Baltimore, Williams & Wilkins, 1965

2. Brenner BM, Dean WM, Roberton CR: Determinants of glomerular filtration rate. Physiol Rev 56:9, 1976

3. Brenner BM, Dean WM, Robertson CR: Glomerular filtration, in Brenner BM, Rector FC (eds): The Kidney. Philadelphia, WB Saunders, 1976

4. Burg MB: Renal handling of sodium and chloride, in Brenner BM, Rector FC (eds): The Kidney. Philadelphia, WB Saunders, 1976

5. Burg M, Green N: Function of the thick ascending limb of Henle's loop. Am J Physiol 224:659, 1973

6. Chantler C: Evaluation of laboratory and other methods of measuring renal function, in Lieberman E (ed): Clinical Pediatric Nephrology. Philadelphia, JB Lippincott, 1976

7. Chantler C, Barratt TM: Estimation of filtration rate from plasma clearance of 51-chromium edetic acid. Arch Dis Child 41:613, 1972

8. Dell RB: Pathophysiology of dehydration, in Winters RW (ed): The Body Fliuds in Pediatrics. Boston, Little, Brown, 1973

9. Dirks JH, Seely JF, Levy M: Control of extracellular fliud volume and the pathophysiology in Brenner BM, Rector FC (eds): The Kidney. Philadelphia, WB Saunders, 1976

10. Fitzsimmons JT: The Physiological Basis of Thirst. Kidney Int 10:3, 1976

11. Giebisch G: Coupled ion and fliud transport in the kidney. N Engl J Med 287:913, 1974

12. Goldberg M, Agus ZS, Goldfarb S: Renal handling of phosphate, calcium and magnesium, in Brenner BM, Rector FC (eds): The Kidney. Philadelphia, WB Saunders, 1976

13. Grantham JS: Renal transport and excretion of potassium, in Brenner BM, Rector FC (eds): The Kidney. Philadelphia, WB Saunders, 1976

14. Gross JB, Imai M, Kokko JP: A functional comparison of the cortical collecting tubule and the distal convoluted tubule. J Clin Invest 55:1284, 1975

15. Hayes RM, Levin SD: Pathophysiology of water metabolism, in Brenner BM, Rector FC (eds): The Kidney. Philadelphia, WB Saunders, 1976

16. Jacobson HR, Kokko JP: Intrinsic differences in various segments of the proximal convoluted tubule. J Clin Invest 57:818, 1876

17. Jamison RL: Urinary concentration and dilution, in Brenner BM, Rector FC (eds): Philadelphia, WB Saunders, 1976

18. Jamison RL, Maffly R: The urinary concentrating mechanism. N Engl J Med 295:1059, 1976

19. Kawamura S, Imai M, Seldin DW, et al: Characteristics of salt and water transport in superficial and juxtamedullary straight segments of proximal tubules. J Clin Invest 55:1269, 1975

20. Kokko JP: Proximal tubule potential difference: Dependence on glucose, HCO_3 and amino acids. J Clin Invest 52:1362, 1973

21. Lewy JE, Windhager EE: Peritubular control of proximal tubular fliud reabsorption in the rat kidney. Am J Physiol 214:943, 1968

22. Schrier RW, de Wardener HE: Tubular reabsorption of sodium ion: Influence of factors other than aldosterone and glomerular filtration rate. N Engl J Med 285:1231, 1292, 1971

23. Schwartz GJ, Haycock MB, Edelmann CM, et al: A simple estimate of glomerular filtration rate in children derived from body length and plasma creatinine. Pediatrics 58:259, 1976

24. Schwartz MM, Venkatachalam MA: Structural differences in thin limbs of henle: Physiological implications. Kidney Int 6:193, 1974

25. Sertel H, Scopes J: Rates of creatinine clearance in babies less than one week of age. Arch Dis Child 48:717, 1973

26. Steel TH, Rieselback: The renal handling of urate and other organic anions,

in Brenner BM, Rector FC (eds): The Kidney. Philadelphia, WB Saunders, 1976

27. Stein JH, Reineck HJ: Effect of alterations in extracellular fliud volume on segmental sodium transport. Physiol Rev 55:127, 1975
28. Valtin H: in: Renal Function: Mechanisms Preserving Fliud and Solute Balance in Health. Boston, Little, Brown, 1973

CHAPTER 4: GENERAL REFERENCES

1. Loeb JN: The hyperosmolar state. N Engl J Med 290:1184, 1974
2. Zeppa R, Drucker WR, Callahan AB: in Malinin TI (ed): Acute Fliud Replacement in the Therapy of Shock. New York, Grune & Stratton, 1974
3. Robertson GL: Vasopression in osmotic regulation in man. Ann Rev Med 25:315, 1974
4. Sharp GWG: Action of cholera toxin on fliud and electrolyte movement in the small intestine. Ann Rev Med 24:19, 1973

CHAPTER 5: GENERAL REFERENCES

1. Balsan S, Garabedian M, Sorgniard R, et al: 1,25-dehydroxyvitamin D_3 and 1,α-hydroxyvitamin D_3 in children: Biologic and therapeutic effects in nutritional rickets and different types of vitamin D resistance. Pediatr Res 9:586, 1975
2. Bordier P, Pechet HM, Hesse R, et al: Response of adult patients with osteomalacia to treatment with crystalline 1α-hydroxy vitamin D_3. N Engl J Med 291:866, 1974
3. Brown DM, Boen J, Bernstein A: Serum ionized calcium in newborn infants. Pediatrics 49:841, 1972
4. Coburn JW, Hartenbower DL, Norman AW: Metabolism and action of the hormone vitamin D—It's relation to diseases of calcium homeostasis. West J Med 121:22, 1974
5. Cohen BD: Uremic toxins. Bull NY Acad Med 51:1228, 1975
6. DeLuca HF: The kidney as an endocrine organ involved in the function of vitamin D. Am J Med 58:39, 1975
7. DeLuca HF: Vitamin D—1973. Am J Med 57:1, 1974
8. DeLuca HF: Vitamin D today, in Dowling HF (ed): Disease-a-Month. Chicago, Year Book, 1975, pp. 1–37
9. Diaz-Buxo JA, Knox FG: Effects of parathyroid hormone on renal function. Mayo Clin Proc 50:537, 1975
10. Fisch C: Relation of electrolyte disturbances to cardiac arrhythmias. Circulation 47:408, 1973
11. Fraser D, Kooh SW, Kind HP, et al: Pathogenesis of hereditary vitamin-D-dependent rickets. N Engl J Med 289:817, 1973
12. Giordano C (ed): Uremia, Proceedings of a Conference. Kidney Int [Suppl 3] 7, 1975
13. Harrison HE, Harrison HC: Rickets then and now. J Pediatr 87:1144, 1975

14. Kodicek E: The story of vitamin D—From vitamin to hormone. Lancet 1:325, 1974

15. Kooh SW, Fraser D, DeLuca HF, et al: Treatment of hypoparathyroidism and pseudohypoparathyroidism with metabolites of vitamin D: Evidence for imparied conversion of 25-hydroxyvitamin D to 1α-dihydroxyvitamin D. N Engl J Med 293:840, 1975

16. Lewis EJ, Magill JW (guest eds): Nutritional aspects of uremia (conference). Am J Clin Nutr vol 21, nos 5 and 6 1968

17. Lewy JE, Potter DE: The management of dialysis and transplantation in children. J Dialysis 1:75, 1976

18. Marks J: The fat-soluble vitamins in modern medicine. Vitam Horm 32:131, 1974

19. Mcneely GR, Battarbee HD: Sodium and potassium. Nutr Rev 34:225, 1976

20. Norman AW: 1,25-Dihydroxyvitamin D_3: A kidney-produced steroid hormone essential to calcium homeostasis. Am J Med 57:21, 1974

21. Raskin NH. Fishman RA: Neurologic disorders in renal failure. N Engl J Med 294:143, 204, 1976

22. Reiss E, Canterbury JM: Spectrum of hyperparathyroidism. Am J Med 56:794, 1974

23. Review: Enhanced efficiency in uremia in re-use of urea N for serum albumin synthesis. Nutr Rev 34:110, 1976

24. Review: Neonatal calcium homeostasis, vitamin D and parathyroid function. Nutr Rev 34:112, 1976

25. Root AW, Harrison HE: Recent advances in calcium metabolism. I. Mechanisms of calcium homeostasis. J Pediatr 88:1, 1976

26. Root AW, Harrison HE: Recent advances in calcium metabolism. II. Disorders of calcium homeostasis. J Pediatr 88:177, 1976

27. Sorell M, Rosen JF: Ionized calcium: Serum levels during symptomatic hypocalcemia. J Pediatr 87:67, 1976

28. Suki WN, Yium JJ, von Minden M, et al: Acute treatment of hypercalcemia with furosemide. N Engl J Med 283:836, 1970

CHAPTER 6: GENERAL REFERENCES

1. Davenport HW: in: The ABC of Acid-Base Chemistry. Chicago, University of Chicago Press, 1974

2. Goldberger E: in: A Primer of Water, Electrolyte and Acid-Base Syndromes. Philadelphia, Lea & Febiger, 1970

3. Kintner EP: Acid-base, blook gas, and electrolyte balances. Prog Clin Pathol 4:143, 1972

4. Masoro EJ, Siegel PD: in: Acid-Base Regulation: Its Physiology and Pathophysiology. Philadelphia. WB Saunders, 1971

5. Muntwyler E: in: Water and Electrolyte Metabolism and Acid-Base Balance. St Louis, CV Mosby, 1968

6. Rector FC (guest ed): Acid-base homeostasis (symposium). Kidney Int 1:273, 1972

7. Robinson JR: in: Fundamentals of Acid-Base Regulation. London, Blackwell Scientific, 1974
8. Winters RW, Engel K, Dell RB, et al: in: Acid-Base Physiology in Medicine. A Self-instruction Program. Cleveland, The London Company, Copenhagen, Radiometer A/S, 1967

PART III: GENERAL REFERENCES

1. Abston S: Burns in children. Clin Symp 28:2, 1976
2. Mason EE: in: Fliud, Electrolyte and Nutrient Therapy in Surgery. Philadelphia, Lea & Febiger, 1974
3. Meng HC, Law DH (eds): in: Parenteral Nutrition. Springfield, Ill, Charles C Thomas, 1970
4. Parsa MH, Ferrer JM, Habif DV: in: Safe Central Venous Nutrition. Springfield, Ill, Charles C Thomas, 1974
5. Young DG: Fliud balance in paediatric surgery. Br J Anaesth 45:953, 1973

Index